Internal Medicine Learning A to Z and 1, 2, 3

Joe Lezama

Internal Medicine Learning A to Z and 1, 2, 3

A High Reliability Approach to Clinical Knowledge and Standardized Testing Success

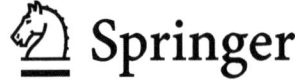 Springer

Joe Lezama
Morsani College of Medicine
University of South Florida
Tampa, FL, USA

ISBN 978-3-031-57545-7   ISBN 978-3-031-57546-4   (eBook)
https://doi.org/10.1007/978-3-031-57546-4

This Springer imprint is published by the registered company Springer Nature Switzerland AG
The registered company address is: Gewerbestrasse 11, 6330 Cham, Switzerland

Paper in this product is recyclable.

This book is dedicated

TO MY WIFE, AMY, AND MY CHILDREN, KAITLYN, DEREK, AND MADDY

whose support has been incredible throughout these years.

Preface

I have spent the last 24 years as a faculty member in the Department of Internal Medicine at the University of South Florida Morsani College of Medicine, developing strategies for teaching internal medicine residents. I have created unique ways to communicate material for retention, which has translated into standardized testing success for the trainees in our department. I have found that auditory and visual cues are helpful in organizing and learning material.

I began a board review series during my first year on the faculty that continues to this day. My teaching techniques were pivotal in our program, which achieved a near perfect pass rate on the internal medicine board exam from 2001 to 2010. To date, our program boasts one of the highest board pass rates for all university programs nationwide over the last 24 years.

Herein I share my methods for successfully preparing trainees for standardized examinations in internal medicine. I have found these methods to be motivational during the challenging times of residency training for my learners. This book intends to set internal medicine and medicine-pediatrics residents up for success on their internal medicine board examination. Still, it is also a valuable resource for internal medicine primary care physicians, hospitalists, and other specialty physicians preparing for recertification examinations. Medical students will also find this book among their go-to references when studying for their internal medicine shelf examination or standardized national examination.

Tampa, FL, USA   Joe Lezama

Acknowledgements

I thank Harold Adelman, Donald Doll, Dennis Ledford, Phil Altus, Ricardo Gonzalez-Rothi, Jay Lynch, and John Sinnott for their unfailing support and mentorship.

Contents

About the Author

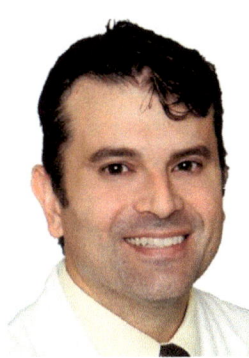

Joe Lezama is a Professor of Medicine and Vice Chair of Education for the Department of Internal Medicine at the University of South Florida (USF) Morsani College of Medicine, a role he has held since 2012. He is a "double Gator," having obtained an undergraduate degree in microbiology and cell science and his MD from the University of Florida. Upon completing his internal medicine residency at USF in 2000, he joined the USF Morsani College of Medicine as a faculty member.

He was instrumental in establishing one of the nation's first Patient Safety and Quality Improvement fellowships nearly 15 years ago. The program has graduated close to 20 trainees who have gone on to leadership roles. His group gained national recognition from the Institute for Safe Medication Practices in 2014. His educational accolades include more than 30 awards and recognitions, including three-time winner of "Teacher of the Year" for the USF College of Medicine and seven-time winner of "Teacher of the Year" for the Department of Internal Medicine. He was inducted into the University of Florida College of Medicine Wall of Fame in 2020 and selected by the American College of Physicians for the Laureate Award in 2021. He was elected to the mastership level of the American College of Physicians in October 2023.

He is married to Amy Abreu Lezama, Pharm D, and has three children, Kaitlyn, Derek, and Maddy.

How to Use This Book

This book is divided into three parts that exemplify the teaching strategies I have developed for internal medicine and medicine-pediatric residents over the past 24 years.

Part I comprises quick teaching tips for standardized test examinations in internal medicine. The tips are created to help with long-term retention. It is vital for those preparing for examinations to use a "road map," such as this, to review topics that can be exhaustive in nature and to be familiar with the design and format of the standardized tests they will encounter. For example, a few strategies focus on the importance of a solid comprehension of pharmacological therapeutics that may be referred to in the examination by the drug itself or the pharmacological family to which it belongs. Other strategies emphasize the "big picture" of cross-content material, such as dermatology or epidemiology.

Part II uses the "A–Z" format for twelve common disciplines in internal medicine. Alongside specialties such as cardiology, gastroenterology, and endocrinology, I so use the "A–Z" approach in areas that must be mastered to succeed in internal medicine standardized testing of psychiatry, dermatology, epidemiology, ophthalmology, and orthopedics. It is suggested that learners in a three-year program focus on one topic per month, allowing for the repetition of the material three times during residency, leading to greater comprehension and retention.

Part III is the most comprehensive section and forms the scaffolding of this learning strategy. It tests grit and resiliency while building the foundation for a dedicated learner. The target is to learn eight to ten "*pearls of knowledge*" each day from conferences and attending rounds. The most demanding time of training is during inpatient medical wards consisting of one day on-call, a day post-call, and 1–2 days of off-duty wellness. Organization is key to allow for three dedicated days each week for intensive review and self-education of materials. As such, this section lays out a detailed three-year, three-day-per-week plan to tackle the often-overwhelming amount of information trainees must learn. The "1,2,3" method is reflected in these three days a week. The *pearls* are of varying length given some material in internal medicine can be addressed quickly, while other material needs development in view of a broader context. The varying patterns of material depth aid learners in preparing for the internal medicine examinations, which feature concise questions and assessment of extensive stems, laboratory methods, and radiological features of conditions. Throughout this three-year study plan, *pearls* are reiterated and presented in different lights, essential for making connections and absorbing information.

© The Author(s), under exclusive license to Springer Nature Switzerland AG 2024
J. Lezama, *Internal Medicine Learning A to Z and 1, 2, 3*,
https://doi.org/10.1007/978-3-031-57546-4_1

Part I
Getting Started with the High-Reliability Journey

Introduction

Having a clear and consistent strategy for standardized testing is one of the strongest concepts I have pushed on my internal medicine residents and medical students over my many years of teaching as an attending internal medicine physician. I have had the experience of watching medical residents and medical students struggle with being uniform on the way they study and approach testing preparation. One of the themes in this section will deal with preparing for two areas that are asked with consistency on standardized testing, namely epidemiology and pharmacology. Another theme will deal with the emphasis on generic medication names and building strong familiarity with those terms not only from the standpoint of the medication itself but also the drug class for which the medication belongs. Yet another theme that is examined in this section involves the emphasis on common diseases much more in a standardized test than rare diseases. This section will provide a very concise yet complete strategic plan for the internal medicine resident or medical student preparing for a standardized internal medicine examination.

Tips for Testing

2

1. Never choose an option for an answer on standardized testing that states "ethics or psychiatry consult." You are expected to be the "complete" clinician and be able to choose a path of action that is listed as one of the choices.

2. If a rare condition such as Fabry disease is the answer to a question. You will be given at least 3–5 clinical clues to the diagnosis.

    Fabry disease is a lysosomal storage disease caused by the deficiency of alpha-galactosidase A. The disease is more prevalent in men than women. It causes a buildup of fat known as globotriaosylceramide in patients. Treatment is enzyme replacement.

3. Uncommon manifestations of common diseases are more likely as an answer than common manifestations of an uncommon diseases.

    Examples: Choose diabetes mellitus over Moyamoya disease when asked about a third nerve cranial palsy. Choose myopia over Leber's hereditary optic neuropathy when asked about cause for retinal detachment.

4. Learn classic disease groupings. You will be given one piece of the puzzle and then be asked to figure out the rest.

    Examples: MEN 1 syndrome—Hyperparathyroidism, pituitary tumors, and pancreatic tumors; MEN 2 syndrome—Hyperparathyroidism, medullary cancer of the thyroid, and pheochromocytoma; MEN 1 and MEN 2—autosomal dominant inheritance

5. Know every drug in a common drug class.

    Examples: Chlorthalidone for thiazide diuretics; Etodolac for NSAIDs; Tirofiban for glycoprotein 2b-3a receptor drugs; Other NSAIDs that appear on standardized exams. Naproxen, ibuprofen, indomethacin, ketoprofen, nabumetone, piroxicam, sulindac, tolmetin

6. Know the family (class) of drugs that medications belong.

    Examples: Metformin is a biguanide; Pioglitazone is a thiazolidinedione; Entacapone is a catechol-O-methyl transferase inhibitor (COMT inhibitor)

7. It is always good to know the second-line agents of treatment for conditions.

    Examples: Amoxicillin for Lyme disease in adults as second line; Anagrelide for second-line treatment essential thrombocytosis; Amiloride for second-line treatment of Conn's syndrome; Clindamycin and pyrimethamine as second-line treatment of toxoplasmosis; Dapsone as second-line prophylaxis for Pneumocystis jirovecii pneumonia

J. Lezama, *Internal Medicine Learning A to Z and 1, 2, 3*, https://doi.org/10.1007/978-3-031-57546-4_2

8. Start low and go slow in the elderly as far as dosing such as with levothyroxine. In younger folks, be aggressive with drugs such as levothyroxine where you start at the 1.6–1.7 micrograms/kg level in a young patient.

9. Smoking cessation always wins as a choice on the test. From CAD to peripheral vascular disease to histiocytosis X (Langerhans cell granulomatosis), smoking cessation is the next step in management.

    About histiocytosis X: Histiocytosis X is seen in predominantly the male population and the condition is marked by restrictive lung disease with high incidence of spontaneous pneumothorax.

10. Always learn the term in *parentheses* associated with many conditions

    Examples: Stein–Leventhal for polycystic ovarian disease; Osler–Weber–Rendu for hemorrhagic hereditary telangiectasia; Eosinophilic granuloma for histiocytosis X

11. Watch out for the "erythema"-like terms.

    Examples: Erythrasma vs. erythema multiforme vs. erysipelas vs. ecthyma vs. erythema marginatum.

12. Learn the details.

    Examples: Don't just learn arrythmias, learn atrial versus ventricular arrythmias. Potassium marked deficiency leads more commonly to ventricular arrythmias; COPD leads to atrial arrythmias

13. Learn issues associated with pregnancy.

    Examples: Hypertension treatment algorithm (alpha-methyldopa then hydralazine then labetalol); blistering disorder such as herpes gestationis; states such as epulis and melasma and meningiomas; issues with hepatitis E and microangiopathic hemolytic anemias.

14. Know the *ACLS* protocol.

    Example: When to do non-pharmacological maneuvers and when to go first to synchronized cardioversion. The commonly tested scenario will be the management of supraventricular tachycardia (SVT). The first step in assessing a patient with SVT is to have them do vagal maneuvers (cough and bear down activities). They resolve most of these arrythmias effectively. If that fails, then move forward with carotid massage as long as there are no carotid bruits auscultated in patients.

15. Know the classic dermatological states.

    Examples: Dermatofibroma, seborrheic dermatitis, seborrheic keratosis, basal cell cancers, melanoma, tinea versicolor, keratoacanthoma, actinic keratosis

16. Know the core neurological diseases of ALS, multiple sclerosis, myasthenia gravis, Parkinson's disease and variants of parkinsonism, West-Nile encephalitis.

17. Non-pharmacological measures beat pharmacological measures if a "tie" is present in the answers as a quest for avoiding medications.

    Examples: Choose foam overlay mattress to prevent decubitus ulcers, using hip protectors to prevent falls, using night lights to prevent falls, etc.

18. Always go back to the beginning of the question in a "question–answer" reconciliation before making a final choice.

    Examples: If a scenario given that the person is a fish handler or meat handler with cellulitis of hand, then likely choose erysipeloid as the cause of infection. If the scenario involves a patient with untreated hepatitis C history, then likely choose porphyria cutanea tarda for cause of blistering disease. If they have a scenario of a farmer going to a silo with fresh silage with acute dyspnea, then likely suspect nitrogen dioxide pneumonitis as the cause.

19. Know all the severe poisonings and antidotes.

    Examples: Know the carbon monoxide and treatment of hyperbaric oxygen, ethanol and similar alcohol poisonings with treatment of acute dialysis in severe life-threatening situations, and the salicylate poisoning with the scenario of respiratory alkalosis and anion gap metabolic acidosis with treatment of systemic alkalinization with monitoring of urine pH values.

20. Review all epidemiology facts.

    Examples: Sensitivity, specificity, negative predictive value, positive predictive value, number needed to treat, relative risk for cohort studies

21. Age and gender often aid in testing choices.

    Examples: On exams, multiple sclerosis new onset diagnosis over age 70 would not be expected; Goodpasture's disease won't be expected as a new onset diagnosis over age 50; temporal arteritis would not be expected as a new onset diagnosis under age 50; histiocytosis X is male driven and lymphangioleiomyomatosis is female driven.

22. If there are numerous medications listed in the first paragraph, then the answer likely involves making a change to the medication profile.

    Examples: Adjustment of dose; discontinuation of medication

23. Diseases such as pancreatitis or celiac sprue or ASD/VSD have numerous manifestations and could be an answer multiple times throughout the test and maybe even in the same session of questions.

24. Always look for the most complete answer in all the choices.

    Example: Aspirin and hydroxyurea as therapy for a patient with essential thrombocytosis

25. If the heart is listed as a choice when asked about the most significant benefit or worst side effect profile of a state, choose the heart!

    Examples: Hemochromatosis with starting phlebotomy having the best benefit for heart failure as disease modification; most patients with rheumatoid arthritis have cardiac disease as their number one cause of mortality; erythroderma can lead to new onset heart failure as the worst presenting clinical feature outside of skin findings; worst effect from scurvy is from systolic dysfunction heart failure.

26. EKG facts are important.

    Examples: Digoxin toxicity should be suspected in any patient with chronic atrial fibrillation who develops a regular junctional rhythm especially if with bigeminy. Low voltage on EKG is associated with hypothyroidism, pericardial effusions, and amyloidosis. The most common cause of left ventricular hypertrophy (LVH) on an EKG is underlying hypertension. Multifocal atrial tachycardia (MAT) is a common arrythmia seen in patients with severe COPD exacerbation.

Introduction

As the internal medicine resident prepares for the difficult task of learning such a broad range of material that encompasses the specialty over 3 years, repetition becomes crucial for the retaining of knowledge. The first "prescription" for internal medicine residents that I work with in this preparation in our program is for selecting a specialty topic per month to devote a large amount of study time over that month and for that specialty topic to be repeated in that same month in each of the three years of residency. This strategy allows that internal medicine resident to focus on a specialty topic in a given month consistently every year. An example would be to review allergy and immunology as the topic for July which is the first specialty by alphabet but fits nicely in July given the material for that specialty is not as voluminous as the other 11 specialty topics and July tends to be a month of transition for internal medicine residents whether it is the first month of residency for interns or the first month as a senior level resident in the second year.

The format of this section is done in A–Z manner so as to help keep the reader engaged and to help with recall of facts in a much easier fashion. An example from the allergy section is from the F letter which leads to fleeting infiltrates headliner that then leads to allergic bronchopulmonary aspergillosis being tied into that phenomenon of that ever-changing radiographic pattern. The 26 pearls or set of pearls for each letter of the alphabet set the stage for the internal medicine resident to pick up on necessary knowledge within that specialty topic in a consistent fashion every year for 3 years such that no stone is left unturned and encourages residents to further read for supplementation on the pearls that are given for each letter.

Allergy and Immunology

3

Alpha 1 Antitrypsin Young patients with advanced COPD, even if they smoke, need to be ruled out for alpha 1 antitrypsin disease. Lung disease is much more predominant than cirrhosis in patients with alpha 1 antitrypsin disease.

Belly Pain from ACEs ACE inhibitors can cause acute abdominal pain by creating a state of small bowel angioedema that is often mistaken for acute pancreatitis.

Candidiasis Heads Up Recurrent oral candidiasis is seen much more often in patients with cell-mediated immunity problems and not those patients with humoral immunity problems (low IGG or IgM). The most common endocrine disorder associated with mucocutaneous candidiasis is primary hypoparathyroidism.

Decongestants Only The first-line treatment of non-allergic perennial rhinitis is low-dose decongestants. Steroids are to be avoided as first-line agents.

Emphysema Emphysema can be distinguished from asthma on a set of PFTs by the DLCO which will be low in emphysema. Emphysema is an obstructive lung disease which means the FEV1 to FVC ratio must be below 70% for diagnosis of obstructive lung disease.

Fleeting Infiltrates Allergic bronchopulmonary aspergillosis is associated with "brown hamburger meat" sputum and will have positive skin tests to mold spore extracts. This condition is associated with fleeting pulmonary infiltrates and will commonly require initiation of steroids or increase in current steroid dose when symptoms worsen. Although an IGE level is helpful, the diagnostic test of choice is skin precipitins to Aspergillus.

Glucagon Glucagon is the treatment of choice in patients on beta-blockers who are not responding to epinephrine in the throes of an anaphylactic attack. Epinephrine is always the first drug to be given. After two doses with no response, then introduce the glucagon.

HIV Testing Issues Do not order HIV antibody serology in patients who have immunological disorders with low or non-existent gamma globulins as it may lead to false negative results. These patients will need lymphocyte subset testing or PCR for HIV viral load.

Ipratropium Nasal ipratropium is an effective treatment of gustatory rhinitis. This is a common finding on test questions involving patients eating at a spicy food location for instance.

Just for You Among the hypersensitivity reactions that are anaphylactoid (non-IGE mediated) are radiocontrast dye reaction, hypersensitivity pneumonitis, sulfite reaction, and reaction to yellow dye number five.

Know your Systemic Manifestations Urticaria pigmentosa is marked by mast cell infiltration of the skin and presents with Darier's sign where stroking of a macule causes formation of a wheal over the macule. Systemic involvement is termed systemic mastocytosis and this spectrum includes mast cell leukemia.

Levamisole Necrosis Patients with cocaine laced with levamisole which is an anti-helminthic drug will have skin necrosis of appendages such as the ears. This is not an allergic reaction!

More Fun with Numbers With deficiency of the late components of the complement pathway (C5b-C9), there is an association with recurrent Neisseria meningitidis infections.

Nasal Blood Flow Rate The definitive treatment of all allergic rhinitis conditions is the use of intranasal steroids. Steroids reduce mucus and nasal blood flow rate.

Oh My NSAID The Cox-2 inhibitors such as celecoxib are the safest to use with patients with the aspirin triad. Salsalate is the Cox-1 inhibitor safest to use if celecoxib is not available to patients.

PPI GERD should be in the differential of chronic cough and treatment-resistant asthma. A trial of portion pump inhibitor (PPI) is reasonable especially if the patient has worsened symptoms after recumbency.

Quiz Time On Delayed Hypersensitivity Delayed hypersensitivity occurs with involvement of T-cells usually 12–24 hours at minimum after the agent comes into contact with classic examples being poison ivy reactions.

Rhinitis Medicamentosa Rhinitis medicamentosa refers to drug-induced rhinitis caused most often by nasal oxymetazoline but also could be caused by alpha-blockers and estrogen-containing compounds.

Swelling (Angioedema) The two most common conditions resulting in acquired angioedema are CLL (chronic lymphocytic leukemia) and Waldenstrom's macroglobulinemia. CLL is also known for "exaggerated" skin responses to insect bites that are mistaken as "allergies" and such a response is truly a sign to rule out the presence of the disease.

Triad The aspirin allergy triad is of asthma, nasal polyps, and aspirin/NSAID intolerance. This has historically been known as Samter's triad.

Unilateral Sinusitis In the differential for unilateral sinusitis, tumor needs to be included. Tumors that can cause this condition include adenoid squamous cell cancer, lymphoma, angiofibromas (more common in adolescents), and inverted papillomas.

Very Important Test Serum tryptase levels are extremely helpful in working up patients with suspected mastocytosis.

When to Order CT in Sinusitis Rhinoscopies and limited sinus CT scans should be considered in patients with unilateral sinusitis findings.

EXtra Syndrome to Learn Granulomatosis with eosinophilia is a vasculitis with presenting signs of eosinophilia and asthma. Obviously, the vasculitis affects the lung. Treatment is with cyclophosphamide.

Yes Roaches! Cockroaches are one of the leading environmental reasons why asthma is felt to be increased in the inner-city population.

Zesty Final Allergy Fact Cromolyn sodium is an effective therapy in the treatment of exercise-induced asthma. Mechanism is mast cell stabilization.

Further Reading

Delves PJ, Roitt IM. The immune system. First of two parts. N Engl J Med. 2000a;343(1):37–49. https://doi.org/10.1056/NEJM200007063430107.

Delves PJ, Roitt IM. The immune system. Second of two parts. N Engl J Med. 2000b;343(2):108–17. https://doi.org/10.1056/NEJM200007133430207.

Fanta CH. Asthma. N Engl J Med. 2009;360(10):1002–14. https://doi.org/10.1056/NEJMra0804579.

Cardiology

4

Aortic Insufficiency/Regurgitation The usual murmur of chronic aortic regurgitation is a high-pitched, decrescendo mid to holo-diastolic murmur best heard with the bell and the patient leaning forward at the end of expiration at the left upper sternal border. There can be an associated Austin-Flint murmur which manifests as rumbling diastolic murmur due to a regurgitant stream hitting the anterior leaflet of the mitral valve. The acute aortic regurgitation murmur is usually a much shorter diastolic murmur.

Beta-blockers Side effects on the non-cardiac side of beta-blockers include nightmares, hyperkalemia, and possible blunted responses to epinephrine in patients on anaphylaxis.

COPD Arrythmias Patients with underlying COPD diagnosis often have multifocal atrial tachycardia marked by three different p-wave-forms on an EKG and is associated with pulmonary disease (especially with use of theophylline) and low potassium and magnesium states. Digoxin is contraindicated due to high risk of creating digoxin toxicity (can be seen with paroxysmal atrial tachycardia (PAT) with block or can be seen with multiform ventricular bigeminy with underlying junctional rhythm). Never cardiovert digoxin toxic patients unless it is truly a last resort as they can degenerate into ventricular fibrillation after cardioversion attempt.

Dobutamine and Dopamine Dobutamine is an inotropic agent that is useful in patients with severe ventricular failure. Unlike dopamine, it has no vasoconstricting effects.

Endocarditis Unique Organisms Patients with *Streptococcus bovis* or *Clostridium septicum* endocarditis will need colonoscopy to rule out colon cancer.

Fun with EKGs The causes of low voltage on an EKG are COPD, amyloidosis, hypothyroidism, and pericardial effusion. Hypothyroidism can cause this phenomenon even in the absence of a pericardial effusion.

Gallops s3 and s4 An s3 gallop can be heard best in the left lateral decubitus position and is heard in CHF exacerbation commonly. An s4 gallop is due to contraction of the atria against a stiffened ventricle and is found in ischemic heart disease, diabetic cardiomyopathy, and hypertensive heart disease with concentric hypertrophy. An s4 gallop is not found in patients with chronic atrial fibrillation as they lose their atrial kick that helps form the S4 gallop.

High Output Heart Failure Diseases with high-output heart failure include multiple myeloma, Paget's disease, hyperthyroidism, beriberi (thiamine or vitamin B1 deficiency), carcinoid syndrome, and anemia. Interestingly, the cardiac output is usually normal at the time of diagnosis because ventricular failure has advanced.

Ibutilide Ibutilide is a class III anti-arrhythmic which is associated with hypokalemia and a risk of torsades des pointes (thus have a magnesium level > 2.0 mg/dl before infusion).

J Wave (Osborne Wave) A slight slurring of the QRS complex on the downside of the complex (as opposed to the slurring on the upside of the complex as seen with Wolff–Parkinson–White patients) seen in patients with hypothermia. Rapid rewarming of patients is indicated with this clinical EKG finding in the setting of severe hypothermia.

Kussmaul Sign In patients with constrictive pericarditis, since the heart is encased in a calcified pericardium, the usual negative pressure associated with inspiration is sent to the venous inflow tract causing increased jugular venous distension during inspiration (known as the Kussmaul sign).

Left Main and Proximal LAD Disease Patients that benefit from CABG as their procedure of revascularization include left main disease, three vessel disease with reduced EF, and two vessel disease with considerable proximal LAD (left anterior descending) artery disease and either a reduced ejection fraction or impressive inducible ischemia during non-invasive testing.

Mobitz Mobitz 1 (second-degree heart block with increasing PR interval then a dropped QRS also known as Wenckebach phenomenon) is most commonly seen with inferior MI when it occurs in the setting of ischemia or infarction. If a patient with an anterior MI is admitted with a Mobitz 2 block (second degree with no increase in PR interval before a beat is dropped) or a new bifascicular or trifascicular block, then that patient will likely need mechanical pacing.

Negative Chronotropic and Inotropic Effect Verapamil is contraindicated in the setting of acute atrial flutter as it may lead to CHF or hypotension. Verapamil is a negative inotrope (meaning decreased oxygen demand but increased potential for heart failure) and a negative chronotropic activity (slowing of the SA and AV nodes). Diltiazem does not have as strong chronotropic or inotropic properties, but it usually is still avoided in acute CHF when ejection fraction is known to be under 35%. Treatment for thoracic aortic dissection distal to the subclavian artery is first accomplished with IV beta-blockers followed by nitroprusside.

Oh My Procainamide Procainamide is the classic member of the class Ia anti-arrhythmias that can lead to QT interval prolongation and the drug-induced lupus state similar to hydralazine. The most common side effects of that medication are GI intolerant effects such as diarrhea, nausea, and vomiting.

Posterior Wall MI Posterior wall myocardial infarctions are associated with large R wave in lead V1 and impressive ST-segment depression of greater than 2 mm along leads V1 and V2. There is usually an associated inferior infarction and there might be a right ventricular infarction (so check right-sided EKG and look for 1 mm ST elevation in lead V4r), especially if there is associated acute tricuspid regurgitation (pansystolic murmur at the lower left sternal border). Right-sided V-waves are large in tricuspid regurgitation and ventricular septal rupture in acute MI. Left sided V-waves are large with acute mitral regurgitation (as in MI) but not with chronic mitral regurgitation.

QRS Widening Widening of the QRS complex is a worrisome sign for patients with tricyclic antidepressant (TCA) poisoning and should lead to even more aggressive measures to enhance alkalinization therapy as this helps clear the TCAs from the system. Arterial blood gas pH should be followed for titration of degree of alkalinization occurring in the patient.

Right Ventricular Infarction Hypotensive patients with right ventricular infarcts need volume expansion with normal saline and the discontinuation of nitrates or furosemide.

Split of S2 The most common cause of a paradoxical split of S2 (split heard in expiration rather than inspiration) is a left bundle branch block. Other causes include right ventricular ectopic beats, IHSS (hypertrophic cardiomyopathy), aortic stenosis, and patent ductus arteriosus.

Tirofiban and Glycoprotein 2b-3a The glycoprotein 2b-3a inhibitors (abciximab, tirofiban, eptifibatide) are indicated in patients with acute coronary syndromes with persistent ST-segment depression and positive Troponin values.

U Wave The U-wave is most commonly seen in patients with electrolyte problems such as hypokalemia and hypomagnesemia.

Valve Issues A patient with symptomatic aortic stenosis should have valve replacement (symptoms usually fall in order of angina, syncope, and heart failure). Percutaneous balloon valvuloplasty is the treatment of choice in patients with symptomatic mitral stenosis, as long as there is not greater than moderate mitral regurgitation (in which case an open surgical procedure to include annuloplasty would have to be done). Complications of the valvuloplasty include severe mitral regurgitation, embolization, and tamponade. Complications of mitral stenosis prevented by the procedure include pulmonary hypertension, left atrial enlargement, and atrial fibrillation.

Wide Fixed Splits A persistently/widely split S2 (split quite noticeable in inspiration as expected but continues not as prominent in expiration) happens with RBBB, ectopic beats of the left ventricle, pulmonary embolism, and pulmonic stenosis. A fixed split S2 is seen with atrial septal defect (ASD) with usually the presence of a holosystolic murmur due to mitral or tricuspid regurgitation.

XTRA Careful with Syncope Patients with structural heart disease for which a cause of syncope is not found and not felt to be vasovagal syncope should undergo electrophysiologic testing.

Y Do We Need to Know This? Patients with supraventricular arrythmias can easily respond to vagal maneuvers that you can have them do such as bearing down or coughing. If that does not work, carotid massage once a carotid bruit is excluded on exam is the next step. Adenosine can work but the reason to know the above is that you will make the patient feel miserable every time that you give adenosine in treating their arrythmia.

Zesty Final Fact in Cardiology Deep symmetrical T-wave inversions over leads V1–V4 are commonly associated with a proximal left anterior descending coronary artery lesion and those patients generally should be taken to cardiac catheterization for immediate life-saving action. The EKG finding is known as Wellens sign.

Further Reading

McGee S. Etiology and diagnosis of systolic murmurs in adults. Am J Med. 2010;123(10):913–21 e911. https://doi.org/10.1016/j.amjmed.2010.04.027.
Neubauer S. The failing heart—an engine out of fuel. N Engl J Med. 2007;356(11):1140–51. https://doi.org/10.1056/NEJMra063052.
Nishimura RA, Holmes DR Jr. Clinical practice. Hypertrophic obstructive cardiomyopathy. N Engl J Med. 2004;350(13):1320–7. https://doi.org/10.1056/NEJMcp030779.
Pinto DS. A 43-year-old man with angina, elevated troponin, and lateral ST depression: management of acute coronary syndromes. JAMA. 2010;303(1):54–63. https://doi.org/10.1001/jama.2009.1870.
Ramanath VS, Oh JK, Sundt TM 3rd, Eagle KA. Acute aortic syndromes and thoracic aortic aneurysm. Mayo Clin Proc. 2009;84(5):465–81. https://doi.org/10.1016/S0025-6196(11)60566-1.
Ramani GV, Uber PA, Mehra MR. Chronic heart failure: contemporary diagnosis and management. Mayo Clin Proc. 2010;85(2):180–95. https://doi.org/10.4065/mcp.2009.0494.
Reimold SC, Rutherford JD. Clinical practice. Valvular heart disease in pregnancy. N Engl J Med. 2003;349(1):52–9. https://doi.org/10.1056/NEJMcp021265.

Geriatrics, Epidemiology, and Ophthalmology

5

Anisocoria Anisocoria that is long standing and present with less than 2 mm difference in the size of the pupils is usually a normal variant. A driver's license photo is a helpful tool in the ER when trying to distinguish whether the anisocoria is old or new if the patient is unaware.

Bias Selection bias is avoided if the randomization of subjects does not allow systematic unbalanced allocation of study subjects with predictive factors for cancer mortality into one of the study groups. This selection bias can be avoided by "intention to treat" analysis, rather than according to whether the subjects received screening or not.

Copper in the Eye Patients with Wilson's disease not only have Kayser-Fleischer rings due to copper deposition in Descemet's membrane but also are notorious for developing "sunflower" cataracts.

Diabetes Mellitus and the Eyes Diabetes mellitus can present with cranial nerve palsies (most commonly cranial nerve 3) that are usually painless and resolve with better control of underlying disease. Suspect if given clinical scenario with Hispanic population or Pima Indian population as both groups have marked increased incidence of diabetes.

Episcleritis Episcleritis refers to a limited inflammation of the superficial conjunctival area and runs a self-limited course with no referral usually needed to ophthalmology. It is not marked by the symptom of eye pain. Scleritis (which is frequently marked by eye pain) has the potential to erode through the sclera and needs to be urgently referred to ophthalmology.

Facts about Incontinence Detrusor hyperreflexia (instability) is the most common cause of incontinence in patients with Parkinson's disease. It is also considered the most common cause of incontinence in the general population. Choices in treatment are giving an anticholinergic to block bladder contraction or giving an alpha-adrenergic agonist to increase urethral resistance (preferred option).

Graves' Disease In Graves' disease, there is thickening of the extraocular muscles with sparing of the tendons. This differs from pseudotumor cerebri where the tendon is also thickened.

Hypopyon Iritis Hypopyon iritis refers to the pooling of white cells in the anterior chamber of the eye and can be seen in patients with Behcet's disease. Patients with this disease can have both posterior and anterior uveitis and the disease is also marked by pulmonary artery aneurysms, skin pathergy, and thrombophlebitis. The eye disease and the arterial disease respond best to chlorambucil.

J. Lezama, *Internal Medicine Learning A to Z and 1, 2, 3*,
https://doi.org/10.1007/978-3-031-57546-4_5

Intention to Treat "Intention to treat" is a method of analysis that involves analyzing data based on initial randomization into treated and untreated groups, regardless of subsequent outcomes such as poor compliance, crossovers, or migration. Thus, it is essential to answering the following question. "Does the decision to treat a certain population improve their outcome?"

Just Making Sure you Know A statistically significant test ($p < 0.05$) rejects the null hypothesis (the null hypothesis states that no differences of effect will be found). Thus, $p < 0.05$ indicates that a difference was found and that there is less than 5% probability that it occurred by chance. Trends in studies usually point to the need for larger, more involved study of a specific association.

Knowledge Check in Epidemiology A cohort would have study subjects categorized based on the exposure or lack of exposure of a risk factor (smoking in pregnancy) and then followed to determine if a particular outcome (low birth weight babies) results. A clinical trial is a prospective study in which an intervention is applied. In a case control study (which is always retrospective), you would select patients that are normal and those that have a unfavorable outcome (low birth weight) and then compare the frequency of a variable (maternal smoking) in both groups. Cross-sectional studies look at exposure and outcome at the same point in time.

Liver Metabolic Reactions in Elderly Phase 2 liver metabolic reactions of glucuronidation, acetylation, and sulfation remain unchanged in activity in elderly patients.

Macular Degeneration Macular degeneration is the most common cause of visual loss in this country and can have drusen seen in the macula on fundoscopic exam.

Neurofibromatosis and the Eye Patients with neurofibromatosis can develop Lisch nodules (hamartomas of the iris) if they have NF-1 disease, whereas patients with NF-2 disease are at risk of a peculiar cataract known as juvenile posterior subcapsular lenticular opacity. NF-1 and NF-2 are carried on different chromosomes. Optic gliomas can be seen in both conditions but remember that the bilateral acoustic neuromas are seen in NF-2.

Oculomotor Palsy An oculomotor palsy will leave the eye appearing "down and out." The lateral rectus is served by CN6, while the superior oblique is served by CN 4. A common scenario for patients with CN4 difficulties is a patient who gives a history of difficulty walking down the stairs due to vision.

Predictive Value Facts Predictive value of a test is dependent on the prevalence of a disease. The positive predictive value of a test is best described as "of those who have a test positive, how many will actually have the disease?" or [TP/(TP + FP)]. The negative predictive value is best described as "of those who have a test negative, how many actually do not have the disease" or [TN/(TN + FN)].

Quiz on Lead-Time Bias Randomized controlled trials with cancer mortality end points are the best way to avoid lead-time bias, because they measure mortality in both screened and non-screened patients from the same point of time, namely when they enter the study rather than when they were diagnosed with the cancer.

RA and the Eye Rheumatoid arthritis can cause scleritis, episcleritis, *Scleromalacia perforans*, corneal melt, corneal ulcers, and perforation of the eye globe. Rheumatoid eye disease responds well to cyclosporine-A.

Sjogren's and the Eye Sjogren's disease patients have dry eyes and dry mouth with positive anti-RO (anti-SS-A) and anti-LA (anti-SS-B) antibodies. The diagnosis of Sjogren's can also be made from a minor salivary gland biopsy showing reticular lymphocytosis.

Temporal Arteritis A pale, swollen, almost "ghost -like" optic disc is seen in patients with temporal arteritis. Treatment is immediate high-dose steroids with bilateral temporal artery biopsy to be scheduled within a week. Biopsy should show giant cells with disruption of the internal elastic lamina-but frequently the pathology is not seen as the disease tends to have skip areas.

Understanding Relative Risk The relative risk can be calculated by dividing the incidence of a disease in exposed individuals by the incidence of the disease in unexposed individuals.

Volunteer Effect Generalizability is a confounding effect that is not addressed by randomization in a definitive cancer-screening trial of volunteer study subjects with cancer mortality end points. The phenomenon introduced by the volunteer subjects is known as the healthy volunteer effect.

Wernicke's Disease Wernicke's disease in alcoholics can present with cranial nerve palsies along with ataxia. CN6 is the most common involved in this scenario.

XTRA Pearl on CMV Retinitis CMV (cytomegalovirus) retinitis can be treated with either daily IV foscarnet or IV ganciclovir or intraocular ganciclovir. Another way of treatment if the patient refuses all above choices is IV cidofovir once a week, which should be avoided in patients with marked chronic renal insufficiency.

Yes to Knowing Geriatric Physiology Among the physiological changes that occur in the normal elderly population are increased half-life of lipophilic drugs (e.g., benzodiazepines), decreased liver blood flow, decreased reductive/hydroxylation/oxidative/demethylation metabolism (phase 1 reactions) by the liver, decreased renal blood flow, tubular function, renal mass, and glomerular filtration rate.

Zesty Facts on Geriatric Cerebral Bleeds A cerebral bleed in elderly patients with a distribution not classic for hypertension-related (the classic hypertension-related areas are the pons, the pulvinar of the thalamus, the putamen, cerebellar poles) is usually due to the entity known as amyloid angiopathy.

Further Reading

Aletaha D, Smolen JS. Diagnosis and Management of Rheumatoid Arthritis: a review. JAMA. 2018;320(13):1360–72. https://doi.org/10.1001/jama.2018.13103.

Brisman JL, Song JK, Newell DW. Cerebral aneurysms. N Engl J Med. 2006;355(9):928–39. https://doi.org/10.1056/NEJMra052760.

Edlow JA, Caplan LR. Avoiding pitfalls in the diagnosis of subarachnoid hemorrhage. N Engl J Med. 2000;342(1):29–36. https://doi.org/10.1056/NEJM200001063420106.

Salvarani C, Cantini F, Boiardi L, Hunder GG. Polymyalgia rheumatica and giant-cell arteritis. N Engl J Med. 2002;347(4):261–71. https://doi.org/10.1056/NEJMra011913.

van der Worp HB, van Gijn J. Clinical practice. Acute ischemic stroke. N Engl J Med. 2007;357(6):572–9. https://doi.org/10.1056/NEJMcp072057.

Wong TY, Scott IU. Clinical practice. Retinal-vein occlusion. N Engl J Med. 2010;363(22):2135–44. https://doi.org/10.1056/NEJMcp1003934.

Endocrinology

6

Amenorrhea Patients with secondary amenorrhea who have withdrawal bleeding with progesterone challenge should have a workup that includes FSH, LH, prolactin, and TSH. Patients that fail this challenge should next receive cyclic estrogen/progesterone birth control pills for at least 2 months and if menses occurs, then a diagnosis of estrogen deficiency is made.

Beta-Hydroxybutyrate Beta-hydroxybutyrate is not detected in urine acetone tests done in patients with DKA. Besides hypokalemia arising with insulin treatment, hypophosphatemia (can cause diaphragmatic paralysis) can also occur.

Cushing's Syndrome Discussion Suppression of serum cortisol to less than 5 mg/dL (or suppression of urinary 17-hydroxycorticosteroids to less than 3 mg/dL) with a high-dose dexamethasone test speaks for the diagnosis of Cushing's disease (pituitary is the problem). If there was not suppression of serum cortisol on the high-dose dexamethasone test, this would leave adrenal adenoma, adrenal cancer, and ectopic ACTH as possibilities. A very high serum ACTH level is seen usually seen only with ectopic ACTH (most commonly with small or oat cell cancer of lung, but also carcinoid disease of the lung). In the patients with low ACTH, the diagnosis of adrenal adenoma is distinguished from adrenal carcinoma by measuring serum dehydroepiandrosterone (DHEA) or dehydroepiandrosterone-sulfate (DHEA-S) level or urinary 17-ketosteroids (which are all elevated in adrenal cancer).

Diabetes Insipidus (DI) Use of water deprivation test or DDAVP challenge (desmopressin acetate) helps distinguish patients with diabetes insipidus. If the ADH (antidiuretic hormone) does not increase with rising plasma osmolality, then the diagnosis is central (or neurogenic) DI. If there is increasing ADH with no concomitant increase in urine osmolality, then the diagnosis of nephrogenic DI is made.

Elevated Serum Calcium State Hyperparathyroidism is marked by elevated calcium and low phosphorus when it is primary, and the most common abnormality is a single adenoma in 85% of cases.

For Clarity on SIADH SIADH (syndrome of inappropriate antidiuretic hormone) that is chronic can be treated with demeclocycline. It decreases the sensitivity of the kidney to ADH. If a patient on this drug develops diarrhea, you must consider *Clostridium difficile* infection as the drug is an antibiotic. Patients should also be warned of photosensitivity with this medication.

G Raves' Disease Graves' disease has an increased radioactive iodine uptake (RAIU) as

J. Lezama, *Internal Medicine Learning A to Z and 1, 2, 3*,
https://doi.org/10.1007/978-3-031-57546-4_6

does toxic multinodular goiter and toxic adenoma. Young adults with Graves' disease (30% presenting with no goiter) should be treated with antithyroid medication first rather than radioactive iodine ablation. TSI antibodies are positive in Graves' disease. The pretibial myxedema in Graves' disease (also can be seen with hypothyroidism) appears peau d' orange due to a lymphocytic infiltrate.

Hashimoto's Disease The anti-microsomal antibodies (also known as antithyroid peroxisomal antibodies) will be elevated in Hashimoto's disease (the most common cause of hypothyroidism).

IGF-2 IGF-2 (insulin-like growth factor 2) or somatomedin C is used to screen patients with possible acromegaly. Confirmation of acromegaly would then require a growth hormone level to be drawn to be followed by a glucose load given. If the growth hormone level does not suppress, then acromegaly is biochemically confirmed.

Just in Time Thyroid Fact Patients with hypothyroidism can present with multiple physical exam manifestations to include alopecia, delayed relaxation phase on tendon reflexes, and muffled heart sounds from a pericardial effusion.

Klinefelter's Syndrome In male patients with primary hypogonadism, the testosterone level will be low and the LH will be high. Klinefelter's syndrome can cause this finding (karyotype XXY) and it is diagnosed with karyotyping from cells from a buccal smear or from peripheral leukocytes in blood.

Low Calcium States Hypocalcemia can be seen with hypomagnesemia (since magnesium is essential for PTH function) and pseudohypoparathyroidism (PTH resistance/congenital condition with adolescents of short stature and with short metacarpals in association with high phosphorus and PTH levels with normal alkaline phosphatase levels).

Macrosomia The risk of unchecked diabetes during pregnancy is of macrosomia of the fetus (birth weight greater than 9 pounds). A patient with diabetes who becomes pregnant will usually need about 50% more insulin administration than usual (due to insulin resistance) but these increased insulin requirements vanish within hours after delivery, thus careful observation is needed of the patient.

Nephrogenic Diabetes Insipidus and Central Too Thiazide diuretics are helpful in the treatment of nephrogenic diabetes insipidus (DI). Cheaper alternatives to DDAVP (desmopressin acetate) in mild to moderate central DI include chlorpropamide use in combination with either carbamazepine or clofibrate.

Osteomalacia Osteomalacia should be considered as a diagnosis in patients with bone pain and proximal muscle weakness. The test of choice is the 25 hydroxyvitamin D level if decreased intake is suspected but the usual cause of vitamin D deficiency is malabsorption (can also check the 25 hydroxyvitamin D level with this). Treatment of the condition is with oral 1,25 dihydroxyvitamin D. It can cause the finding of Looser's zones or Looser's lines on bone films which appear as fractures when none is present.

PTU PTU (Propylthiouracil) is the preferred drug of choice of hyperthyroidism during pregnancy as methimazole can cross the placenta and cause aplasia cutis of the fetus.

Quest for Adrenal Knowledge Patients with Conn's syndrome due to bilateral adrenal hyperplasia should respond nicely to medical therapy for hypertension with therapy that includes aldosterone receptor blocking agent (such as spironolactone or eplerenone).

Real-Time Skin Manifestation of Diabetes Necrobiosis lipoidica diabeticorum is characterized usually by a large plaque with overlying telangiectasias and can frequently be found in the anterior leg area of patients. This rash does not improve with hemoglobin A1c improvements and will often need local therapy such as steroid injections or laser therapy. It can also be found in about 30% of cases in the absence of any underlying diabetes mellitus.

Surgery Parathyroidectomy Time Indications for parathyroidectomy in primary hyperparathyroidism include 24-h urinary calcium excretion greater than 400 mg (usually seen with nephrocalcinosis of the kidney on ultrasound), serum calcium level above 11.0 mg/dL, and peak bone mass greater than or equal to 2 standard deviations below the mean for age, sex, and race. Luckily, this disease usually causes cortical rather than trabecular bone loss, thus vertebral fractures are rare. Other indications to take out parathyroid adenomas are urolithiasis, age less than 50, and creatinine clearance less than 70% of normal. Hyperparathyroidism is also associated with pancreatitis, peptic ulcer disease, and hypertension.

Thalamus Issues Causes of hypothalamic amenorrhea (decreased GNRH) include anorexia, bulimia (examine knuckles of patients for erosions and oral cavity for increased dental caries), and long-distance running. The prolactin level will be normal in these patients. Women with other types of hypothalamic amenorrhea can be treated with a GNRH pulsatile release pump which restores fertility.

Understanding Acromegaly Screening The best test for acromegaly screening is the somatomedin C level (also known as insulin growth factor level 1 (IGF-1)).

Vanillylmandelic Acid (VMA) The sensitivity of urine VMA levels for pheochromocytoma is lower than that seen for metanephrines testing but the specificity is quite high and can approach nearly 99% in non-familial cases of pheochromocytoma.

WHDA Syndrome VIP-OMAS (vasoactive intestinal peptide tumors) present with watery diarrhea, hypokalemia, and achlorhydria which has been termed the WHDA syndrome.

XTRA on CAH Late-onset congenital adrenal hyperplasia occurs with partial 21-hydroxylase deficiency most commonly and the screening test to differentiate it from polycystic ovarian disease is to measure for an elevated serum 17-hydroxyprogesterone level (seen with CAH). There is another type of late-onset congenital adrenal hyperplasia that involves 11-hydroxylase deficiency (thus serum 11-deoxycortisol will be elevated) and this can be seen in patients presenting with amenorrhea, hirsutism, hypertension, and hypokalemia.

Y Not Surgery Right Away? Treatment of pheochromocytoma is surgery but you need to delay surgery until there is initial proper pharmacological medical treatment initiated. The patients are given alpha blockade initially with phenoxybenzamine with an eventual transition to a concomitant beta-blocker (or just switched to labetalol monotherapy) to control tachycardia prior to surgery.

Zesty Pheochromocytoma Facts Pheochromocytoma (adrenal medulla tumor) is associated with MEN IIA (hyperparathyroidism and medullary carcinoma of thyroid) and MEN IIB (mucosal neuromas and the mentioned thyroid cancer). A clonidine suppression test is helpful to measure serum catecholamines after inconclusive urinary catecholamines as clonidine will suppress serum norepinephrine in essential hypertension but not with pheochromocytoma.

Further Reading

Chakera AJ, Vaidya B. Addison disease in adults: diagnosis and management. Am J Med. 2010;123(5):409–13. https://doi.org/10.1016/j.amjmed.2009.12.017.

Cooper DS. Antithyroid drugs. N Engl J Med. 2005;352(9):905–17. https://doi.org/10.1056/NEJMra042972.

Eisenbarth GS, Gottlieb PA. Autoimmune polyendocrine syndromes. N Engl J Med. 2004;350(20):2068–79. https://doi.org/10.1056/NEJMra030158.

Ismail-Beigi F. Clinical practice. Glycemic management of type 2 diabetes mellitus. N Engl J Med. 2012;366(14):1319–27. https://doi.org/10.1056/NEJMcp1013127.

Melmed S. Medical progress: acromegaly. N Engl J Med. 2006;355(24):2558–73. https://doi.org/10.1056/NEJMra062453.

Rosenfield RL. Clinical practice. Hirsutism. N Engl J Med. 2005;353(24):2578–88. https://doi.org/10.1056/NEJMcp033496.

Gastroenterology

7

Acetaminophen Acetaminophen is the most common cause of acute liver failure in the USA. A patient with acute fulminant hepatic failure should be transferred to a center with expertise in liver transplantation.

Bleeding Time The most common causes of lower GI bleeding include diverticulosis of the large intestine and angiodysplasia of the upper and lower gastrointestinal tract.

Celiac Sprue Celiac sprue is associated with lymphoma, and sometimes iron deficiency anemia will be the first and only clinical manifestation. The skin disease associated with this condition is dermatitis herpetiformis. If antibodies remain positive in this disease during treatment, then suspect non-compliance with dietary regimen.

D-Xylose D-xylose test checks for malabsorption involving the jejunum (small bowel). The test is abnormal if after 2 hours there is less than 20 mg/dL in serum or less than 5 g in 5 h in urine.

ETOH Alcohol is the most common cause of chronic pancreatitis. It is associated with calcifications of the pancreas that can often be seen with plain abdominal radiography.

Fat Malabsorption A qualitative screen for fat malabsorption is the fecal fat stain (Sudan Black). The diagnostic test is a 72-hour stool collection showing a fat output of greater than 7% of intake (between 60 g and 100 g).

Gaucher Disease Gaucher disease and Fabry disease are the two most common lysosomal storage disorder. Gaucher disease causes hepatosplenomegaly in nearly all patients afflicted with this disorder.

Hemangiomas Hemangiomas can be detected with tagged, pooled RBC nuclear scan. Only large hemangiomas (usually larger than 10 cm) will usually require surgical excision due to risk for spontaneous bleeding.

Irritable Bowel Syndrome Treatment of irritable bowel syndrome includes fiber supplementation with psyllium if constipated, loperamide if having diarrhea, exercise, lactose restriction, fluids, and anticholinergic medications if having spasms.

Just in Time. SBP Facts Spontaneous bacterial peritonitis is caused most commonly by *Escherichia coli*. *Streptococcus pneumoniae* is second most common pathogen on the list in many series. The treatment of choice is cefotaxime or ceftriaxone which are third-generation cephalosporins.

Kidneys in Cirrhosis Hepatorenal syndrome is marked by a urine sodium commonly less than

J. Lezama, *Internal Medicine Learning A to Z and 1, 2, 3*,
https://doi.org/10.1007/978-3-031-57546-4_7

5 mg/dL, and there is a very poor prognosis associated with the condition. There are no lesions that can be proven in histology of affected kidneys, and the kidneys may even be donated to transplant if the cause of the liver failure is not hepatitis B or C.

Lymphoma in GI   *Helicobacter pylori* is associated with a low-grade non-Hodgkin's lymphoma called MALToma, in which nearly 80% will regress just with antibiotics and might be diagnosed by biopsy of an area of redundant mucosal folds.

Mesalamine   Mesalamine (5-ASA) is considered first-line therapy for patients with mild to moderate active ulcerative colitis. Patients who have acute flares should be treated with intravenous corticosteroids.

Neoplasm GI   An adenocarcinoma neoplasm at the Ampulla of Vater will lead to silvery colored stools due to the combination of bile and blood entering the GI tract. These neoplasms can occur especially in patients with underlying Gardner's syndrome and thus why an esophagogastroduodenoscopy (EGD) is recommended as part of screening and surveillance of these patients.

Opisthorchis   *Opisthorchis viverrini* and *Clonorchis sinensis* are two of the worms highly associated with cholangiocarcinoma especially in the Southeast Asia corridor.

Peritonitis   The most common feared complication after cholecystectomy is for bile duct injury that would manifest as a bile peritonitis. It is particularly painful. In fact, it is considered the peritonitis is most often associated with severe pain on presentation.

Q-Fever and Liver   Q-Fever (*Coxiella burnetii*) is a common cause of acute liver failure with associated endocarditis. It is the most common culture-negative endocarditis cause of Europe and titers are needed in order to make the diagnosis. The treatment includes doxycycline.

Right Heart Failure in GI   Patients with right heart failure will have ascites that has a serum/ascites albumin gradient (calculated by subtraction of values) greater than 1.1 (similar value also seen in portal hypertension, myxedema, and Budd-Chiari syndrome) with total protein greater than 2.5 mg/dL (similar value also seen in tuberculous peritonitis, peritoneal carcinomatosis, pancreatitis, and nephrotic syndrome).

Swallowing Issues   Achalasia is associated with hypertensive lower esophageal sphincter with increased contractions of the esophageal body and abnormal contractions of the esophagus. "Bird's beak" is seen on barium swallow. Scleroderma is the opposite as it has a hypotensive lower esophageal sphincter. Patients with diffuse esophageal spasm will have a "corkscrew "appearance to their barium swallow and have normal lower esophageal sphincter pressure.

Tumor Necrosis Factor   Infliximab is superior to 6-mercaptopurine and metronidazole combination therapy for treatment of fistulas in Crohn's disease. Infliximab works against tumor necrosis factor-alpha.

Urea Breath Test   Patients felt to have recurrence of *Helicobacter pylori* need to be tested with urea breath test and should be off proton inhibitor pump therapy for at least 1 week and off antibiotics for at least 2 weeks.

Viruses   Patients who have been vaccinated for hepatitis B will not show a positive anti-HBc IgM or IgG (no core antibodies). The hepatitis B-e antigen ("e-antigen") usually reflects active viral replication and is positive in most cases of acute hepatitis B. Often the core IgM antibody of hepatitis B will be positive in acute cases (window period).

Watch out Clots!   Mesenteric artery embolus is associated with atrial fibrillation or rheumatic heart disease and presents with acute central belly pain—next test is mesenteric angiogram with embolectomy if possible. In contrast, ischemic colitis is associated with low-flow state and presents with rectal bleeding and lower abdominal pain with flexible sigmoidoscopy for diagnosis and surgery only if peritonitis develops.

XTRA Facts with Sprue Among the antibodies found in celiac sprue are the antiendomysial, anti-reticulin, and antigliadin antibodies. Patients with celiac sprue have small bowel biopsies showing blunting or atrophy of villous structures with hypertrophy of the crypts.

Yes Important Facts for Travelers! Patients with tropical sprue have similar lesions to celiac sprue except the former has a lymphocytic infiltrate rather than a monocytic infiltrate. Treatment of tropical sprue can be carried out with tetracycline therapy four times daily and folic acid daily therapy. Suspect if recent trip to the Caribbean or India or sub-Saharan Africa. Most patients present with mild eosinophilia and a megaloblastic anemia. They can have fat globules in stool.

Zesty Final Side Effects Fact Hypomagnesemia and tubular interstitial nephritis are among the side effects that can be seen with proton pump inhibitor therapy.

Further Reading

Kaplan MM, Gershwin ME. Primary biliary cirrhosis. N Engl J Med. 2005;353(12):1261–73. https://doi.org/10.1056/NEJMra043898.

Krawitt EL. Autoimmune hepatitis. N Engl J Med. 2006;354(1):54–66. https://doi.org/10.1056/NEJMra050408.

Lee WM. Drug-induced hepatotoxicity. N Engl J Med. 2003;349(5):474–85. https://doi.org/10.1056/NEJMra021844.

Leffler D. Celiac disease diagnosis and management: a 46-year-old woman with anemia. JAMA. 2011;306(14):1582–92. https://doi.org/10.1001/jama.306.14.1582.

Oxentenko AS, Bundrick JB, Litin SC. Clinical pearls in gastroenterology 2011. Mayo Clin Proc. 2011;86(11):1104–8. https://doi.org/10.4065/mcp.2011.0399.

Pratt DS, Kaplan MM. Evaluation of abnormal liver-enzyme results in asymptomatic patients. N Engl J Med. 2000;342(17):1266–71. https://doi.org/10.1056/NEJM200004273421707.

Whitcomb DC. Clinical practice. Acute pancreatitis. N Engl J Med. 2006;354(20):2142–50. https://doi.org/10.1056/NEJMcp054958.

Hematology and Oncology

8

Antibodies Antibodies in the antiphospholipid syndrome are directed against beta-2-glycoprotein-1. Livedo reticularis is a skin rash that can be seen in this disorder (rash also seen with cholesterol emboli syndrome).

Burkitt's Lymphoma Burkitt's lymphoma is the solid tumor version of ALL subtype L3 and is associated with a "starry-sky" appearance in bone marrow due to multiple vacuoles (filled with fat) that encompass the nucleus of these cells.

Colon Cancer Patients with Dukes' stage C colon cancer will have positive lymph nodes and should receive systemic chemotherapy with regimens such as 5-FU (fluorouracil) and leucovorin.

Drugs Time Drugs acceptable in treatment of heparin-induced thrombocytopenia (HIT) include hirudin, lepirudin, argatroban, ancrod, and danaparoid sodium. Note that low molecular weight heparin is contraindicated. Patients with HIT can present with thrombotic disease (white clot syndrome).

Erythromelalgia Erythromelalgia describes the redness, pain, and swelling of the digits seen with essential thrombocythemia and polycythemia vera. It is characteristically relieved with aspirin (some consider the immediate relief with aspirin as diagnostic of erythromelalgia).

Fun with Mixing The two causes of a PTT that does not correct in a 1 to 1 mixing study most commonly encountered in clinical medicine include the presence of a factor inhibitor and the antiphospholipid syndrome.

Gardner's Syndrome Gardner's syndrome is associated with colon polyps (with high malignant potential) and osteomas of the jaw. After colectomy, there is a high chance of recurrence in the ampulla of Vater which can present with "silvery stools."

HCC Hepatocellular carcinoma (HCC) is a risk factor in all patients with liver cirrhosis and is associated with a high AFP level. Patients with Wilson's disease have the lowest risk of proceeding to this state (felt to be due to somewhat protective effects of copper).

I Better Know this Benzodiazepines are the treatment of choice for anticipatory nausea and vomiting of chemotherapy. Decadron is quite effective for delayed nausea and vomiting of chemotherapy.

Just in Time Lymphoblastic lymphoma tends to have mediastinal involvement (anterior), presents in young patients with HIV, and CSF should be sampled to rule out involvement.

Knowledge Check Thymomas are associated with pure red cell aplasia and myasthenia gravis.

© The Author(s), under exclusive license to Springer Nature Switzerland AG 2024
J. Lezama, *Internal Medicine Learning A to Z and 1, 2, 3*,
https://doi.org/10.1007/978-3-031-57546-4_8

Leukemia AML M4 (myelomonocytic) and AML M5 (monocytic) need a lumbar puncture as part of workup due to high incidence of CNS involvement. An inversion of chromosome 16 with bone marrow eosinophilia imparts a good prognosis for AML m4 patients.

More Leukemia Facts AML M2 with 8,21 translocation and AML M3 with 15.17 translocation (promyelocytic leukemia) patients also have an excellent prognosis. In general, age greater than 60 is a poor prognosis for patients with AML.

Neoplastic Therapy Vincristine is associated with a peripheral neuropathy. Bleomycin leads to pulmonary fibrosis. Doxorubicin at cumulative doses of at least 450 mg/m^2 can potentially lead to cardiomyopathy.

Osmotic Fragility Test Osmotic fragility test used in the diagnosis of hereditary spherocytosis.

Prostate Cancer Pain Patients with prostate cancer who have multiple metastatic bone sites with pain not responding to appropriate opioid doses should be considered for strontium-89 therapy as an option for pain relief.

Quiz Time Patients with stage I prostate cancer have equal outcomes with surgery versus radiation therapy. Patients with metastatic disease should be considered for hormonal therapy (single agent as good as combination in most studies). Patients who have had orchiectomies in the past for prostate cancer do not need LH-RH analogue therapy and these patients should be placed on nuclear receptor blocking agents (flutamide) instead if the decision is made to treat with hormonal therapy.

R You Ready for This A prolonged bleeding time (as well as abnormal platelet factor assay testing) is NOT seen in hemophilia but rather with von Willebrand's disease. Remember that hemophilia B is also X-linked but that it involves factor 9 assay. Also, ristocetin cofactor assays are abnormal in von Willebrand's disease and not in hemophilia.

Small Bowel Most small bowel tumors are benign. A common histology type is a leiomyoma (although leiomyomas are usually found in the stomach most commonly). Small bowel tumors can serve as leading edges ("lead points") in adult intussusception.

Tylosis Tylosis of the hands (hyperkeratosis) is a finding associated with squamous cell cancer of the esophagus. Barrett's esophagus is not implicated in this histology type (only adenocarcinoma is associated with Barrett's).

Unknown Primary A woman with adenocarcinoma of unknown primary should have an axillary node dissection and if cancer is found in the lymph nodes, then she should be treated with chemotherapy targeted for breast cancer.

Very Important Pearl Turcot's syndrome is the only colon polyp syndrome that is felt by most authorities to be inherited in an autosomal recessive fashion. This syndrome is also associated with parenchymal brain lesions.

Watch Out Patients with a "bird's beak" appearance on a barium swallow should not be assumed to have achalasia *until* an EGD is performed to rule out infiltrating gastric cancer which can mimic achalasia on a barium swallow.

XTRA Good Pearl Spherocytes are seen in autoimmune hemolytic anemia and with hereditary spherocytosis (pigment gallstones common in this condition). When autoimmune hemolytic anemia is seen with idiopathic thrombocytopenia (ITP), it is called Evan's syndrome.

Yes Know This Polyps in Peutz-Jeghers syndrome (melanosis of lips and oral mucosa most commonly) are most commonly found in the small bowel, although they can be found in large bowel and stomach. Endometrial, ovarian, pancreatic, and breast cancer is associated with this syndrome as well.

Zesty Amyloid Facts AL amyloid is seen with multiple myeloma and primary amyloidosis.

AA amyloid is seen with inflammatory diseases such as rheumatoid arthritis. An enlarged tongue and "shoulder pad" sign can be seen with amyloidosis. Hypercalcemia is still the most common cause of renal failure in multiple myeloma. A subcutaneous fat pad aspiration is the best test to diagnose amyloid and is very non-invasive.

Further Reading

Bain BJ. Diagnosis from the blood smear. N Engl J Med. 2005;353(5):498–507. https://doi.org/10.1056/NEJMra043442.

Menon KV, Shah V, Kamath PS. The Budd-Chiari syndrome. N Engl J Med. 2004;350(6):578–85. https://doi.org/10.1056/NEJMra020282.

Moake JL. Thrombotic microangiopathies. N Engl J Med. 2002;347(8):589–600. https://doi.org/10.1056/NEJMra020528.

Olivieri NF. The beta-thalassemias. N Engl J Med. 1999;341(2):99–109. https://doi.org/10.1056/NEJM199907083410207.

Pelosof LC, Gerber DE. Paraneoplastic syndromes: an approach to diagnosis and treatment. Mayo Clin Proc. 2010;85(9):838–54. https://doi.org/10.4065/mcp.2010.0099.

Schafer AI. Thrombocytosis. N Engl J Med. 2004;350(12):1211–9. https://doi.org/10.1056/NEJMra035363.

Tefferi A, Hanson CA, Inwards DJ. How to interpret and pursue an abnormal complete blood cell count in adults. Mayo Clin Proc. 2005;80(7):923–36. https://doi.org/10.4065/80.7.923.

Infectious Disease

Asplenia State The mnemonic "SBED" can help you remember infections that afflict a patient with asplenia state. (S) Salmonella, (B) Babesiosis, (E) Encapsulated organisms such as Streptococcus, Neisseria, and Haemophilus, and (D) dog fermentor 2 infection, which is now referred to as *Capnocytophaga canimorsus* (pathogen from dog bite that can cause necrosis, purpura, sepsis, adrenal infarction, and subsequent hypotension).

Bullous Hemorrhagic Lesions Bullous hemorrhagic lesions can occur with infections due to *Vibrio vulnificus* or *Vibrio parahemolyticus*. Look out for liver disease patients that eat raw seafood or oysters or who come into contact with sea water. Liver disease leads to very high baseline ferritin levels that allow these organisms to thrive. Management is IV doxycycline plus possibly IV cefepime in addition if severe. A surgical consultation should be obtained in these cases as well given fasciitis is a common occurrence.

Cellulitis Review the common states and their treatments.

1. Diabetic foot ulcers requiring inpatient treatment should be treated with piperacillin-tazobactam or ticarcillin-clavulanic acid.
2. Usual cases of cellulitis in an immunocompetent non-diabetic patients requiring hospital-ization should be treated IV cefazolin or IV ampicillin-sulbactam or IV nafcillin.
3. Erysipelas infections should be treated with IV ampicillin-sulbactam.
4. Erysipeloid (caused by *Erysipelothrix rhusiopathiae*) should be treated with oral trimethoprim-sulfamethoxazole, oral clindamycin, oral fluoroquinolone, or oral penicillin (this infection common with fish handlers and meat handlers).
5. Cellulitis marked by streaking erythema is almost always caused by Streptococcus species and IV ampicillin-sulbactam is the drug of choice for those patients requiring hospitalization and one can add short-term IV clindamycin to further bid toxin.

Dengue and Malaria Dengue fever causes "break bone fever" and can lead to hemorrhagic variant if you have had previous dengue fever. The cerebral variant of malaria is caused by *Plasmodium falciparum* and you will often need red blood cell exchange transfusions for patients with heavy parasitemia load. For malaria infections with *Plasmodium vivax* or *Plasmodium ovale,* clinicians must add primaquine treatment to standard malaria treatment for liver phase eradication.

Erythrasma and Tinea Erythrasma is caused by *Corynebacterium minutissimum*. It mimics

J. Lezama, *Internal Medicine Learning A to Z and 1, 2, 3*, https://doi.org/10.1007/978-3-031-57546-4_9

tinea but it is a bacterial infection. A Wood's lamp will fluoresce coral red. Treat with oral erythromycin preferred. Tinea is a dermatophyte. It responds to terbinafine. It does not respond to nystatin, which treats only Candidiasis. Tinea does not generally have satellite lesions as seen in Candidiasis. *Trichophyton* is the most common genus causing tinea infections in the adult.

Fun with Endocarditis MSSA (methicillin sensitive *Staphylococcus aureus*) endocarditis is treated with IV beta-lactam (generally nafcillin or oxacillin) plus or minus aminoglycoside therapy. If vancomycin initially started due to fears of MRSA (methicillin resistant *Staphylococcus aureus*) but cultures return with MSSA as causative agent, then you must switch to IV nafcillin or oxacillin even if clinical improvement is occurring.

Great Pneumonia Facts Oral macrolide or doxycycline therapy is generally considered first-line treatment of outpatient community-acquired pneumonia in immunocompetent patients.

HIV Disease Prophylaxis If a patient has a CD 4 cell count which is at the threshold to start *Pneumocystis jirovecii* prophylaxis, then one should start with trimethoprim-sulfamethoxazole and may use dapsone if allergic to sulfa-based antibiotics. One may have to use atovaquone if a patient has glucose 6 phosphate dehydrogenase (G6PD) deficiency, and if reaching the threshold to start *Toxoplasmosis gondii* prophylaxis, then trimethoprim-sulfamethoxazole will also be effective but dapsone as a single agent therapy will not be effective alone. Pyrimethamine twice weekly will need to be added to dapsone for effective prophylaxis in those cases.

Infectious Diarrhea The most common traveler's diarrhea cause is ETEC (*Escherichia coli* toxigenic). The most common bacterial pathogen found in the USA is *Campylobacter jejuni*. Clinicians need to watch out for reactive arthritis weeks after patient has Salmonella, Shigella, Yersinia, or Campylobacter infections.

Just to Review Acute infections in HIV are treated as follows: *Pneumocystis jirovecii* infections are treated with IV trimethoprim-sulfamethoxazole and add steroids if AA gradient greater than 35 or PAO2 at room air less than 70 mmHg, and Toxoplasmosis infections are treated with IV trimethoprim-sulfamethoxazole plus daily pyrimethamine with clindamycin used with pyrimethamine in case of sulfa allergies.

Knowledge Effects on HIV Medications Abacavir can cause an acute hypersensitivity syndrome that can lead to death. Protease inhibitors increase likelihood of lipodystrophy changes although HIV itself can cause lipodystrophy without any medication effect.

Liver Disease Patient Infections Infections in patients with underlying liver disease can be referred to by the mnemonic "LYVA." "L" for Listeria meningitis (IV ampicillin first-line therapy), "Y" for Yersinia enterocolitica which can cause pseudoappendicitis infections (IV ceftriaxone as first-line therapy), "V" for Vibrio parahemolyticus and vulnificus (oral doxycycline as first-line therapy with addition of IV cefepime if severe infection present), and "A" for Aeromonas infection which is an aggressive cellulitis from freshwater exposure (IV penicillin as first-line therapy).

Meningitis Initially start with a broad-spectrum treatment with IV vancomycin plus IV ceftriaxone in all patients, adding IV ampicillin if the patient is pregnant, over age 65, has leukemia/lymphoma, or is a transplant patient. Once CSF is obtained, tailor according to the results as follows:

1. Gram-negative diplococci (Neisseria). Stop everything except IV ceftriaxone.
2. Gram-positive diplococci (Strep pneumonia). Continue IV vancomycin and IV ceftriaxone until the results of the oxacillin disc diffusion test return. If adequate susceptibility is noted, then stop IV vancomycin. IV ampicillin is discontinued as soon as that gram stain returns with gram-positive diplococci.

3. Gram-positive rod (Listeria). Continue IV ampicillin alone.

Nodular Lymphangitis Also referred to as the "sporotrichoid pattern" as it mimics the classic infection sporotrichosis and can be seen with the following causative organisms: Sporotrichosis, Nocardia braziliensis, Tularemia, and Leishmaniasis.

Oral Infections Oral hairy leukoplakia is a synergism of HIV and EBV (Ebstein Barr virus) infections.

Parotiditis and Head and Neck Diseases Almost all acute bacterial parotiditis are MSSA. Clinicians should treat with oral dicloxacillin or if severe, IV oxacillin or nafcillin. Watch out for Lemierre's syndrome. It is caused by Fusobacterium Necrophorum and starts in the submental space but then spreads to cause internal jugular vein thrombophlebitis followed by septic pulmonary emboli. Treat with IV beta-lactam and aminoglycoside.

Q-Fever and Other Diseases that Affect GI Tract Q-fever is caused by Coxiella burnetii which is notorious for endocarditis and liver failure. Treat with doxycycline. Tropical sprue can be seen in travelers to Caribbean or sub-Saharan Africa or India/Malaysia and should be treated with high-dose tetracycline and folinic acid for 4–6 months. Whipple disease is caused by *Tropheryma whipplei* and can cause hyperpigmentation, dementia, arthritis, and endocarditis. Treat with sulfa-based drug as first line for 12–18 months. PAS laden macrophages on biopsy tissue will be seen in this disease.

Rapid Infections MRSA fasciitis can be very aggressive and treatment should include surgical consultation early in the process as well as drugs that cover MRSA such as daptomycin and vancomycin. Mild MRSA infections with associated cellulitis can be treated with oral trimethoprim-sulfamethoxazole.

SBP First-line treatment for spontaneous bacterial peritonitis (SBP) is IV cefotaxime or ceftriaxone. Second line is IV fluoroquinolone therapy. One time episode of SBP equals lifelong prophylaxis with sulfa-based medication (first choice) twice weekly or fluoroquinolone once weekly.

Tick Bites
1. Lyme disease is associated with a rash called erythema chronicum migrans. It can also cause encephalitis and carditis (PR interval prolongation on EKG). First-line treatment is oral doxycycline in adults, and if allergic use amoxicillin therapy. For severe cases of carditis and neurological disease manifestations, one must use IV ceftriaxone,
2. Ehrlichiosis can lead to splenomegaly, hepatitis, thrombocytopenia, WBC inclusions and treat with doxycycline.
3. Babesiosis can lead to hemolytic anemia with RBC inclusions. Treat with azithromycin and atovaquone, OR treat with quinine and clindamycin.

Urinary Tract Infections Emphysematous pyelonephritis is most commonly caused by *E. Coli* in diabetics and first line is still IV ceftriaxone or fluoroquinolone, but patient may need nephrectomy if it does not clinically improve. Incidence is markedly increased in patients with diabetes mellitus.

Vibrio Infections *Vibrio vulnificus* and *Vibrio parahemolyticus* infections should be treated with doxycycline and adding a fourth-generation cephalosporin for severe disease states. All patients should get surgical consultations given the high degree of fasciitis.

Wuchereria *Wuchereria bancrofti* causes an infection that can lead to marked leg swelling. This occurs over years of exposure in an endemic area.

X Marks the Spot Disseminated gonorrheal disease with skin and joint manifestations can occur in which case you should extend to IV ceftriaxone for up to 4 weeks if severe. Gonorrhea classically causes a hemorrhagic pustular rash on erythematous base most often seen in the back of the hand.

Yersinia Infections Yersinia enterocolitica infections can mimic appendicitis and are best treated with ceftriaxone.

Zesty Final Facts on Nocardiosis Treatment of disseminated nocardiosis should be with oral trimethoprim-sulfamethoxazole for 3–6 months. Nocardia can cause brain abscess disease which may need a few weeks of IV amikacin as well as adjunctive therapy. Clinicians should look for disseminated subcutaneous nodules in the skin. Nocardia can cause cavitary lung disease which is partially AFB positive (but look for gram stain to be weakly gram positive as well which would not be seen in tuberculosis cases).

Further Reading

Jacoby GA, Munoz-Price LS. The new beta-lactamases. N Engl J Med. 2005;352(4):380–91. https://doi.org/10.1056/NEJMra041359.

Keller EC, Tomecki KJ, Alraies MC. Distinguishing cellulitis from its mimics. Cleve Clin J Med. 2012;79(8):547–52. https://doi.org/10.3949/ccjm.79a.11121.

Khawcharoenporn T, Tice A. Empiric outpatient therapy with trimethoprim-sulfamethoxazole, cephalexin, or clindamycin for cellulitis. Am J Med. 2010;123(10):942–50. https://doi.org/10.1016/j.amjmed.2010.05.020.

Mylonakis E, Calderwood SB. Infective endocarditis in adults. N Engl J Med. 2001;345(18):1318–30. https://doi.org/10.1056/NEJMra010082.

Oehler RL, Velez AP, Mizrachi M, Lamarche J, Gompf S. Bite-related and septic syndromes caused by cats and dogs. Lancet Infect Dis. 2009;9(7):439–47. https://doi.org/10.1016/S1473-3099(09)70110-0.

Swartz MN. Clinical practice. Cellulitis. N Engl J Med. 2004;350(9):904–12. https://doi.org/10.1056/NEJMcp031807.

Taege AJ. Tick trouble: overview of tick-borne diseases. Cleve Clin J Med. 2000;67(4):245–9. https://doi.org/10.3949/ccjm.67.4.241.

van de Beek D, de Gans J, Tunkel AR, Wijdicks EF. Community-acquired bacterial meningitis in adults. N Engl J Med. 2006;354(1):44–53. https://doi.org/10.1056/NEJMra052116.

Vannier E, Krause PJ. Human babesiosis. N Engl J Med. 2012;366(25):2397–407. https://doi.org/10.1056/NEJMra1202018.

Wenzel RP, Fowler AA 3rd. Clinical practice. Acute bronchitis. N Engl J Med. 2006;355(20):2125–30. https://doi.org/10.1056/NEJMcp061493.

AIP Acute intermittent porphyria (AIP) is associated with abdominal pain, hyponatremia, urine that turns dark on prolonged exposure with light, and is associated with a deficiency in HMB synthase (formerly known as PBG deaminase). This disease sometimes is misdiagnosed as familial Mediterranean fever due to abdominal pain complaint. Urine porphyrins should be obtained to help elucidate diagnosis.

Back Pain in Young Folks Ankylosing spondylitis is associated with apical pulmonary fibrosis, aortic insufficiency, arthritis, anterior uveitis, Ig A deposition in the kidney, and with increased incidence of amyloid in the kidney (note all the A's). Aortic insufficiency is also seen in relapsing polychondritis. Initial presentation of these folks can be back pain.

Cricoarytenoid Joint Involvement Hoarseness in a patient with rheumatoid arthritis (RA) should raise suspicion of cricoarytenoid joint involvement. C1-C2 sensory/motor findings in a patient with RA should raise suspicion of atlantoaxial subluxation. Patients with C1-C2 symptoms before an elective surgery should have preoperative lateral C-spine X-rays in flexion and extension to evaluate the degree of subluxation.

Drug-Induced Lupus Arthritis and pleuropericardial symptoms are commonly seen in drug-induced lupus (positive anti-histone antibodies). Renal disease is not associated with this syndrome, thus complement levels and anti-ds-DNA antibody levels should remain unchanged.

Extra Good Stuff on FMF Familial Mediterranean fever (FMF) is seen in patients of Turkish and Armenian descent and in the Sephardic Jewish population. Patients lack the inhibitor to C5a and tend to have episodes of peritonitis (#1 symptom noted), pleuritis, arthralgias, and even a rash near the ankles resembling erysipelas (sharp heaped-up, well demarcated borders). These patients are at risk of AA amyloid deposition in the kidneys. Treatment of choice for prophylaxis of attacks and to prevent the amyloidosis and proteinuria is colchicine in doses of at least 1.5 mg daily, which is theorized to work best if the creatinine of these patients is less than 1.5 mg/dL.

Felty's Syndrome Among the findings in Felty's syndrome (RA, neutropenia, and splenomegaly) are an association with large granular lymphocyte (LGL) syndrome, pretibial hyperpigmentation, and malleolar ulcers.

Gout Probenecid should not be used in patients with gout when the patient feels he or she will not be able to drink at least 1 gallon of water daily, when there is chronic renal insufficiency, and when there is a history of nephrolithiasis.

© The Author(s), under exclusive license to Springer Nature Switzerland AG 2024
J. Lezama, *Internal Medicine Learning A to Z and 1, 2, 3*,
https://doi.org/10.1007/978-3-031-57546-4_10

Hemochromatosis Hemochromatosis is associated with an arthritis of the second and third MCP joints. The joint pain does not tend to improve even after phlebotomy.

Iridocyclitis Iridocyclitis is a uveitis-type finding that can be found in patients who have Behcet's syndrome and ankylosing spondylitis.

Joints In over 90% of cases with *Staphylococcus aureus* septic joint (the most common cause of septic arthritis in RA and the general population), the organism will grow from synovial cultures.

Knowledge Check There must be at least 6 weeks of symptoms present before the diagnosis of rheumatoid arthritis is entertained, as many viral arthritides present very similar to rheumatoid arthritis but generally run their course in a month. Palindromic rheumatism is an entity of migrating oligoarticular arthritis that eventually flourishes into rheumatoid arthritis.

Levels of Complement in Lupus Complement levels (decrease of C3 and C4) and rising titers of anti-ds-DNA antibody are seen when there is exacerbation of renal disease with lupus. One-third of patients with SLE presenting with hypo-complementemia and nephritis will have a high titer of autoantibodies to C1q. All complement deficiencies can be screened with a CH50 assay.

Methotrexate Methotrexate is indicated as first-line treatment of rheumatoid arthritis (RA) in patients with erosive bone disease, which also tend to have positive rheumatoid factor and active deformities.

Not Gout Fact (Pseudogout) Pseudogout, which is associated with hyperparathyroidism and hemochromatosis, can give an X-ray finding of chondrocalcinosis of the affected joint. The clinical scenario usually given for pseudogout is that of knee arthritis in an elderly patient post-operatively after receiving crystalloid and colloid products which may have induced total body fluid changes.

Osteoarthritis Arthritis of the first carpometacarpal joint is most common in osteoarthritis.

Polyarteritis Nodosum Polyarteritis nodosa is a vasculitis associated with mononeuritis multiplex (commonly seen as foot drop), microaneurysms in a mesenteric angiogram in patients with abdominal pain, and with sparing of the lung.

Quiz on CPK The CPK level is normal in patients with temporal arteritis or polymyalgia rheumatica.

RA and Rheumatoid Nodules Methotrexate can cause a paradoxical increase in the formation of rheumatoid nodules.

Spinal Stenosis Spinal stenosis patients have pain worse with hyper-extension, while patients with sciatica tend to have pain worse with hyper-flexion.

Temporal Arteritis Vs. PMR The main symptoms noted in polymyalgia rheumatica (PMR) are pain and stiffness but classically there is *no* weakness. Steroid use of no more than 15 mg daily should bring about relief. Higher dose of steroids (usually 60 mg daily) is used in temporal arteritis.

U Better Know This The saddle nose deformity is seen in granulomatosis with polyangiitis (generally C-ANCA positive), congenital syphilis, relapsing polychondritis (red ears with redness sparing the lower non-cartilaginous lobe and with tracheochondritis as cause of respiratory failure), and lethal idiopathic granuloma of the midline.

Vasculitis The most common vasculitis is a drug-induced vasculitis, and it tends to be at the level of the post-capillary venule.

Wrists Carpal tunnel syndrome is seen in patients with RA, beta-2 microglobulin amyloid (patients with this condition have had hemodialysis for at least 5 years), acromegaly, pregnancy, and hypothyroidism. There also seems to be an increased incidence in diabetes mellitus but not as strongly as in the first five conditions mentioned.

X-Ray Findings Among the X-ray findings in osteoarthritis can be joint space narrowing, osteophyte formation, subchondral sclerosis or cyst formation, and prominence of tibial plateaus (usually in early knee disease).

You Look at the Nails in Rheumatology Nailfold capillaroscopy should be done in all patients with Raynaud's phenomenon.

Zesty Final Fact on Rheumatology A very high rheumatoid factor may be a clue to rheumatoid lung disease or rheumatoid vasculitis, and it tends to be also associated with rheumatoid nodule formation.

Further Reading

Sakane T, Takeno M, Suzuki N, Inaba G. Behcet's disease. N Engl J Med. 1999;341(17):1284–91. https://doi.org/10.1056/NEJM199910213411707.

Scott DL, Kingsley GH. Tumor necrosis factor inhibitors for rheumatoid arthritis. N Engl J Med. 2006;355(7):704–12. https://doi.org/10.1056/NEJMct055183.

Trentham DE, Le CH. Relapsing polychondritis. Ann Intern Med. 1998;129(2):114–22. https://doi.org/10.7326/0003-4819-129-2-199807150-00011.

Shekelle PG, Newberry SJ, FitzGerald JD, Motala A, O'Hanlon CE, Tariq A, Okunogbe A, Han D, Shanman R. Management of Gout: a systematic review in support of an American College of Physicians Clinical Practice Guideline. Ann Intern Med. 2017;166(1):37–51. https://doi.org/10.7326/M16-0461.

Stone JH. Polyarteritis nodosa. JAMA. 2002;288(13):1632–9. https://doi.org/10.1001/jama.288.13.1632.

Nephrology

11

A List for FSGS Causes of focal segmental glomerulosclerosis include HIV disease, chronic heroin use, chronic vesicoureteral reflux, obesity, Charcot-Marie-Tooth disease (associated with sensorimotor neuropathies and "stork" calves), and Fabry's disease (a lysosomal storage disorder that is X-linked recessive and associated with angiokeratomas).

Berger's Disease The most common of the acute glomerulonephritis syndromes is Berger's disease which involves mesangial deposition of IgA. Hematuria can occur after viral illness or after exercise. There is no effective treatment.

Calcium Stones Patients with idiopathic hypercalciuria have calcium oxalate renal stones and should be treated with thiazide diuretics and a low-sodium diet to decrease urine calcium. Low calcium diets do not work and are not practical with risk of osteoporosis.

Drugs Tips Among the rheumatological drugs that can lead to proteinuria are gold and penicillamine. NSAIDs can also cause proteinuria with a nephritic sediment. NSAIDs also decrease the release of renin which can lead to hyperkalemia in patients with hyporeninemic hypoaldosteronism.

Extra Lithium Fact Lithium can cause a nephrogenic diabetes insipidus. Treatment in severe intoxications is with emergent hemodialysis.

FENA Exceptions to the Rule The fractional excretion of sodium is always less than 1% in glomerulopathies. Acute glomerulopathies are associated with sodium retention due to intrarenal hemodynamic factors.

Glomerulonephritis Goodies Post-infectious glomerulonephritis is associated with diffuse cellular proliferation and subepithelial humps on kidney biopsy. This is a type 3 reaction causing granular deposits of IGG and C3. The skin infection and pharyngitis *both* lead to this condition but the skin infection is usually present well before the renal disease occurs. Group A beta-hemolytic strep infections are usually considered the common cause, and malaria and toxoplasmosis are two parasitic causes. Complement levels will return to normal after a short period of time.

Helpful Test at Times The urine chloride is a helpful test in metabolic alkalosis. If the level is less than 20 mg/dl, then the process can be treated with normal saline infusion.

J. Lezama, *Internal Medicine Learning A to Z and 1, 2, 3*,
https://doi.org/10.1007/978-3-031-57546-4_11

Interstitial Nephritis Chronic interstitial nephritis is associated with papillary necrosis and chronic analgesic abuse (especially mixed analgesics and those that have NSAIDs) with an incredible cumulative ingestion of the analgesic of greater than 6 pounds. It can also be caused by sickle cell disease, multiple myeloma, Sjogren's disease, and lead/cadmium poisoning.

Just Lie Down There is an entity known as benign orthostatic proteinuria in which proteinuria will revert to near-normal value once the patient becomes supine.

Knowledge Check If a patient with nephrotic syndrome range proteinuria is found to have an idiopathic cause (no underlying disease detected), the most common histology on kidney biopsy will be membranous glomerulopathy in Caucasian patients. A solid tumor can arise years after diagnosis of membranous nephropathy especially in the gastrointestinal tract. If minimal change disease is found in an adult as a cause of nephrotic syndrome, consideration to Hodgkin's disease should be given.

Level with Me Nephrotic syndromes usually have a normal C3 level. The C3 level is usually low in post-infectious glomerulonephritis and is low about half the time in membranoproliferative glomerulonephritis.

Medullary Kidney Disease There are two types of medullary kidney disease—medullary sponge kidney (usually diagnosed by IVP and not clinically significant unless kidney stones form) and medullary cystic kidney disease (in which there is usually a normal urinalysis with mild to no proteinuria, hyperkalemia, and hyperchloremic metabolic acidosis).

Nephrotic Syndrome Nephrotic syndrome patients tend to get edema, hypoalbuminemia, hypogammaglobulinemia (increased infections with Streptococcus and Haemophilus), loss of thyroid and iron binding globulins (low total thyroxine and iron levels), and loss of antithrombin III (leading to pulmonary emboli and renal vein thrombosis). They also have hyperlipidemia and despite the fact they can get pulmonary effusions and ascites, they usually do not get pulmonary edema unless they also have CHF.

Oh Kidney Stones Struvite stones (magnesium-ammonium-phosphorus stones) can be seen with staghorn calculi and are caused by recurrent Proteus infections with urinary pH generally above 8.0 value. Cystine stones have strong family history component and appear as a hexagonal crystal. Hyperoxaluria as a mechanism for calcium oxalate stones is seen in patients with Crohn's disease who have had terminal ileum resections. The radiolucent stones are the cystine and uric acid stones. Probenecid is contraindicated in patients with history of uric acid kidney stones.

PCKD Polycystic kidney disease (usually a mutation in short arm of chromosome 16) can present with progressive renal failure, hematuria, and hypertension. Proteinuria may be absent and if present is usually minimal. In adults, it is inherited in autosomal dominant fashion.

Quiz on Renal Failure in Pregnancy Patients with renal failure are not at increased risk of abortion of fetus or malformation in fetus nor is there a risk of progression of kidney disease during the pregnancy. There is an increased risk of pre-eclampsia. As renal failure worsens in a woman, her chance of becoming pregnant significantly decreases and most patients on dialysis cannot become pregnant.

RTAs RTA type 1 (distal) is the RTA associated with kidney stones, and the RTA type 1 is marked by a urine pH usually greater than 5.5 (unlike the other RTAs), has less than 10% bicarbonate filtered, is not associated with the Fanconi syndrome (distinguishes it from type 2 RTA), and is marked by a positive urine anion gap (unlike the process of GI bicarbonate loss) with low serum potassium (similar to RTA type 2 but unlike RTA type 4).

Syndromes Bartter's syndrome refers to the state of increased renin and aldosterone associated with hypokalemia and metabolic alkalosis in patients with normal blood pressure. This disease is due to hyperplasia of juxtaglomerular apparatus with prominence of medullary interstitial cells. Treatment is with *both* potassium and magnesium supplements (magnesuria is common) and patients are encouraged to have a liberal sodium dietary intake as they can get hypotensive. Spironolactone is the drug of choice to stop potassium wasting.

Top Five List The five diseases most closely associated with low complement levels are postinfectious glomerulonephritis, lupus, membranoproliferative glomerulonephritis, cholesterol emboli syndrome, and cryoglobulinemia.

Urinary Alkalinization Urinary alkalinization is used in all stones except struvite and calcium phosphate stones. Citrate therapy is useful in all calcium stones as it chelates calcium.

Very Conn Time Conn's syndrome is primary hyperaldosteronism and is associated with urine potassium and chloride levels above 30, hypokalemia, hypertension, and a metabolic alkalosis. Treatment is with spironolactone, or amiloride if patients cannot tolerate spironolactone. Potassium supplements are generally needed.

What Should I Know? Membranous nephropathy is associated with renal vein thrombosis and is marked by subepithelial deposits. It is the most common type of nephropathy after diabetes mellitus.

Xcellent Pearl Young women suspected to have renal artery stenosis should have a renal arteriogram to confirm the diagnosis (beading of the renal artery) and respond to interventional radiologic therapy.

Yes It's Poison! Ethylene glycol can cause calcium oxalate stones if taken in large amounts. Methanol (like ethylene glycol) can cause an osmolar gap and an anion gap metabolic acidosis but it does not cause oxalate crystals but it does cause a papillitis with acute visual loss. Isopropyl alcohol (rubbing alcohol) is not associated with a marked anion gap metabolic acidosis and can have hypoglycemia and a falsely elevated creatinine level. Treatment of all the alcohol-related ingestions when severe is with emergent hemodialysis.

Zesty Facts About Rapidly Progressive Glomerulonephritis Causes of rapidly progressive glomerulonephritis include SLE (systemic lupus erythematosus), granulomatosis with polyangiitis, Goodpasture's syndrome, and polyarteritis nodosa. This is marked by severe renal failure of recent onset. Cryoglobulins is also a cause, and treatment of the cryoglobulinemic glomerulonephritis will be with plasmapheresis and then an alkylating agent. It is marked by crescentic deposits in the kidney biopsy.

Further Reading

Chandrashekar KB, Fulop T, Juncos LA. Medical management and prevention of nephrolithiasis. Am J Med. 2012;125(4):344–7. https://doi.org/10.1016/j.amjmed.2011.10.022.

D'Agati VD, Kaskel FJ, Falk RJ. Focal segmental glomerulosclerosis. N Engl J Med. 2011;365(25):2398–411. https://doi.org/10.1056/NEJMra1106556.

Grantham JJ. Clinical practice. Autosomal dominant polycystic kidney disease. N Engl J Med. 2008;359(14):1477–85. https://doi.org/10.1056/NEJMcp0804458.

Himmelfarb J, Ikizler TA. Hemodialysis. N Engl J Med. 2010;363(19):1833–45. https://doi.org/10.1056/NEJMra0902710.

Psychiatry

12

Akathisia Akathisia is a term used to describe motor restlessness and is considered one of the extrapyramidal symptoms of anti-psychotics. Useful in treatment is anticholinergic drugs (such as benztropine) and beta-blockers.

Bupropion Bupropion is generally contraindicated in patients with a seizure disorder.

Clozapine Time Clozapine can cause agranulocytosis when used in the treatment of schizophrenia and patients will require weekly CBCs in the first few months of treatment.

Dyskinesia—Tardive Dyskinesia Tardive dyskinesia refers to the generally irreversible automatisms that develop due to long-standing anti-psychotic treatment, and it can be marked by dramatic lip smacking in patients.

Extrapyramidal Side Effects Among the extrapyramidal side effects of several anti-psychotics is pseudo-Parkinson's syndrome (resting tremor, cogwheel rigidity, shuffling gait). Treatment is with anticholinergic drugs and stopping or lowering the dose of the anti-psychotic drug.

Forget Me Not Pearl Early morning awakening is a usual finding in most cases of typical depression.

Great Pearl to Remember MAO-inhibitors and meperidine are contraindicated to be given in the same patient as there is a marked increase in seizures and hypertensive crises in patients that have received these medications concomittantly.

Haldol Haldol is useful in the treatment of tics and coprolalia associated with Tourette's syndrome.

Insomnia Early morning awakening is a classic hallmark feature of depression's effects on the sleep cycle.

Just for Emergency Acute serious lithium toxicity is treated with emergent hemodialysis.

Knowledge Check The stages of grief in a patient who is dying are the following five stages in order of presentation. Denial (shock), anger, bargaining, depression, and acceptance.

Lithium Lithium is associated with hypothyroidism. Lithium is associated with nephrogenic diabetes insipidus, which means there will be no response of the urine osmolality with administration of DDAVP.

Manic Disorder Treatment Valproic acid is used in the treatment of bipolar disorder (particu-

© The Author(s), under exclusive license to Springer Nature Switzerland AG 2024
J. Lezama, *Internal Medicine Learning A to Z and 1, 2, 3*,
https://doi.org/10.1007/978-3-031-57546-4_12

larly if rapid cycling) and has associated side effects of alopecia, pancreatitis, and weight gain.

Neuroleptic Malignant Syndrome Among the signs of neuroleptic malignant syndrome are fever greater than 105 degrees Fahrenheit, rigidity, hypertension, seizures, metabolic acidosis, and myoglobinuria. It tends to occur within the first 30 days of treatment and is more common in young adults. Treatment is in an ICU with bromocriptine (first line) or even dantrolene with close monitoring of potassium and numerous supportive measures to decrease fever including gastric lavage with cool ice water if needed. If patients persist in hyperthermia for a prolonged time, there is a risk of development of a permanent cerebellar syndrome.

Oh My MAO (Monoamine Oxidase Inhibitor) Selegiline is an MAO-B inhibitor that at usual doses for Parkinson's disease will cause seizures when given with meperidine.

Psychoses Severe depression in the elderly could present with psychoses and paranoid delusions. A diagnosis of new onset schizophrenia in a patient over age 65 is unlikely.

Quiz Time Clomipramine is a tricyclic antidepressant that is efficacious in the treatment of obsessive-compulsive disorder. It is second line after selective serotonin inhibitor (SSRI) therapy.

Really Nice Buspirone Pearl Buspirone is a non-sedating anxiolytic that is efficacious in the treatment of generalized anxiety disorder.

SSRI SSRI therapy is the first-line treatment of OCD, PTSD, social phobias (if drug therapy needed), and generalized anxiety disorder.

TCAs The tricyclic antidepressants with the fewest cholinergic side effects are the secondary amine compounds, which are desipramine and nortriptyline.

U Better Know This: Side Effect Time Side effects of trazadone therapy include sedation, priapism, and orthostatic hypotension.

Venlafaxine Side effects of venlafaxine include increased pulse and blood pressure as it is has noradrenergic/adrenergic effects.

Widening of QRS Widening of the QRS complex is a poor prognostic sign in patients with tricyclic antidepressant overdose.

XTRA Good Pearl Thorazine (Chlorpromazine) has been used in the treatment of chronic hiccups. It also can cause cholestatic liver disease.

Yes I Would Like Another Pearl on Hyponatremia Hyponatremia is a known lab abnormality that may occur during treatment of depression with SSRIs (such as paroxetine, fluoxetine).

Zesty Final Fact on Psychiatry Most serotonin syndrome episodes are marked by fever, along with confusion, diaphoresis, and seizures. Clonus is noted on neurological exam more than rigidity in serotonin syndrome episodes.

Further Reading

Boyer EW, Shannon M. The serotonin syndrome. N Engl J Med. 2005;352(11):1112–20. https://doi.org/10.1056/NEJMra041867.

Freedman R. Schizophrenia. N Engl J Med. 2003;349(18):1738–49. https://doi.org/10.1056/NEJMra035458.

Fricchione G. Clinical practice. Generalized anxiety disorder. N Engl J Med. 2004;351(7):675–82. https://doi.org/10.1056/NEJMcp022342.

Jenike MA. Clinical practice. Obsessive-compulsive disorder. N Engl J Med. 2004;350(3):259–65. https://doi.org/10.1056/NEJMcp031002.

ABPA Treatment of allergic bronchopulmonary aspergillosis (brown hamburger meat sputum) usually includes corticosteroids.

Biopsy Pleural biopsy is needed in many cases of pleural effusions to make a diagnosis of tuberculosis and mesothelioma.

Churg-Strauss Vasculitis Churg-Strauss vasculitis or granulomatosis with eosinophilia is associated with necrotizing small vessel vasculitis with eosinophilia. Patients have pre-existing symptoms of asthma and there is peripheral blood eosinophilia. Treatment is with both steroids and cytotoxic agents.

D-Vitamin Levels with Sarcoid Sarcoidosis is comprised of non-caseating granulomas which can cause hypercalcemia by increased hydroxylation of 25-hydroxyvitamin D to 1,25 OH2D3 which leads to increased calcium reabsorption from the intestine.

Extra-Thoracic Restriction Pure extra-thoracic restriction on PFT testing (will appear with attenuated flow-volume area on inspiration, which is the bottom of the flow-volume loop) is seen with kyphoscoliosis, obesity, and status post-CABG with cold cardioplegia (due to bilateral diaphragm paralysis). These patients will have low FVC value but FEV1/FVC value is above 80% because this is restrictive lung disease.

Flow-Volume Loops Patients with COPD will have attenuated area under their expiratory portion of the flow-volume loop (the upper part) and will have FEV1/FVC value below 70%. Treatment of choice is with anticholinergic agents (ipratropium).

Goodpasture's Syndrome Goodpasture's syndrome is a pulmonary-renal syndrome associated with hemoptysis usually seen in young male patients (ages 20–40) and associated with anti-glomerular basement membrane antibodies. Treatment in acute disease is with plasmapheresis.

Hypertension, Pulmonary The best diagnostic test for pulmonary hypertension is the right-sided heart catheterization which shows an elevated right atrial pressure and a pulmonary diastolic blood pressure greater than pulmonary capillary wedge pressure (which is usually over 20).

Intrathoracic Restriction Intrathoracic restrictive lung disease is distinguished from extra-thoracic lung disease by a disproportionately lower DLCO than TLC in the intrathoracic type. Intrathoracic restriction is seen with interstitial lung diseases.

Just So You Know About Methacholine A negative methacholine challenge test reliably excludes the diagnosis of asthma. A positive methacholine challenge test can be seen with other conditions and with 7% of the normal population.

Knowledge Check The best test for diagnosing *Pneumocystis jirovecii* lung infection is bronchoalveolar lavage.

Lungs Continued A pH above 7.4 and mesothelial cells above 5% in pleural fluid are two diagnostic findings that speak highly against a diagnosis of tuberculosis in patients with such findings.

Most Common Time Among the most common causes of hypersensitivity pneumonitis are moldy hay (due to thermophilic actinomycetes—also called "farmer's lung"), isocyanates, grain dust, and air-conditioning systems. These patients can have "fleeting" infiltrates.

Not Going to Be Tricked The most common cancer of the lung associated with asbestos exposure is adenocarcinoma/squamous cell lung cancers, *not* mesothelioma. Risk is synergistic with smoking. Most patients with mesothelioma will recall a history of having been exposed to asbestos in significant fashion or working an occupation with that risk factor. Smoking does not increase the risk for mesothelioma among those exposed to asbestos but it does increase the risk for lung cancer among those with asbestos exposure greater than those who smoke and do not have asbestos exposure.

On BOOP The treatment of choice of BOOP (bronchiolitis obliterans organizing pneumonia), which can be seen with patchy bilateral infiltrates in a patient with insidious onset of symptoms, is corticosteroids. Open lung biopsy is the diagnostic test.

Polyarteritis Nodosum Generally, polyarteritis nodosum is the most common vasculitis syndrome that spares the lung. It causes a non-granulomatous vasculitis of medium-sized arteries.

Quiz on Exudative Effusions Lupus, RA, pancreatitis, Boerhaave's syndrome (esophageal rupture), cancer, and infection are among the causes of exudative pleural effusions.

RA and Lung Effusions A pleural fluid analysis that has a low glucose (less than 40 mg/dl) and no sign of infection could be caused by rheumatoid arthritis.

Sarcoidosis Sarcoidosis can be diagnosed with a CXR showing bilateral hilar adenopathy if symptoms of erythema nodosum and ankle arthritis are present (Lofgren's syndrome).

Triglyceride Pleural Effusions Chylous pleural effusions (triglyceride level above 110 mg/dl) are seen with trauma to thoracic duct, lymphoma, mediastinal cancer/fibrosis, and lymphangioleiomyomatosis (a disease of premenopausal women also associated with spontaneous pneumothorax).

Under the Weather on Monday Workers in the cotton textile industry are at risk of byssinosis associated with chest tightness toward the end of the first day of the workweek.

Ventilator Permissive hypercapnea is often used in ARDS patients to keep peak pressures no higher than 35 cm H_2O. This avoids barotrauma and helps to avoid oxygen toxicity (FIO_2 should be below 60%).

Want Another One for ARDS? ARDS pearl again. Acute respiratory distress syndrome (ARDS) is defined as an acute lung injury where the Pao_2/Fio_2 value is less than 300 and is usually seen with bilateral pulmonary infiltrates and a wedge (PCWP) less than or equal to 18.

X-Factor for Cavitating Lesion Treatment of an aspergilloma (crescent sign on CXR or CT scan) that is heavily bleeding is with lobectomy of affected area not antifungal agents.

Yes, Know This Fact Tracheal stenosis presents with horizontal flattening of the top of both the expiratory and inspiratory portions of the flow-volume loop giving an appearance of a pentagon.

Zesty Facts on Secondary Pulmonary Hypertension Secondary pulmonary hypertension could be caused by chronic hypoxia, polycythemia vera, scleroderma (through intimal proliferation), chronic pulmonary emboli, filariasis/schistosomiasis, and any parenchymal lung disease.

Further Reading

Barker AF. Bronchiectasis. N Engl J Med. 2002;346(18):1383–93. https://doi.org/10.1056/NEJMra012519.

Laffey JG, Kavanagh BP. Hypocapnia. N Engl J Med. 2002;347(1):43–53. https://doi.org/10.1056/NEJMra012457.

Light RW. Clinical practice. Pleural effusion. N Engl J Med. 2002;346(25):1971–7. https://doi.org/10.1056/NEJMcp010731.

Ryu JH, Olson EJ, Midthun DE, Swensen SJ. Diagnostic approach to the patient with diffuse lung disease. Mayo Clin Proc. 2002;77(11):1221–7; quiz 1227. https://doi.org/10.4065/77.11.1221.

Ware LB, Matthay MA. Clinical practice. Acute pulmonary edema. N Engl J Med. 2005;353(26):2788–96. https://doi.org/10.1056/NEJMcp052699.

Dermatology and Neurology

14

Actinic Keratosis Actinic keratoses are the precursor lesions to squamous cell cancer of the skin. Cryotherapy is used in treatment of actinic keratoses but other therapies can be used for widespread disease.

Basal Cell Cancer Basal cell carcinoma is the most common skin cancer in immunocompetent individuals. Patients with solid organ transplant will have a marked increase in squamous cell cancer formation.

Carbamazepine Carbamazepine is the preferred treatment of trigeminal neuralgia.

Dopamine Receptor Agonists Dopamine agonist receptor drugs such as ropinirole or pramipexole can cause increased gambling behavior and mania-type symptoms (such as starting numerous jobs but never finishing any of them).

EEG Monitoring Inpatient video EEG monitoring should be done as next step in all patients with history of questionable seizures, particularly if "pelvic thrusts" are part of the movements described in the seizure (as these are unusual movements in true seizure episodes).

Fabry's Disease Skin Manifestations Fabry's disease is associated with angiokeratomatosis diffusum corporis as one of its leading skin manifestations.

Gold Side Effects Dermatology Gold is associated with an exfoliative dermatitis in treatment very similar to the exfoliative state that can be seen in patients taking lamotrigine.

Hemorrhagic Stroke A patient having a hemorrhagic cerebellar stroke should be evaluated by the neurosurgery team in urgent fashion for a decompression surgery.

Important Medication Note Methotrexate patients must take folic acid daily to avoid neuropathy along with prevention of oral ulcerations that can occur with folic acid deficiency.

JC Virus Look out for progressive multifocal leukoencephalopathy (PML) caused by the JC virus in patients with HIV disease who have low CD 4 counts and present with mental status changes and visual field deficits with ataxia.

Knowledge Check A serum ceruloplasmin measurement is the first step in management when suspecting a patient with Wilson's disease who has had seizures, liver disease, hemolytic anemia, and psychic overtones.

J. Lezama, *Internal Medicine Learning A to Z and 1, 2, 3*,
https://doi.org/10.1007/978-3-031-57546-4_14

Light Therapy UV light therapy can be used in management for patients with psoriasis. Ensure that the patient does not have a mimicker of this condition which is subacute cutaneous lupus erythematosus which will worsen with UV Light therapy by checking to make sure anti-Ro (anti-SS-A) antibodies are negative.

Metoclopramide Metoclopramide can cause a myriad of neurological issues to include tardive dystonia, akathisia, and drug-induced Parkinsonism.

Neurodermatitis Watch out for manifestations of patients with chronic scratch-itch cycle to include lichen simplex chronicus and prurigo nodularis.

ORF Orf is a skin rash caused by the poxvirus which can come about from handling of sheep and other livestock.

Progressive Supranuclear Palsy Patients with progressive supranuclear palsy will present with a "Parkinson's plus" type picture with bradykinesia, cogwheel rigidity, difficulty making turns, and tremor.

Q-Fever *Coxiella burnetii* can cause palpable purpura skin changes if there is associated endocarditis from the infection. Q-fever also likes to cause liver failure as well.

Rigidity in Serotonin Syndrome Rigidity is seen in less than half of cases of serotonin syndrome. More common neurological manifestations include hyperreflexia (clonus can be seen).

Startle Myoclonus Look for "startle myoclonus" in patients with rapidly progressive dementia when suspecting Creutzfeldt-Jacob disease.

Torticollis Botulinum toxin injections are used in the treatment of torticollis conditions.

Ulcers of the Skin The most common ulcerative skin lesion state associated with ulcerative colitis is pyoderma gangrenosum.

Very Important Association Look for multiple sclerosis if a patient has repeated episodes of trigeminal neuralgia or optic neuritis.

Wilson's Disease Wilson's disease which can be marked by seizures as part of its presentation is treated with D-penicillamine in acute stages and then treatment transitions to zinc for chronic therapy.

X-CESS of Pyridoxine Pyridoxine deficiency and excess can *both* cause a peripheral neuropathy.

Youthful Seizure Disorder Juvenile absence epilepsies may have an onset as late as age 16 and may have up to a quarter of patients suffer from myoclonic jerks. Valproic acid is first-line therapy for treatment of seizures from this condition.

Zinc Deficiency Acrodermatitis enteropathica is an inherited form of zinc deficiency with lifelong complications of alopecia, dermatitis, and secondary bacterial and fungal infections that can occur if zinc supplementation is not sustained.

Further Reading

Morison WL. Clinical practice. Photosensitivity. N Engl J Med. 2004;350(11):1111–7. https://doi.org/10.1056/NEJMcp022558.

Nestle FO, Kaplan DH, Barker J. Psoriasis. N Engl J Med. 2009;361(5):496–509. https://doi.org/10.1056/NEJMra0804595.

Purdy RA. The most important neurologic reflex! Am J Med. 2010;123(9):793–5. https://doi.org/10.1016/j.amjmed.2010.03.023.

Stam J. Thrombosis of the cerebral veins and sinuses. N Engl J Med. 2005;352(17):1791–8. https://doi.org/10.1056/NEJMra042354.

Part III

Internal Medicine Learning in the 1,2,3 Methodology: A Dedicated Three Days Per Week Approach

Year 1: Internal Medicine Learning Using "1,2,3 Methodology"

15

15.1 Introduction

While tackling a general specialty topic per month as pointed out earlier in this book, it is extremely important for the internal medicine resident to have a full balance of topics throughout all 3 years of internal medicine training. In particular, the first year should have a stronger blend of pearls material in the areas of cardiology, gastroenterology, and infectious diseases but needs to still introduce the concepts in endocrinology, rheumatology, and other outpatient electives. The pearls have been designed during the first year to have a greater emphasis on inpatient concepts given the fact that residents will spend more time on the wards and the ICUs during their first year than their next 2 years in general. In taking on this strategy, this will engage the internal medicine resident with this "prescription" for 3 days of every week of the first year.

The 3 days of pearls per week is based on the structure of the most difficult work structure usually present for a resident which is the ward week structure. During the ward week structure at most health care facilities, the resident is on a day of "long call" where they are taking admissions and thus a day not very negotiable for reading pearls of medicine in a structured fashion. Similarly the day after "long call," often called "post-call" is one where the ward team is usually at its highest census of the week. The resident then may also have either 1 or 2 days off during the week, and therefore in this book we decided to block out 4 days of the week for reading required pearls and push the requirement to read the pearls to the other 3 days of the week that are not "long call," "post call," or potential "off" days.

15.2 Year 1—Week 1—Day 1

1. In the differential diagnosis of tall R-waves in lead V1 of an EKG, be sure to include Wolff–Parkinson–White (WPW) syndrome, Duchenne's muscular dystrophy, posterior myocardial infarction, and right ventricular hypertrophy as possible underlying causes.
2. Methadone is the analgesic most associated with QT interval prolongation. The class IA anti-arrhythmic agent most associated with anticholinergic symptoms is disopyramide. Dapsone and metoclopramide are among the drugs that can cause methemoglobinemia.
3. The treatment of methemoglobinemia caused by dapsone includes activated charcoal for up to 3 days due to the enterohepatic cycling of the drug.
4. The most common toxicity of nitroprusside is thiocyanate toxicity, not cyanide toxicity.
5. Azathioprine is associated with drug-induced pancreatitis.

6. L-asparaginase is used in many treatment regimens for acute lymphocytic leukemia (ALL) and it is also associated with drug-induced pancreatitis.

7. Azithromycin and atovaquone, as well as clindamycin and quinine, are acceptable treatment regimens for Babesiosis. Treatment is short in duration in most cases with average being for about 5–7 days.

8. White blood cell inclusion bodies can be noted in the peripheral smear with Ehrlichia infections. Other lab abnormalities include thrombocytopenia and transaminitis in this infection.

15.3   Year 1—Week 1—Day 2

1. The treatment of mild methemoglobinemia is with oral methylene blue or with oral ascorbic acid. Life-threatening complications begin to occur with methemoglobin levels above 30%.

2. Inferior-lateral Q waves with no ischemia present can be seen on EKG in patients with hypertrophic cardiomyopathy.

3. The usual murmur of chronic aortic regurgitation is a high-pitched, decrescendo mid- to holo-diastolic murmur best heard with the bell and the patient leaning forward at the end of expiration at the left upper sternal border. There can be an associated Austin-Flint murmur (rumbling diastolic murmur due to a regurgitant stream hitting the anterior leaflet of the mitral valve). The acute aortic regurgitation murmur is usually a much shorter diastolic murmur.

4. Serum fructosamine levels can be measured in patients who have unreliable hemoglobin A1C levels due to hemoglobinopathies, such as sickle cell anemia. The fructosamine level reflects control over the preceding 30–45 days.

5. Beta-blockers are the anti-hypertensive agents most linked to nightmares.

6. There is a link noted between restless leg syndrome and iron deficiency anemia.

7. Scarring alopecia and follicular plugging in the ears are signs seen with discoid lupus.

8. The anti-Ro antibody will be positive in many cases of subacute cutaneous lupus erythematosus.

9. Dapsone is useful in treatment of lupus skin manifestations that do not respond initially to first-line medication of hydroxychloroquine.

10. Hemorrhagic bullous lesions can be seen with systemic lupus erythematosus (SLE).

15.4   Year 1—Week 1—Day 3

1. Pancytopenia, splenomegaly, and an unusual predilection for Legionella infections are hallmarks of hairy cell leukemia.

2. Hairy cell leukemia is treated with cladribine, also known as 2-CDA (2-chlorodeoxyadenosine).

3. Fludarabine and Rituxan (anti-CD20 monoclonal antibody) are among the more popular treatments for aggressive chronic lymphocytic leukemia (CLL).

4. Basal cell carcinoma may need Mohs microsurgery if it is sclerosing and located in places such as the nose or nasolabial fold.

5. The most common type of melanoma is superficial spreading type.

6. A pure seminoma tumor of the testicle will be AFP (alpha fetal protein) stain negative always.

7. A pinealoma is associated with Parinaud's syndrome, which includes obstructive hydrocephalus, papilledema, and inability for upward gaze.

8. An ACTH stimulation test for 17-hydroxyprogesterone is a useful test in working up congenital adrenal hyperplasia.

9. Idiopathic hirsutism in women can be treated with spironolactone.

10. Lidle's syndrome, which mimics Conn's syndrome in presentation but is not associated with elevated aldosterone, is best treated with amiloride.

15.5 Year 1—Week 2—Day 1

1. Insulin resistance and platelet dysfunction are among the problems associated with coronary artery bypass grafting (CABG).
2. Two other complications from CABG include cold cardioplegia syndrome (phrenic nerve paralysis) and a possible sympathetic injury mechanism leading to an exudative pleural effusion, usually on the left side.
3. Theophylline can cause multifocal atrial tachycardia similar to that seen in patients with chronic obstructive pulmonary disease (COPD).
4. To check on dietary compliance in patients with celiac sprue, check antibody titers regularly as they should go negative with dietary (gluten-free diet) compliance.
5. Cholesterol emboli syndrome can be caused by both post-cardiac catheter procedure setting and during an early period of initiation of anticoagulation treatment.
6. Coumadin can cause adrenal insufficiency by causing bilateral adrenal hemorrhages.
7. Gram-negative septicemia can occur in patients with *Strongyloides stercoralis* infections.
8. Mitoxantrone is indicated in secondary progressive multiple sclerosis. Glatiramer acetate has only been approved generally for use in relapsing-remitting multiple sclerosis.
9. A patient on a beta-blocker may not respond to epinephrine when it is given in the setting of anaphylaxis.
10. The first line treatment for the development of anaphylaxis in a patient taking a beta blocker medication will be epinephrine. Glucagon is given as rescue medication if no response to epinephrine.

15.6 Year 1—Week 2—Day 2

1. Amiodarone and D-penicillamine are among the drug-induced causes of BOOP (bronchiolitis obliterans with organizing pneumonia).

2. Dry, "Velcro-like" rales are auscultated in patients with idiopathic pulmonary fibrosis.
3. Patients with silicosis are at marked increased risk of tuberculosis.
4. Pulmonary alveolar proteinosis is treated with total lung lavage.
5. Sweet's syndrome is marked by an increased risk of acute myelogenous leukemia (AML) in the future as well as other hematological disorders.
6. Cimetidine and trimethoprim-sulfamethoxazole (due to the trimethoprim portion) are known to cause false elevations in serum creatinine in patients with unchanged glomerular filtration rates.
7. Diffuse esophageal spasm will cause a "corkscrew" pattern on a barium swallow.
8. Achalasia and tylosis are underlying risk factors to develop squamous cell carcinoma of the esophagus.
9. Cyclophosphamide is the treatment of choice for patients with polymyositis with interstitial fibrosis (these patients can be anti-JO-1 positive or anti-histidyl TRNA synthetase positive).
10. Bleomycin can cause scleroderma-like changes of the skin.

15.7 Year 1—Week 2—Day 3

1. The two drugs to especially avoid in patients with accessory pathway conduction are digoxin and verapamil.
2. Lown–Ganong–Levine syndrome is similar to Wolff–Parkinson–White (WPW) syndrome except there are no delta waves seen and conduction is by the Bundle of James (Bundle of Kent is the one in WPW).
3. Syncope is a cause of convulsions that may resemble seizures (felt to be due to sudden hypoxia to the brain).
4. Syringomyelia is the most common cause of upper extremity Charcot joints.
5. Treatment of tricyclic antidepressant poisoning is systemic alkalinization, which is followed by pH of the arterial blood gas.

6. Widening of the QRS complex portends the poorest prognosis in patients with tricyclic antidepressant (TCA) poisoning.

7. One of the possible complications in correcting acidosis in patients with diabetic ketoacidosis is the development of hypophosphatemia, which theoretically could lead to respiratory failure by diaphragmatic dysfunction.

8. Cyclobenzaprine and oxybutynin are causes of mental status changes, especially in the elderly, due to the anticholinergic nature of the drug.

9. Hypertrophic cardiomyopathy and mitral stenosis are cardiac causes of syncope.

10. The two types of neurocardiogenic syncope are vasodepressor and cardioinhibitory (where asystole greater than 3 s may be seen).

15.8   Year 1—Week 3—Day 1

1. Sulfasalazine, cyclosporine, and infliximab are treatment options for pyoderma gangrenosum.

2. *Streptococcus* is the most common infectious agent to cause erythema nodosum. Other infectious causes include *Yersinia, Coccidiomycosis*, and tuberculosis.

3. Aphthous ulcers can be seen in patients with inflammatory bowel disease.

4. Acrodermatitis enteropathica is the rash that is seen with zinc deficiency.

5. Scurvy is seen with perifollicular plugging and corkscrew hair formation. Treatment is ascorbic acid and complications include left ventricular dysfunction leading to heart failure.

6. Dermatitis herpetiformis and lichen planus lesions are pruritic.

7. Tissue transglutaminase is felt to be the most sensitive and most specific antibody to detect celiac sprue.

8. Oral beta-carotene is the treatment of variegate porphyria, which demonstrates features of both porphyria cutanea tarda and acute intermittent porphyria.

9. Urticaria and vasculitis can be seen with hepatitis A infections.

10. There has been an association in the literature between hepatitis C and lichen planus. The better known dermatological association of hepatitis C is porphyria cutanea tarda, which is caused by lack of activity or by deficiency of uroporphyrinogen decarboxylase. The abnormal enzyme in acute intermittent porphyriahas has two names used in the literature for description which are hydroxymethylbilane (HMB) synthase or porphobilinogen (PBG) deaminase.

15.9   Year 1—Week 3—Day 2

1. The three essential components to preoperative clearance for a non-cardiac surgery are (a) functional capacity, (b) the type of surgery being done, and (c) the clinical predictors of coronary artery disease.

2. The most common cause of a paradoxical split of S2 (split heard in expiration rather than inspiration) is a left bundle branch block. Other causes include right ventricle ectopic beats, hypertrophic cardiomyopathy, aortic stenosis, and patent ductus arteriosus.

3. Carotid endarterectomy is considered an "intermediate risk" vascular surgery in the perioperative risk assessment literature.

4. Most abdominal surgeries (including radical prostatectomies) are considered as intermediate risk surgeries for cardiac events as well.

5. Most breast surgeries are considered low risk surgeries for cardiac events.

6. A patient with intermediate clinical risk factors for coronary artery disease (CAD) and with good functional capacity going for an intermediate risk surgery (such as hip or knee replacement) can go straight to the operating room without any further cardiac

workup under most pre-operative risk assessment models.

7. A good functional capacity implies the ability to do activities that include walking up one flight of stairs, walking up a hill, or walking on flat ground at 4 miles/h without chest pain or shortness of breath.

8. A patient with CAD with increasing dyspnea on exertion in a crescendo pattern should be treated just as if it was crescendo angina (as the dyspnea is an anginal equivalent) and cardiac catheterization should be strongly considered.

9. A hospitalized patient with trifascicular heart block and syncope should be strongly considered for pacemaker placement before discharge from hospital.

10. Smoking cessation within 6–8 weeks of surgery has not been shown to improve surgical outcomes as far as pulmonary complications, and some studies have even shown worse outcomes.

15.10   Year 1—Week 3—Day 3

1. Manifestations of acute pancreatitis include lobular panniculitis, Grey-Turner's sign, and Cullen's sign (periumbilical hemorrhage).

2. Essential thrombocytosis is associated with erythromelalgia (redness and burning of the extremities that are relieved with aspirin).

3. Syphilis is associated with generalized lymphadenopathy and oral mucous patches when it is secondary. Treatment is benzathine penicillin G for three treatments (separated by 1 week).

4. Lemierre's syndrome is associated with *Fusobacterium* infections marked by septic pulmonary emboli and internal jugular vein thrombophlebitis.

5. A persistent widely split S2 (split quite noticeable in inspiration as expected but continues not as prominent in expiration) happens with right bundle branch block, ectopic beats of the left ventricle, pulmonary embolism, and pulmonic stenosis. A fixed split S2

is seen with atrial septal defect (usually there is also a holosystolic murmur due to mitral or tricuspid regurgitation).

6. Multiple sclerosis can cause blurry vision with hot showers due to decreased nerve conduction with heat.

7. Lichen planus is associated with a pruritic rash usually at the wrist that can have oral lesions.

8. Parvovirus infections can be seen with livedo reticularis.

9. Parvovirus infections are associated with aplastic anemia and giant pronormoblasts can be seen in the bone marrow aspirate/biopsy.

10. Myasthenia gravis has an association with thymoma and thymic hyperplasia. Computed tomography (CT) of thorax should be done in these patients.

15.11   Year 1—Week 4—Day 1

1. Livedo reticularis and mental status changes are among the manifestations of antiphospholipid antibody syndrome.

2. Antibodies against beta-2-glycoprotein 1 should be considered in patients suspected to have antiphospholipid antibody syndrome who have negative anticardiolipin antibodies and negative lupus anticoagulant panel.

3. Nailfold capillaroscopy should be done in all patients with Raynaud's phenomenon. Changes can be seen with scleroderma and dermatomyositis patients.

4. Anti-RO (anti-SSA) antibody is positive in patients with subacute lupus erythematosus.

5. Splenic rupture can occur spontaneously in patients with infectious mononucleosis, even from something as simple as a Valsalva maneuver.

6. Do not forget that cytomegalovirus virus (CMV) can also cause an infectious mononucleosis picture.

7. *Salmonella* joint infections are increased in incidence in patients with sickle cell disease due to gut microinfarction.

8. Eosinophilic fasciitis will have a *peau d'orange* appearance and is a mimicker of scleroderma. It usually arises after vigorous physical exertion.

9. Other conditions associated with a *peau d'orange* appearance include pretibial myxedema (most commonly seen with hyperthyroidism and inflammatory breast cancer).

10. Patients with linear scleroderma, also known as morphea, are not at increased risk of visceral involvement. This disease is purely skin-limited.

15.12 Year 1—Week 4—Day 2

1. Monkey bite patients should receive treatment with acyclovir even if no acute infection is seen due to a marked incidence in Herpes infections.

2. Cat and dog bite patients should receive Augmentin (amoxicillin-clavulanic acid). If you are PCN allergic, fluoroquinolone therapy is acceptable second-line treatment.

3. *Pasteurella multocida* is the usual causative agent of most cat bite infections. Pasteurella is also found in dogs, but not to the extent as in cats.

4. *Eikenella corrodens* is a pathogen of concern in human bites. Treatment initially in substantial infections should comprise debridement and IV beta-lactam therapy.

5. *Aeromonas hydrophilia* is a freshwater pathogen with increased incidence in patients with liver disease. It is important to note that it can cause a gas-producing cellulitis, similar to *Clostridium, E. coli, and Klebsiella.*

6. Methicillin-resistant *Staphylococcus aureus (MRSA)* cellulitis can be treated with sulfamethoxazole-trimethoprim or doxycycline.

7. Chronic hidradenitis suppurativa can lead to squamous cell cancer of the skin, similar to chronic erythema ab igne process.

8. If a patient is found to have non-tuberculous *Mycobacterium* pneumonia, one should ask about exposure to hot tubs and indoor swimming pools as risk factors.

9. Hypersensitivity pneumonitis can occur from saunas (Sauna takers lung) and is usually caused by *Aureobasidium* species.

10. *Erysipelothrix rhusiopathiae* is the pathogen responsible for erysipeloid, which affects fish handlers. Treat with amoxicillin-clavulanate as first line but you can use doxycycline in penicillin-allergic patients.

15.13 Year 1—Week 4—Day 3

1. Patients with cat and dog bites should be placed on amoxicillin-clavulanate therapy if being discharged home. Use fluoroquinolones if penicillin allergy present.

2. Cephalosporin therapy does not work on *Enterococcus and Listeria* infections.

3. Low molecular weight heparin should not be used for deep venous thrombosis prophylaxis (DVT) in patients with creatinine clearance that are markedly decreased. Use unfractionated heparin three times daily for DVT prophylaxis of medical patients in this setting.

4. Argatroban and lepirudin are agents that can be safely used for anticoagulation in patients with heparin-induced thrombocytopenia.

5. Recognize that chlorthalidone is a thiazide diuretic that works for hypertension treatment.

6. Non-steroidal anti-inflammatory drug (NSAID) medications include sulindac, mefenamic acid, etodolac, and phenylbutazone.

7. Patients with granulomatosis with polyangiitis are best treated with cyclophosphamide and steroids for therapy.

8. Among one of the best tests for lupus anticoagulant is a sensitive partial prothrombin time (PTT) assay.

9. The lesions of lichen planus are very pruritic. Patients with lichen planus will occasionally have hepatitis B or hepatitis C so it is worth testing for these entities.

10. Hepatitis B is strongly associated with polyarteritis nodosum. Hepatitis C is strongly associated with porphyria cutanea tarda.

15.14 Year 1—Week 5—Day 1

1. If surgery is planned on a medullary carcinoma of the thyroid, then the diagnosis of pheochromocytoma must be ruled out as it could lead to hypertensive crisis during surgery. The screening test for pheochromocytoma is 24-h urinary collection for metanephrines, catecholamines, and VMA. Patients with medullary carcinoma of the thyroid will have elevated serum calcitonin levels.

2. To distinguish patients with TSH below 0.003 who have low to zero radioactive iodine uptake obtain a thyroglobulin level. The thyroglobulin level will be elevated in subacute thyroiditis, while it will be low in surreptitious use of Synthroid (also known as thyrotoxicosis factitia).

3. Among the potential causes of hirsutism in females, a marked elevation occurs in the DHEA (or DHEA-S) level and urinary 17-ketosteroids with the diagnosis of adrenal cancer. These patients generally have a near-normal testosterone level, as opposed to the marked elevation in testosterone in stromal ovarian cancers (which is another cause of hirsutism).

4. Polycystic ovarian disease (Stein-Leventhal) syndrome is marked by a LH to FSH ratio greater than 3, and the disease is marked by obesity/hirsutism/amenorrhea (may be primary) and is also marked by conversion of androgens to estrogens in peripheral tissues.

5. Dysbetalipoproteinemia syndrome is the type 3 of the hyperlipoproteinemia syndromes and is marked by a high IDL (thus high triglycerides and LDL). There is abnormal apolipoprotein E in this disease.

6. Type 2a syndrome of the hyperlipoproteinemia syndromes is marked by a high LDL only and is generally caused by decreased LDL receptors. It has the strongest association of all the syndromes with CAD and LDL levels generally above 250 mg/dl at a young age. Tendon xanthomas are common with this syndrome, but eruptive skin xanthomas (associated more with high triglycerides) are not usually seen.

7. Clofibrate fell out of favor in treatment of hyperlipidemias as it can cause abnormal LFTs, cholelithiasis, and even hepatic cancer. Gemfibrozil is the preferred drug of the fibric acid derivatives as it increases the activity of lipoprotein lipase on VLDL, thus causing a decrease in triglycerides and an increase in HDL with an occasional increase in LDL also that can occur.

8. Chylomicrons are the main reason triglycerides are elevated in hyperlipoproteinemia syndromes type 1 and 5. In type 1, there is either a lipoprotein lipase deficiency or APO CII deficiency, and after serum is spun down and cooled there will be a creamy layer with clear infranatant. In type 5, there is also elevated VLDL so there will be a creamy layer (the chylomicrons) and a milky infranatant (the VLDL).

9. Treatment of prolactin-secreting macroadenomas is with bromocriptine which can restore both menses and fertility in women. Failures to bromocriptine (or patients that cannot tolerate the drug) will need transsphenoidal surgery followed by irradiation.

10. Patients with diabetes mellitus type 2 who initially present with high triglyceride levels can be given insulin which activates lipoprotein lipase and brings down the triglyceride level impressively without use of gemfibrozil, even if the triglyceride levels are over 1000 mg/dl.

15.15 Year 1—Week 5—Day 2

1. *Vibrio vulnificus or parahemolyticus* infected patients (usually with underlying liver disease) will have hemorrhagic bullae present in the lower extremities.

2. Besides those *Vibrio* species, *Listeria, Yersinia, and Aeromonas* are frequent pathogens in patients with underlying liver disease.

3. Patients with Listeria meningitis must receive ampicillin IV for treatment as cephalosporins are ineffective in treating this disease.
4. If a patient has decerebrate posturing, then the midbrain has likely suffered injury. If patient has decorticate posturing (marked by hands to the heart), then the thalamus had likely suffered injury.
5. Patients with elevated prolactin level must be ruled out for pregnancy. In addition, amitriptyline, phenothiazines, and metoclopramide can cause an elevated prolactin level.
6. Severe hypothyroidism can also cause an elevated prolactin level. The treatment is to treat the underlying hypothyroidism.
7. Non-functioning pituitary adenomas can elevate the prolactin level by "stalk effect," whereby dopamine levels are decreased and prolactin subsequently rises.
8. Women who are having irregular periods or are truly amenorrheic and are noted to have clitoromegaly on physical exam need to be ruled out for androgen secreting tumor of the adrenal gland or the ovary.
9. Patients with polycystic ovarian disease will have acne, hirsutism, and obesity.
10. Acanthosis nigricans has a high association with insulin resistance.

15.16 Year 1—Week 5—Day 3

1. There has never been a historical need for endocarditis prophylaxis in patients with ostium secundum ASD (atrial septal defect) or pulmonic valve stenosis.
2. A VSD (ventricular septal defect) may cause a diastolic rumble if it is large or if the left to right shunt is greater than 2.5–1.0 value.
3. Most VSDs are small and cause harsh, holosystolic murmurs which are best heard at the left sternal border and radiate to the right sternal border at times.
4. EKG finding of ASD ostium secundum is the following. Right bundle branch block pattern over lead V1 with a right axis deviation.

5. Coarctation of the aorta can cause a harsh holosystolic murmur that is heard over the back. Rib notching on a CXR may be seen due to development of collateral circulation over the years.
6. Thrombolytic therapy can be used in pregnant patients when the pros of treatment outweigh the cons of treatment.
7. Papillary muscle rupture is usually seen in the setting of inferior myocardial infarction due to a poor supply of the posteromedial aspect of the muscle. A high wedge pressure without a step-up of oxygen saturation between the atria/ventricle would be expected.
8. All mechanical complications after myocardial infarction will require consultation to the thoracic surgery service.
9. An increase in preload or afterload will increase the murmur of hypertrophic cardiomyopathy. Maneuvers or events that will cause this increase include a post-extrasystolic beat, Valsalva maneuver, amyl nitrate infusion, standing from a squat position, isoproterenol infusion, and exercise.
10. S3 gallop or JVD presence is the factor with the highest risk of post-operative cardiac complications per Goldman's criteria.

15.17 Year 1—Week 6—Day 1

1. Cefotaxime is the first-line treatment of choice of spontaneous bacterial peritonitis.
2. Primaquine is used to treat the "liver phase" of *Plasmodium vivax* and *Plasmodium ovale*.
3. Pentoxifylline can be used in the adjunctive treatment of cerebral malaria. Red cell exchange transfusions are more definitive in the treatment.
4. Hypothyroidism can cause transudative pleural effusions and pericardial effusions.
5. Besides its use in CML (chronic myelogenous leukemia), imatinib mesylate is used in the treatment of gastrointestinal stromal tumors (GIST).

6. The most common causes of Conn's syndrome are adrenal adenoma and bilateral adrenal hyperplasia.
7. IGF-1 (insulin-like growth factor 1), which is also known as somatomedin C, is used to screen for acromegaly.
8. Osteomalacia can cause bone pain and pseudofractures on radiology films, and the condition is due to vitamin D deficiency.
9. The test of choice to screen for osteomalacia is a 25-hydroxyvitamin D level.
10. Among the various causes of hypercalcemia is adrenal insufficiency, vitamin A toxicity, vitamin D toxicity, lithium toxicity, and Zollinger-Ellison syndrome.

15.18 Year 1—Week 6—Day 2

1. Fluoroquinolones have been linked to a false positive opioid assay on drug screen.
2. Phentermine is associated with a false positive amphetamine assay on drug screen.
3. Morbid obesity may lead to obstructive sleep apnea, atrial fibrillation, and even nephrotic syndrome.
4. Surgery is needed for only the most severe cases of typhlitis. First-line treatment is metronidazole or beta-lactam therapy with anaerobic coverage.
5. Multiple myeloma was associated with a low anion gap in older lab instrument assays (due to unaccounted cationic charges from proteins).
6. Basophilia is strongly associated with chronic myelogenous leukemia (CML).
7. Eosinophilia may occasionally be associated with leukemia so consider bone marrow biopsy when no diagnosis is uncertain.
8. Splenic and renal infarcts should heighten the suspicion for endocarditis.
9. Gram-negative sepsis is a common complication of patients with *Strongyloides stercoralis* intestinal infections.
10. Actinomycosis is a risk factor in female patients who use intrauterine devices (IUDs). Penicillin is the first-line treatment.

15.19 Year 1—Week 6—Day 3

1. Most patients with severe aortic stenosis and pregnancy will face bed rest throughout their pregnancy.
2. Primary pulmonary hypertension and Eisenmenger's syndrome are absolute contraindications to pregnancy.
3. Think of mitral stenosis in a pregnant patient who comes in with new onset pulmonary edema during pregnancy.
4. Cardiomyopathy can also occur during pregnancy as a cause of pulmonary edema. Patients are at risk of cardiomyopathy in subsequent pregnancies as well.
5. The first step in evaluating a prolonged PT (after repeat testing) is administration of vitamin K.
6. The first step in evaluating a prolonged PTT (after repeat testing) is ruling out heparin effect. Once heparin is eliminated as a possible cause, the next step is a mixing study.
7. If on the mixing study there is a correction of the PTT, then the cause is a factor deficiency. If on the mixing study there is no correction of the PTT, then the cause is either factor inhibitor if they present with bleeding or bruising (most common is factor 8 inhibitor) or antiphospholipid antibody syndrome (if they present with thrombotic events).
8. The best way to manage hyperglycemia post-CABG is with an insulin drip.
9. Lupus tends to flare during pregnancy, whereas rheumatoid arthritis tends to remit during pregnancy (remember the phrase "R.A. remits" and lupus will be the opposite).
10. Thrombotic thrombocytopenia purpura (TTP) can strike during the second trimester of pregnancy, whereas entities such as acute fatty liver, intrahepatic cholestasis, HELLP syndrome, and HUS tend to strike in the third trimester of pregnancy.

15.20   Year 1—Week 7—Day 1

1. High output heart failure can occur from an AV fistula at any site.
2. Paget's disease, beriberi, and multiple myeloma also cause high output congestive heart failure (CHF).
3. Patients with diastolic heart failure have abnormalities in active relaxation and passive stiffness accounting for their CHF.
4. Both *Bartonella quintana and Bartonella henselae* have been associated with cat scratch disease, bacillary angiomatosis, bacillary peliosis, splenitis, endocarditis, and osteomyelitis.
5. The diagnostic stain for Bartonella is the Warthin-Starry silver stain.
6. A Fite stain or Ziehl-Nielsen stain is a modified AFB stain that is useful in detecting *Nocardia* species.
7. Chlorambucil and alpha interferon are among the drugs that have been used to treat erythroderma associated with mycosis fungoides.
8. Secondary syphilis can cause oral mucous patches and a lichenoid rash.
9. Helicobacter pylori infection seems to double the risk of GI bleed in NSAID users.
10. Tiotropium is the name of a once-daily COPD anticholinergic inhaler.

15.21   Year 1—Week 7—Day 2

1. Sudden death, RSR prime pattern in the V1–V3 leads, and ST elevation pattern diffuse are findings in Brugada syndrome.
2. Jugular venous distension, muffled heart sounds, and clear lungs are hallmarks of right heart failure.
3. Hypotension, loud murmur at sternal border, and being having had a myocardial infarction at least 3 days ago are hallmarks of new onset ventricular septal defect.
4. Loud murmur at the apex of heart and post-MI state 3–7 days ago especially with an inferior myocardial infarction are associated with the finding of papillary muscle dysfunction.

5. Prolonged QT syndrome, deafness, and use of beta-blockers for first-line treatment are associations that are seen with Lown-Ganong-Levine syndrome.
6. PR segment depression, diffuse ST elevation, and chest pain are hallmarks of pericarditis.
7. Very fast atrial fibrillation in young patient, delta waves when in sinus rhythm, and short PR intervals are hallmarks of Wolff–Parkinson–White syndrome.
8. COPD, amyloidosis, and hypothyroidism are three common causes of low voltage on an EKG.
9. Pulmonary fibrosis, bluish skin discoloration, and liver function test abnormalities are side effects of amiodarone therapy.
10. Wolff–Parkinson–White, hypertrophic cardiomyopathy, hypothyroidism are three causes of Q waves in the inferior leads not due to ischemia.

15.22   Year 1—Week 7—Day 3

1. Causes of an increased TBG (thyroid binding globulin) and therefore a decreased T3 resin uptake (T3RU) include estrogen (including OCP), pregnancy, tamoxifen, clofibrate, narcotics, hepatitis, and primary biliary cirrhosis.
2. Causes of a decreased TBG and therefore an increased T3RU are androgens, glucocorticoids, and nephrotic syndrome.
3. Among the drugs that block the peripheral conversion of T4 substance to T3 substance are propranolol, glucocorticoids, propylthiouracil (note that methimazole does not), and amiodarone. Lithium and iodine block the thyroidal release of T4 and T3.
4. PTU is the preferred drug of choice of hyperthyroidism during pregnancy as methimazole can cross the placenta and cause aplasia cutis of the fetus.
5. Graves' disease has an increased radioactive iodine uptake (RAIU) as does toxic multinodular goiter and toxic adenoma. Young adults with Graves' disease (30% presenting with no goiter) should be treated with

antithyroid medication first rather than radioactive iodine ablation. TSI antibodies are positive in Graves' disease. The pretibial myxedema in Graves' disease (also can be seen with hypothyroidism) appears peau d' orange due to a lymphocytic infiltrate.

6. In general, the initial test of choice for solitary thyroid nodules is a fine needle aspiration.

7. Among the causes of low RAIU (radioactive iodine uptake) in patients with hyperthyroidism besides those that have already been listed include struma ovarii (thyroid tissue in an ovarian teratoma), recent use of iodine for contrast (Jod-Basedow phenomenon), and lymphocytic thyroiditis (usually painless thyroid as opposed to subacute thyroiditis which is painful).

8. Hyperparathyroidism is marked by elevated calcium and low phosphorus when it is primary, and the most common abnormality is a single adenoma in 85% of cases.

9. Indications for parathyroidectomy in primary hyperparathyroidism include 24 h urinary calcium excretion greater than 400 mg (usually seen with nephrocalcinosis of the kidney on ultrasound), serum calcium level above 11.0 mg/dl, and peak bone mass greater than or equal to 2 standard deviations below the mean for age, sex, and race. This disease usually causes cortical rather than trabecular bone loss, thus vertebral fractures are rare. Other indications to take out parathyroid adenomas are urolithiasis, age less than 50, and creatinine clearance less than 70% of normal. Hyperparathyroidism is also associated with pancreatitis, peptic ulcer disease, and hypertension.

10. Osteomalacia should be thought of in patients with bone pain and proximal muscle weakness. The test of choice is the 25 hydroxyvitamin D level if decreased intake is suspected but the usual cause of vitamin D deficiency is malabsorption (can also check the 25 hydroxyvitamin D level with this). Treatment of the condition is with oral 1,25 dihydroxyvitamin D. It can cause the finding of Looser's zones or lines on bone films which appear as fractures when none is present.

15.23 Year 1—Week 8—Day 1

1. Lymphangioleiomyomatosis is associated with an estrogen-driven lung vessel smooth muscle proliferation leading to chylous pleural effusions and spontaneous pneumothorax. High-resolution CT scanning shows cystic lung disease. The patients are initially tried on progesterone and ultimate treatment is lung transplant.

2. Histiocytosis X (Langerhans cell granulomatosis or eosinophilic granuloma) is a process of cystic lung disease and spontaneous pneumothorax can arise. Treatment is smoking cessation.

3. Pulmonary embolus is associated with transudative and exudative pleural effusions.

4. Pancreatitis and Boerhaave's syndrome are causes of exudative effusions.

5. Lupus and rheumatoid arthritis both cause exudative effusions, but only RA is associated with effusions with low glucose levels.

6. Urticaria pigmentosa is skin-limited mastocytosis. Patients have brown macules that urticate upon stroking (Darier's sign).

7. Psoriasis and pityriasis rubra pilaris are associated with erythroderma.

8. NSAIDs can lead to pseudoporphyria and even mimic bullous pemphigoid.

9. Keratoacanthomas can arise rapidly and are described as "dome-shaped with keratin-filled centers."

10. Hepatocellular carcinomas can cause hypercalcemia, low glucose by IGF-2 secretion, diarrhea, and erythrocytosis by paraneoplastic mechanisms.

15.24 Year 1—Week 8—Day 2

1. The first step in management of a patient suspected of drug-induced lupus is to stop the offending medication and check an ANA

titer. If the ANA is negative, then there is no need to order the anti-histone antibody.

2. Ace-inhibitors are the first-line therapy of hypertensive crises in patients with underlying scleroderma.

3. Cyclophosphamide is the treatment of choice with patients with pulmonary involvement from scleroderma, lupus, or polymyositis.

4. Dermatomyositis can present with dermatological signs that include the heliotrope rash, the shawl sign (erythema of the necks and shoulders), and Gottron's papules or macules (violaceous coloration directly over the joints of finger).

5. There is still controversy over whether there is a true malignancy relationship between dermatomyositis and cancer.

6. Ovarian cancer has been associated with paraneoplastic pemphigus vulgaris.

7. Hydroxychloroquine is the first-line treatment of all skin findings of systemic lupus erythematosus.

8. Among the stranger findings of lupus skin disease are panniculitis, hemorrhagic bullous lesions, psoriasiform skin disease (usually seen in subacute cutaneous lupus erythematosus), and plaque like lesions (discoid lupus).

9. Lupus pernio is a disfiguring skin rash that is associated with Sarcoid not lupus.

10. Steroids are indicated in sarcoid if there is cardiac or neurological involvement, severe systemic disease (such as with uveitis and parotitis), hypercalcemia, lupus pernio, and nephrocalcinosis.

15.25 Year 1—Week 8—Day 3

1. There is a 10% incidence of berry aneurysms (involving the circle of Willis) in patients with polycystic kidney disease (adult form is autosomal dominant with defect found on chromosome 16).

2. Uhthoff's effect refers to decreased nerve conduction in the presence of heat seen in patients with multiple sclerosis.

3. Acute demyelinating encephalopathy may occur after immunization, especially after MMR (measles-mumps-rubella) administration.

4. Beta-interferon and glatiramer (side effect of transient chest pain during infusion of medication) are two drugs used in patients with relapsing-remitting multiple sclerosis to prevent recurrence of disease.

5. Anserine bursitis, seen in greater incidence in patients with osteoarthritis, causes pain a few inches below the medial surface of the patella. First-line treatment is corticosteroid injection into bursae.

6. A ruptured Baker's cyst, seen in osteoarthritis and rheumatoid arthritis, may resemble a DVT and may even lead to DVT formation by promoting venous stasis.

7. The sign of Leser-Trelat is associated with gastrointestinal malignancy, and it involves the rapid appearance of hundreds of seborrheic keratosis and telangiectasias.

8. Pemberton's sign is the event of flushing/erythema of the facial area seen in patients with substernal goiter within minutes of them raising their hands above their head (due to compression of subclavian vasculature by the substernal goiter).

9. The two most common causes of hyperthyroidism with a high radioactive iodine uptake are Graves' disease and toxic multinodular goiter. A thyroid bruit will often be auscultated in Graves' disease patients due to increased vasculature associated with the condition.

10. The two most common causes of hyperthyroidism with a low radioactive iodine uptake are thyrotoxicosis factitia and subacute thyroiditis.

15.26 Year 1—Week 9—Day 1

1. The first-line treatment of choice for patients with trigeminal neuralgia is carbamazepine.

2. NSAIDs are a common cause of lithium toxicity when both drugs are concomitantly used.
3. Olanzapine is associated with a risk of hyperglycemia much more remarkable than other medications in its class of drugs.
4. Dihydropyridine calcium channel blockers (like felodipine) are associated with a risk of gingival hyperplasia and lower extremity edema.
5. D-Penicillamine, still used in many patients with scleroderma, can cause a nephrotic syndrome and a myasthenia gravis-like syndrome.
6. Methotrexate may paradoxically worsen rheumatoid nodules in patients with rheumatoid arthritis (usually the small nodules in the hands). Continue treatment in patients that this occurs, as it is only a minor nuisance in most cases.
7. Metronidazole is the drug of choice in treating patients with inflammatory bowel disease who develop pouchitis.
8. Hypermagnesemia is associated with a loss of deep tendon reflexes, ataxia, lethargy, and mental status changes.
9. Treatment of hypermagnesemia is similar to hyperkalemia with IV furosemide and calcium gluconate for cardiac protection.
10. In patients with inferior myocardial infarction, look for reciprocal ST-segment depression in the "high" lateral leads, which are lead I and lead AVL.

15.27 Year 1—Week 9 – Day 2

1. Always look for an anion gap in acid–base problems. You could be given a patient with a high bicarbonate value, but if the patient has an anion gap greater than 20, there is definitely a hidden metabolic acidosis with anion gap.
2. Pregnancy causes a chronic respiratory alkalosis.
3. It is important to remember that even in compensated acid–base disorders, the pH never goes back to 7.40 (the only exception is possibly chronic respiratory alkalosis).
4. If a metabolic acid–base disorder is not compensated by the correcting formula, such as the Winter's formula, there is likely a hidden respiratory acid–base disorder concomitantly present.
5. The urine chloride level is the most helpful lab test to get in patients with metabolic alkalosis.
6. If the urine chloride level is greater than 30 meq/L, the metabolic alkalosis will *not* correct with normal saline infusion.
7. Whenever you see a PACO2 level that is below 40 mm HG in a patient with a clear-cut metabolic alkalosis, suspect a concomitant respiratory alkalosis is present.
8. Hyperventilation is a common cause of respiratory alkalosis. It can be seen in patients with anxiety disorder, with acute pain syndromes, or patients with pulmonary embolism.
9. The change in bicarbonate level compared to the change in anion gap level is a very useful tool in acid–base disorder management. If a patient has a marked anion gap for a minimal drop in bicarbonate level, suspect a concomitant metabolic alkalosis is present.
10. For each 10 mm HG drop of PACO2 in the setting of respiratory alkalosis, expect the bicarbonate level to drop acutely by 2.0–2.5 meq/L.

15.28 Year 1—Week 9—Day 3

1. Patients with high rheumatoid factor titers are at risk of vasculitis, rheumatoid lung disease, and rheumatoid nodules.
2. In lupus, there is erythema between the joints of the hands as opposed to dermatomyositis which has discoloration only over the joints itself with sparing of interphalangeal area.
3. First-line treatment of patients with Raynaud's phenomenon is a calcium channel blocker; alpha blockers are second-line therapy.

4. Bronchiolitis obliterans can be the end-target damage in the lung in patients with graft versus host disease.

5. Distal renal tubular acidosis is associated with Sjogren's syndrome and kidney stones can occur due to hypocitraturia.

6. Proximal RTA can be seen with multiple myeloma and kidney stones are not common in these patients.

7. Polycystic kidney disease patients with urinary tract infections need longer treatment than usual for UTI (2–4 weeks). Ciprofloxacin and trimethoprim-sulfamethoxazole are good empiric choices for treatment in these patients.

8. Listeria meningitis needs to be treated with IV ampicillin. Use trimethoprim-sulfamethoxazole if the patient has a severe penicillin allergy.

9. *Enterococcus* (group D streptococcus) is increasing in incidence as a causative agent of endocarditis in the elderly.

10. Q-Fever is caused by *Coxiella burnetii*. Treatment is doxycycline. Endocarditis and liver failure may be seen.

15.29 Year 1—Week 10—Day 1

1. Hypocalcemia can be seen with hypomagnesemia (since magnesium is essential for PTH function) and pseudo-hypoparathyroidism (PTH resistance/congenital condition with adolescents of short stature and with short metacarpals in association with high phosphorus and PTH levels with normal alkaline phosphatase levels).

2. The risk of unchecked diabetes during pregnancy is of macrosomia of the fetus (birth weight greater than 9 lbs.). A patient with diabetes who becomes pregnant will need 50% more insulin than usual (due to insulin resistance) but these increased insulin requirements vanish within hours after delivery; thus, careful observation is needed of the patient.

3. Beta-hydroxybutyrate is not detected in urine acetone tests done in patients with DKA. Besides hypokalemia arising with insulin treatment, hypophosphatemia (can cause diaphragm paralysis) can also occur.

4. Patients with secondary amenorrhea who have withdrawal bleeding with progesterone challenge should have a workup that includes FSH, LH, prolactin, and TSH. Patients that fail this challenge should next receive cyclic estrogen/progesterone birth control pills for at least 2 months and if menses occurs, then a diagnosis of estrogen deficiency is made.

5. Causes of hypothalamic amenorrhea (decreased GNRH) include anorexia, bulimia (examine knuckles of patients for erosions and oral cavity for increased dental caries), and long-distance running. The prolactin level will be normal in these patients.

6. Use of water deprivation test or DDAVP helps distinguish patients with diabetes insipidus. If the ADH does not increase with rising plasma osmolality, then the diagnosis is central (or neurogenic) DI. If there is increasing ADH with no concomitant increase in urine osmolality, then the diagnosis of nephrogenic DI is made.

7. Thiazide diuretics are the only helpful treatment for nephrogenic DI (diabetes insipidus).

8. SIADH that is chronic can be treated with demeclocycline. It decreases the sensitivity of the kidney to ADH. If a patient on this drug develops diarrhea, you must consider *Clostridium difficile* infection as the drug is an antibiotic.

9. In male patients with primary hypogonadism, the testosterone level will be low and the LH will be *high*. Klinefelter's syndrome can cause this finding (karyotype XXY) and it is diagnosed with karyotyping from cells from a buccal smear or from peripheral leukocytes in blood. These patients have gynecomastia and an increased risk of male breast cancer.

10. In males with gynecomastia and a testicular mass, two tests can be very helpful. A low LH level is very suggestive of a Leydig cell cancer. An elevated HCG level is very suggestive of a germ cell cancer. The LH level is

elevated by artifact in germ cell cancers because there is a cross-reaction between high levels of HCG and the LH test.

15.30 Year 1—Week 10—Day 2

1. Patients with chronic renal disease who become pregnant have a greater risk of pre-eclampsia than those with no history of renal insufficiency who become pregnant.
2. Among the clues for renal artery stenosis are (1) the presence of a systolic-diastolic abdominal bruit, (2) difficult to treat hypertension (more than 2 agents), and (3) onset of significant hypertension over a relatively short period of time (1–2 years) in a patient above age 50.
3. The sulfosalicylic acid test will be positive in patients with multiple myeloma, while the urine dipstick for albumin will be negative.
4. The most common histology seen in patients with HIV disease who have nephrotic syndrome is focal and segmental glomerulonephritis.
5. HAART therapy can have an impact in the kidney function of patients with HIV chronic kidney disease.
6. An alkaline phosphatase level over 1000 mg/dl with an elevated GGT level and minimal transaminitis and total bilirubin elevation should raise suspicion of a space-occupying lesion in the liver (infiltrative process, malignancy, etc.).
7. *Plasmodium malariae* can cause nephrotic syndrome.
8. Patients with sickle cell disease are LESS prone to get malarial infections compared to the general population.
9. The biggest risk factor for dengue hemorrhagic fever is previous infection to any dengue virus.
10. Patients with *Strongyloides stercoralis* can have super-infection with gram-negative organisms (think of this in situations such as a patient with *E. coli* meningitis).

15.31 Year 1—Week 10—Day 3

1. *Trichinella spiralis* causes eosinophilia, myalgias, and periorbital edema. The diagnostic test is muscle biopsy. Treatment is mebendazole and steroids.
2. Treatment of tropical sprue is with high-dose doxycycline for 3–6 months until malabsorption picture has resolved. Folinic acid supplementation is needed in this situation.
3. *Ancylostoma braziliense* is the likely cause of cutaneous larval migrans in the Caribbean. Treat with albendazole.
4. *Wuchereria bancrofti* (filariasis) can cause chyluria (milk-colored urine). This disease can only be acquired by repeated infection over a 1-year time period at least (thus not a concern to tourists of area).
5. Praziquantel and niclosamide can be used to treat *Diphyllobothrium latum* infections, which can cause megaloblastic anemia (by B12 and folate deficiency).
6. Mebendazole or albendazole and adjunctive steroids are the treatment of choice for neurocysticercosis.
7. *Schistosoma haematobium* infection of the bladder leads to squamous cell carcinoma of the bladder. Treatment is with praziquantel.
8. Protozoans do not give eosinophilia, except rarely Isospora belli (which causes a diarrheal illness in patients with HIV; treat with sulfamethoxazole-trimethoprim similar to Cyclospora). Thus, there is no eosinophilia noted in patients with malaria and Giardia.
9. *Entamoeba histolytica* infections should be treated with metronidazole and a luminal agent to eliminate cysts, such as paromomycin or iodoquinol.
10. *Microsporidia* infections can only be diagnosed by small bowel biopsy (ova and parasite will not reveal organism).

15.32 Year 1—Week 11—Day 1

1. Patients with essential thrombocytosis are at risk of thrombotic events.

2. In reactive thrombocytosis (as in cases of cancer and infection), there is no platelet function abnormalities as opposed to patients who have thrombocytosis from essential thrombocytosis or other myeloproliferative disorders.

3. About 40% of patients with thrombocytosis from a myeloproliferative disorder will have splenomegaly detected.

4. Interferon alpha is the treatment of choice for women with essential thrombocytosis who are contemplating pregnancy as hydroxyurea and anagrelide are contraindicated due to teratogenic risk.

5. Low-dose aspirin was effective in controlling thrombotic complications in patients with polycythemia vera without increasing the risk of major bleeding.

6. Very early post-operative wound infection is usually due to group A streptococcus.

7. Buccal cellulitis, appearing in the cheek, is most commonly due to *Haemophilus influenzae.*

8. Bacteremia is very rare in cellulitis with less than 5% of cellulitis cases having positive blood cultures in general.

9. Oral moxifloxacin can be effective similar to cephalexin for uncomplicated skin and soft tissue infections.

10. Patients with peripheral edema are predisposed to cellulitis, thus in these patients, use support stockings, enforce good skin hygiene, and recognize and rapidly treat tinea pedis infections when they occur to prevent recurrent episodes of cellulitis.

15.33 Year 1—Week 11—Day 2

1. *Yersinia pestis* is the cause of the plague. When treating these patients, droplet and standard precautions are used (no airborne isolation needed). Treatment is with streptomycin or gentamicin, although high-dose tetracycline is also acceptable.

2. Q-Fever is caused by *Coxiella burnetii* and is associated with a wide range of clinical manifestations including liver failure, pneumo-

nia, and endocarditis. Treatment is with doxycycline.

3. Patients with anthrax will usually not feature pulmonary infiltrates and a widened mediastinum is the most likely X-ray manifestation. These patients would not need droplet precautions as the disease is not transmitted person to person. Hemorrhagic mediastinitis is a mechanism of death in these patients.

4. Tularemia can cause oculoglandular syndrome. *Francisella tularensis* is commonly described in patients traumatizing rabbits with lawn equipment causing skin disruption of the animals.

5. Patients with chronic atrial fibrillation usually do fine when in need of a pacemaker with the VVIR pacemaker type as they have long lost their atrial kick (thus no real need for DDDR pacemaker).

6. Sweet's syndrome can mimic cellulitis. The syndrome is also known as acute neutrophilic febrile dermatitis and some series have listed a risk for hematological malignancy (highest risk—AML) as high as 20% over the next 5 years.

7. The histology causing nephrotic syndrome most associated with solid tumor appearance in the next 5 years is membranous nephropathy.

8. Itraconazole can lead to QT interval prolongation. If a patient with sporotrichosis cannot use itraconazole, saturated solution of potassium iodide (SSKI) would be acceptable treatment.

9. Tumor lysis syndrome may occur spontaneously even without chemotherapy treatment, such as in large B-cell lymphomas that begin to become necrotic.

10. Among the most culprit medications causing drug-induced pancreatitis are azathioprine, DDI, DDC, pentamidine, valproic acid, and tetracycline.

15.34 Year 1—Week 11—Day 3

1. Seminomas are radiosensitive similar to CNS dysgerminomas.

2. Seminomas should always be AFP negative. If you have a seminoma by pathology and AFP positive, there are two possibilities—the pathologist is wrong or you have a mixed tumor.

3. All poorly differentiated midline carcinomas that have no characteristics of any tumor that can be identified should be treated as if they are germ cell tumors with bleomycin, etoposide, and cisplatinum as this is the most chance for cure for the patient.

4. Klinefelter's syndrome is associated with an increased risk of both male breast cancer and testicular cancer.

5. Diagnosis of Klinefelter's syndrome is made by karyotyping using material from a buccal smear.

6. Low ceruloplasmin levels along with neuropsychiatric history should raise concern for Wilson's disease.

7. Acutely, Wilson's disease patients are treated with D-penicillamine and then switched over to zinc for chronic copper chelation therapy.

8. Lead poisoning can be treated with several agents, including succimer and EDTA.

9. ATN is marked by isosthenuria (inability to concentrate or dilute urine with specific gravity usually 1.010) and muddy brown casts in the urinalysis.

10. Urinary eosinophils are seen usually only in about 20% of cases of allergic interstitial nephritis, but you may notice a busy urinary sediment with leukocytes with lack of infection.

15.35   Year 1—Week 12—Day 1

1. The organisms that cause emphysematous cholecystitis include *Escherichia coli* (most common), *Klebsiella, and Clostridium welchii.*

2. Porcelain gallbladder, seen as a dense calcification of the gallbladder on abdominal plain film, is still felt to be a risk factor for development of gallbladder adenocarcinoma.

3. Mitotane is the chemotherapeutic agent of choice in treatment of adrenal carcinomas.

4. 10% of pheochromocytomas are extra-adrenal, 10% are bilateral, and 10% are malignant. A network of ganglia near the inferior mesenteric artery's takeoff from the aorta is felt to be the most common place for extra-adrenal pheochromocytoma (that ganglia network is also known as the organ of Zuckerkandl).

5. Histoplasmosis is known to cause splenic and adrenal calcifications, as well as posterior mediastinitis.

6. The left lateral abdominal decubitus film is a helpful view when trying to decide whether free air is present.

7. All the fungal agents ending in "–azole" can cause transaminitis and prolong the QT interval.

8. Among the causes of deeply inverted T-waves in the precordial leads especially are subarachnoid hemorrhage (cerebral T-waves).

9. Short PR interval can be seen in patients with glycogen storage diseases (no other endocrine or metabolic disorder boast such an EKG finding).

10. The anti-epileptic most associated with the complex of weight gain, alopecia, LFT problems, pancreatitis, and thrombocytopenia is valproic acid.

15.36   Year 1—Week 12—Day 2

1. The 5-year survival of liver disease patients with ascites is 30–40% compared to 70–80% if they receive a liver transplantation.

2. Circulatory dysfunction after large volume paracentesis is associated with a high rate of ascites recurrence, hepatorenal syndrome, and dilutional hyponatremia. Albumin needs to be given as a plasma expander to avoid these complications.

3. Refractory ascites is defined as a lack of response to high-dose oral diuretics (300–400 mg spironolactone and 120–160 mg furosemide daily as goal of therapy).

4. Hepatorenal syndrome is characterized by renal failure due to severe vasoconstriction

of the renal circulation (extreme underfilling of arterial circulation). It occurs in up to 10% of patients with cirrhosis and ascites.

5. There are two types of hepatorenal syndrome. Type 1 is marked by progressive oliguria and a rapid rise in serum creatinine with spontaneous bacterial peritonitis (SBP) as a common precipitant of this state.

6. Optic neuritis and trigeminal neuralgia are often herald signs of underlying multiple sclerosis especially when occurring in recurrent fashion.

7. *Escherichia coli* is still the most common organism causing spontaneous bacterial peritonitis (SBP) and third-generation cephalosporins are still first line for treatment.

8. Mechanism of SBP is felt to be translocation of bacteria from intestinal lumen to lymph nodes, leading to bacteremia and infection of ascites.

9. The most severe complication of SBP is hepatorenal syndrome.

10. Without initiation of long-term antibiotic prophylaxis after one episode of SBP, the recurrence rate can be as high as 70% in the first year.

5. Cardiac herniation can occur in the setting of pneumonectomy.

6. The coronary vessel that can get involved often in aortic dissection is the right coronary artery, so always include aortic dissection in the differential of a patient presenting with chest pain and ST-segment elevation over the inferior leads.

7. The high lateral leads (I and AVL) will show the reciprocal ST depression changes to a true inferior myocardial infarction.

8. Right ventricular infarction can occur in the setting of an inferior myocardial infarction. Right-sided EKG showing a 1 mm ST-segment elevation over lead V4R is helpful in making the diagnosis.

9. The capillary wedge pressure on Swan-Ganz measurements is helpful in distinguishing congestive heart failure from acute respiratory distress syndrome (ARDS). There should be a normal wedge pressure in ARDS.

10. A patient with septic shock will have an increased cardiac index, low wedge pressure, and low systemic vascular resistance on Swan-Ganz measurement.

15.37 Year 1—Week 12—Day 3

1. Carbamazepine can be associated with a Stevens-Johnson/toxic epidermal necrolysis syndrome which often occurs within the first 7–14 days of initiation of the medication.

2. Behcet's disease is marked by not only pulmonary artery aneurysms but also the ability to form right atrial thrombi. Chlorambucil is a medication that has been used for the vascular features of Behcet's disease.

3. Constrictive pericarditis is seen less often nowadays due to a change in the way radiation is delivered to the chest to patients with malignancy involving the thorax.

4. Rheumatoid arthritis is the rheumatological disease most associated with cases of constrictive pericarditis.

15.38 Year 1—Week 13—Day 1

1. Consider underlying von Willebrand's disease in female patients with history of dysfunctional uterine bleeding.

2. Vertical nystagmus should raise a concern for a central lesion, and further studies with MRI/MRA should be performed.

3. Chlorpromazine is helpful for patients with difficulty with hiccups.

4. If a patient receives chlorpromazine and has an acute dystonic reaction, the treatment of choice is diphenhydramine.

5. The preferred route of epinephrine nowadays is intramuscular route. The anterior lateral thigh seems to be the most popular place to give the medication.

6. Consider lymphoproliferative disorders (such as CLL or lymphoma) in patients presenting later in life with angioedema.

7. Metformin is helpful for the acne that occurs with polycystic ovarian disease. First-line treatment of PCOD or polycystic ovarian syndrome (Stein-Leventhal syndrome) is still oral contraceptives.

8. Danazol has been used for hereditary angioedema. It is important to recognize that the medication is a teratogen, so contraception methods need to be well documented.

9. Patients presenting with widespread open and closed comedones as part of their acne would likely benefit from starting with topical isotretinoin rather than the usual topical clindamycin/benzoyl peroxide.

10. Among the side effects of oral isotretinoin are pseudotumor cerebri and marked increase of triglyceride level.

15.39   Year 1—Week 13—Day 2

1. Mesenteric artery embolus is associated with atrial fibrillation or rheumatic heart disease and presents with acute central belly pain. Next test in management is mesenteric angiogram with embolectomy if possible. In contrast, ischemic colitis is associated with low-flow state and presents with rectal bleeding and lower abdominal pain with flexible sigmoidoscopy for diagnosis and surgery only if peritonitis develops.

2. Achalasia is associated with hypertensive lower esophageal sphincter with increased contractions of the esophageal body and abnormal contractions of the esophagus. "Bird's beak" is seen on barium swallow. Scleroderma is the opposite as it has a hypotensive lower esophageal sphincter. Patients with diffuse esophageal spasm will have a "corkscrew" appearance to their barium swallow and have normal lower esophageal sphincter pressure.

3. Avoid propafenone (class Ic agent) for antiarrhythmic therapy in patients with underlying structural heart disease.

4. Spontaneous bacterial peritonitis is commonly caused by *E. coli* in most cases. *Streptococcus pneumoniae* is second on the list in many series. The treatment of choice is cefotaxime which is a third-generation cephalosporin.

5. Hepatorenal syndrome is marked by a urine sodium less than 5 mg/dl, and there is a very poor prognosis associated with the condition. There are no lesions that can be proven in histology of affected kidneys, and the kidneys may even be donated to transplant if the cause of the liver failure is not hepatitis B or C.

6. TPN can cause liver function abnormalities. These should be monitored, and therapy does not need to be changed or discontinued as long as they are mild. Deficiencies associated with TPN include zinc (acral dermatitis), selenium (hemolytic anemia and muscle pain), and chromium (glucose intolerance).

7. Patients who have cholecystectomies for history of gallstones and who 1 week later develop pancreatitis should be suspected to have retained common bile duct stone and should go for ERCP.

8. Cronkite-Canada syndrome is a colon polyp syndrome associated with fingernail dystrophy, alopecia, and cutaneous hyperpigmentation. It can degenerate into colon cancer. It is marked by diarrhea similar to villous adenomas which can cause hypokalemia and a secretory diarrhea.

9. Non-alcoholic steatohepatitis (NASH) is associated with diabetes mellitus, obesity, and hyperlipidemia. There is large droplet steatosis and inflammation like that seen in alcoholic hepatitis. The disease can progress to cirrhosis and need for liver transplant.

10. Among the drugs causing cholestatic liver disease are halothane, estradiol, erythromycin estolate, chlorpromazine, captopril, and sulfonamides. Granulomatous hepatitis can be caused by allopurinol, procainamide, and phenytoin. Nitrofurantoin, methyldopa, isoniazid (continue with treatment until AST or ALT is three times normal), and trazadone are associated with chronic hepatitis.

15.40 Year 1—Week 13—Day 3

1. Double-stranded DNA antibodies and Smith antibodies should be ordered in patients suspected of SLE who have a positive ANA test.
2. Complement levels and a urinalysis (checking for RBCs) should also be ordered in patients suspected of having SLE.
3. Disseminated gonorrhea can cause a migratory arthritis, a skin rash with hemorrhagic pustules, and is treated with IV ceftriaxone for 1 week.
4. Sulfasalazine works well for the arthritis of inflammatory bowel disease.
5. The X-ray findings of rheumatoid arthritis usually follow in the order of (1) juxta-articular osteoporosis, (2) marginal joint erosions, and (3) loss of joint space.
6. Hydroxychloroquine may take up to 6 months to take effect for relief of arthritis in patients with rheumatoid arthritis and lupus.
7. Dapsone and thalidomide if dapsone fails are helpful in lupus patients with hydroxychloroquine-refractory skin disease.
8. Bleomycin can cause Raynaud's phenomenon.
9. Rheumatoid factor can be found positive in diagnostic testing in patients with cryoglobulinemia.
10. Mixed connective tissue disease will have positive U1-ribonucleoprotein assay (generally a good prognosis).

15.41 Year 1—Week 14—Day 1

1. Patients with scleroderma may initially present solely with puffy fingers (edema with no sclerodactyly).
2. CREST syndrome patients will have positive anti-centromere antibodies, whereas those with diffuse scleroderma will have positive SCL-70 antibodies (anti-topoisomerase antibodies).
3. Lupus patients can have false positive RPR on lab testing.
4. CH-50 is the first lab test to check in a patient who one feels may have a complement defi-

ciency. If the test is normal, there is no need to do individual complement level testing.
5. Visceral angioedema has been described in patients with or without other sites of angioedema.
6. Diffuse alveolar hemorrhage can be seen in patients with lupus and presents with diffuse infiltrates, hemoptysis in 75% of patients, increased DLCO on PFTs, and is treated with IV Cytoxan.
7. Rheumatoid arthritis goes into remission in pregnancy, whereas SLE is unpredictable and may flare in the final trimester.
8. SS-A/anti-Ro antibodies may be seen in patients with SLE or with subacute cutaneous lupus erythematosus (SCLE) besides the known finding in Sjogren's syndrome.
9. Antiphospholipid antibody syndrome may present with both arterial and venous clots.
10. Eruptive xanthomas can be seen in patients with familial hypertriglyceridemia (tan to flesh colored papules throughout the body). They resolve as the triglyceride level comes down with drug therapy.

15.42 Year 1—Week 14—Day 2

1. DILS (Diffuse infiltrative lymphocytosis syndrome) is seen in patients with HIV disease and mimics Sjogren's syndrome (keratoconjunctivitis sicca, chipmunk facies due to parotid gland enlargement are among physical exam features).
2. Sjogren's syndrome can cause RTA type 1 and can cause lymphoma and pseudolymphoma.
3. Patients with rheumatoid arthritis are also at increased risk of lymphoma.
4. Keratoacanthomas arise rapidly and are dome-shaped with keratin-filled centers. They should be completely excised.
5. Hypertension is a common cause of recurrent epistaxis in the elderly.
6. Wegener's granulomatosis patients may present with hearing loss (as CN-8 is affected as part of a mononeuritis multiplex).

7. Amiodarone may cause corneal toxicity; tamoxifen may cause both corneal and retinal toxicity; hydroxychloroquine causes only retinal toxicity.
8. The most common cause of retinal detachment in the general population is myopia.
9. Hyperopia (far-sightedness) is a risk factor for subsequent development of glaucoma.
10. Amiodarone can also cause pulmonary fibrosis, hyper- or hypothyroidism, LFT abnormalities, and bluish skin discoloration.

15.43 Year 1—Week 14—Day 3

1. Leflunomide is a pyrimidine nucleotide inhibitor which should be used after methotrexate for treatment of rheumatoid arthritis. Its main limiting side effect is diarrhea.
2. Among the causes of pseudo-infarction Q waves are: (1) hypothermia, (2) hypertrophic cardiomyopathy (IHSS), and (3) Wolff–Parkinson–White syndrome.
3. Chronic eosinophilic pneumonia is associated with peripheral infiltrates with central sparing on CXR. Steroids are part of the treatment of this condition.
4. The treatment of membranoproliferative glomerulonephritis in the setting of lupus is IV cyclophosphamide.
5. L-Asparaginase (used often in chemotherapy treatment of ALL) and azathioprine can cause drug-induced pancreatitis.
6. Cyclophosphamide can lead to hemorrhagic cystitis which in turn leads to bladder cancer.
7. Polymyalgia rheumatica can initially present with a symmetrical arthritis of the small joints of the hands before the more familiar symptoms begin.
8. Membranous nephropathy is associated with an increased risk of renal vein thrombosis as well as increased risk of solid tumor malignancy compared to other histology findings found with nephrotic syndrome (in other words, compared to minimal change disease, focal segmental glomerulosclerosis, membranoproliferative glomerulonephritis, etc.).

9. The treatment of lupus cerebritis (best diagnosed with a SPECT scan of brain, which is a nuclear medicine test) is cyclophosphamide IV.
10. Behcet's syndrome patients have painful mouth ulcers. The mouth ulcers of lupus patients are classically painless.

15.44 Year 1—Week 15—Day 1

1. Among the medications that can cause gingival hyperplasia, one finds phenytoin (dilantin), cyclosporine, and the dihydropyridine calcium channel blockers (felodipine, amlodipine, etc.).
2. The medications most linked to drug-induced gout are the following: Niacin, thiazide diuretics (includes chlorthalidone), cyclosporine, and pyrazinamide.
3. The medications most linked to drug-induced pancreatitis include the following: Valproic acid, tetracyclines, L-asparaginase, azathioprine, DDI, DDC, and pentamidine.
4. Clozapine is still useful for hallucinations associated with Huntington's disease but beware of the risk for agranulocytosis (need frequent complete blood count checks).
5. Clopidogrel has been implicated as a drug-induced cause of TTP, similar to ticlopidine.
6. Mitomycin C is the most common chemotherapeutic agent associated with hemolytic-uremic syndrome.
7. All class Ia anti-arrhythmics (quinidine, disopyramide, procainamide) have gastrointestinal side effects of nausea, abdominal pain, and diarrhea.
8. Glatiramer acetate is associated with a transient chest tightness syndrome that usually occurs near the time of infusion of the medication.
9. Colchicine can lead to a drug-induced myopathy/myositis, especially if the dose is not adjusted in renal failure patients.
10. Steroids are associated with the development of a proximal myopathy (usually type 2 muscle fiber atrophy). CPK levels are usually not elevated in these patients.

15.45   Year 1—Week 15—Day 2

1. Beta-blockers can cause drug-induced hyperkalemia. High-dose sulfa antibiotics, as used in treatment of patients with *Pneumocystis jirovecii*, can also lead to hyperkalemia.
2. Thiazide diuretics are the most common class of drugs to cause drug-induced hyponatremia.
3. Other culprits that can cause drug-induced hyponatremia include carbamazepine (Tegretol) and SSRI medications.
4. Among the medications with drug-induced anti-cholinergic side effects are the following: oxybutynin, cyclobenzaprine, mirtazapine, and disopyramide (the class Ia anti-arrhythmic).
5. Avoid dapsone as well as sulfa drugs in patients who have G-6PD deficiency as they will undergo hemolysis if challenged with these medications.
6. Metoclopramide and dapsone are among the medications that can cause methemoglobinemia. Also remember the topical anesthetic medications can also cause this condition.
7. Valproic acid can cause alopecia, weight gain, LFT abnormalities, and pancreatitis.
8. Both gold and lamotrigine can cause an exfoliative dermatitis.
9. Boerhaave syndrome (esophageal rupture) may be seen in a weightlifter who develops sudden chest pain during his workout and is found to have a large pleural effusion, usually on the left side and exudative in nature. Treatment is emergent surgical correction once diagnosis is proven (such as with radiological swallow study).
10. Minoxidil and hydralazine can both cause a reflex tachycardia. Recall that hydralazine therapy is contraindicated in patients with acute aortic dissection.

15.46   Year 1—Week 15—Day 3

1. HAPE (high-altitude pulmonary edema) occurs above 8000 feet (2400 m). If it occurs or recurs at a lower altitude, workup for cardiac shunts, pulmonary hypertension, and valvular heart disease should be considered.
2. Ataxia is a clinical sign of HACE (high-altitude cerebral edema). This is a clinical diagnosis (HACE); thus, MRI or CT is not needed.
3. Among the factors for getting HACE or HAPE are (a) rapidity of ascent, (b) absolute altitude, (c) duration at altitude, (d) sleeping altitude ("climb high, sleep low" motto).
4. Besides altered taste of carbonated beverages, retinal hemorrhages and flatus may be more common at higher altitudes.
5. Acetazolamide (250 mg) is a useful drug for the treatment of sleep disturbances associated with acute mountain sickness.
6. Painful urination and sensory stocking and glove deficits are among the clinical manifestations of ciguatera poisoning (risk fish include barracuda and red snapper).
7. Both autoimmune hepatitis and primary biliary cirrhosis can have an associated inflammatory, symmetrical arthritis associated with them.
8. The anti-smooth muscle antibodies and anti-liver-kidney-microsomal antibodies (anti-LKM) are among the positive antibodies in autoimmune hepatitis. There can be autoimmune hepatitis with no antibodies detected.
9. Check an RPR to rule out secondary syphilis in all patients with pityriasis rosea or any other extensive lichenification rash.
10. Pinch purpura (discoloration around eyelids due to bleeding) may be seen with systemic amyloidosis in the patient's status post colonoscopy.

15.47 Year 1—Week 16—Day 1

1. ARDS (acute respiratory distress syndrome) may occur in patients status post-trauma and status post-burn state.
2. High-frequency ventilation has shown no benefit in patients with ARDS. Low tidal volumes have shown benefit in patients with ARDS.
3. TTP (thrombotic thrombocytopenic purpura) may be induced by medications such as chemotherapy (bleomycin given as example), but it may be caused as well by clopidogrel and ticlopidine. Pregnancy and HIV disease are two other situations where the disease can strike.
4. The only 2 components of the classic pentad required to entertain a diagnosis of TTP are microangiopathic hemolytic anemia and thrombocytopenia. The other three components are fever, renal dysfunction, and neurological changes.
5. The treatment of TTP is plasmapheresis.
6. The most common type of non-Hodgkin's lymphoma in the general population is diffuse large B-cell lymphoma.
7. Rituximab is a monoclonal antibody against CD-20 which has been used for patients with non-Hodgkin's lymphoma, TTP, and ITP, among several diseases.
8. The most common drug eruption is a morbilliform exanthematous drug eruption (measles-like appearance) which can be delayed up to 2 weeks after the last dose of the medication and can be seen with multiple medications to include short course oral antibiotics (macrolides, fluoroquinolones).
9. 2-Chlorodeoxyadenosine (2-CDA) is also used for Waldenstrom's macroglobulinemia treatment along with its known use for treating hairy cell leukemia.
10. Nocardiosis can be treated with amikacin, minocycline, or trimethoprim-sulfamethoxazole.

15.48 Year 1—Week 16—Day 2

1. Nodular lymphangitis is also known as sporotrichoid pattern dermatitis. A distal ulcerative lesion is mimicked up the lymphatic chain of the arm or leg by similar lesions. Causes include sporotrichosis, *Mycobacterium marinum*, tularemia, other atypical mycobacteria, and *Nocardia braziliensis* infections.
2. Sporotrichosis is treated first-line with itraconazole. Use SSKI (potassium iodide) if LFTs or QT-interval prolongation does not allow for use of itraconazole.
3. Do not use isoniazid to treat *Mycobacterium marinum* as it is very ineffective. Medications such as rifabutin, clarithromycin, and ethambutol will work.
4. A side effect of ethambutol is optic neuritis. Color vision loss is the first warning sign of this phenomenon. It can cause gout as well, but to a lesser degree than pyrazinamide.
5. Although the anti-histone antibody is classically linked to drug-induced lupus, patients with SLE can also have a positive antibody.
6. Autoimmune hemolytic anemia is marked by the presence of spherocytes and a positive direct Coombs test. No schistocytes are seen with this disease.
7. Atovaquone can be used for prophylaxis of both toxoplasmosis and *Pneumocystis jirovecii* pneumonia. Dapsone covers only *Pneumocystis jirovecii* prophylaxis.
8. The most common type of vasculitis seen is a leukocytoclastic vasculitis (at the level of post-capillary venule usually).
9. Methylene blue is first-line treatment of methemoglobinemia. Mild cases can be treated with oral therapy.
10. Vitamin C can be used in cases of methemoglobinemia refractory to methylene blue (due to antioxidant properties).

15.49 Year 1—Week 16—Day 3

1. Amoxicillin and erythromycin are the medications approved for treatment of Chlamydia in pregnant patients.
2. Trichomonas vaginitis is not a cause of upper genital tract disease.
3. Asymptomatic *Chlamydia trachomatis* infections are the most common cause of infertility in the USA.
4. Mirtazapine is an anti-depressant agent that can cause weight gain and has anticholinergic side effects.
5. Clindamycin (900 mg every 8 h) and gentamicin (2 mg/kg initially, then 1.5 mg/kg every 8 h) is a combination that can be used to treat patients with pelvic inflammatory disease who are penicillin allergic.
6. After six infections with HSV in 1 year, prophylaxis is recommended. There are several regimens such as acyclovir 400 mg bid, valacyclovir 500–1000 mg daily, and famciclovir 250 mg bid.
7. Chancroid, caused by a gram-negative organism which can mimic "boxcars" or "sausage links" or "school of fish" called *Haemophilus ducreyi*, can cause suppurative inguinal lymphadenopathy along with tender ulcers.
8. For non-pregnant, penicillin-allergic patients with primary or secondary syphilis, one can use doxycycline 100 mg bid for 14 days or tetracycline 500 mg QID for 14 days.
9. The RPR should decrease by four-fold within 6 months once treated for syphilis. If the titer does not increase, consider treatment failure versus possible CNS involvement.
10. Bacterial vaginosis is the most common cause of vaginal discharge. It has a pH above 4.5 and is associated with PROM (premature rupture of membranes) and preterm labor. Treatment regimens include metronidazole 250 mg bid or clindamycin 300 mg bid for 7 days. There is no need to treat the male sexual partner.

15.50 Year 1—Week 17—Day 1

1. Patients with second-degree heart block Mobitz type 1 can be watched if they are asymptomatic with no therapy.
2. Patients with Lewy body dementia may have marked hallucinations and they can have a rapid decline.
3. Patients with corticobasal ganglion degeneration can have the "alien hand syndrome."
4. Reglan (metoclopramide) can cause drug-induced Parkinsonism and methemoglobinemia.
5. Patients with Parkinson plus syndromes have extra added features besides the usual Parkinson's symptomatology, such as having impaired upgaze (supranuclear palsy progressive) or marked autonomic dysfunction (multiple systems atrophy).
6. Methylene blue can cause methemoglobinemia if it is given at an excessive dose. Vitamin C can be added in such cases.
7. Pyridoxine can lead to B6 deficiency if given in excessive doses (recommended dose is 50–100 mg in patients taking isoniazid therapy).
8. Vitamin C is the treatment of patients with scurvy.
9. Legionella pneumonia is treated with azithromycin as first-line therapy.
10. Rifampin can cause lowering of drugs that work through the cytochrome P450 3A4 system, such as dilantin.

15.51 Year 1—Week 17—Day 2

1. Vancomycin is the first-line oral agent for the treatment of *Clostridium difficile* infections.
2. Ezetimibe may be added to any statin therapy to help best lower the LDL level. There is no significant effect on HDL or triglycerides with this medication.
3. Rosuvastatin and pravastatin are the HMG-CoA reductase inhibitors with no significant activity on the cytochrome p450 3A4 system.
4. Patients with oral retin A (isotretinoin) are at risk of markedly increased triglyceride levels

and pseudotumor cerebri and hypercalcemia.

5. Among the numerous findings in adrenal insufficiency are eosinophilia, normochromic normocytic anemia, and hypercalcemia.

6. Patients should not be labeled with "cryptogenic cirrhosis" until formal testing has occurred to rule out hemochromatosis.

7. Patients with neuropsychiatric history and liver disease should be ruled out for Wilson's disease. Start with a serum ceruloplasmin level, which should be low.

8. Patients with non-alcoholic steatohepatitis (NASH) can progress to fibrosis and cirrhosis.

9. Patients with celiac sprue are at theoretical risk of T-cell lymphoma of the small bowel but there is no evidence that screening for lymphoma in celiac sprue patients is cost-effective or even clinically effective.

10. Patients with pernicious anemia are at increased risk of developing gastric carcinoid lesions.

15.52   Year 1—Week 17—Day 3

1. Essential tremor not responding to beta-blockers could be helped by an old anti-seizure medication known as primidone.

2. Ibutilide is effective in terminating atrial flutter at times, but always either give magnesium sulfate or check a magnesium level before administration of the medication.

3. Dapsone can be effective in attenuating the effects of the sphingomyelinase toxin of the brown recluse spider bite if medication started within 48 h of the attack.

4. Dapsone can also be used for ITP and for autoimmune hemolytic anemia, besides its better known uses in management of PCP, leprosy, and the pruritis of dermatitis herpetiformis.

5. The usual cause of Lemierre's syndrome (septic internal jugular vein thrombophlebitis) is *Fusobacterium necrophorum*. Use clindamycin if a patient is penicillin allergic.

6. Erythromycin is usually ineffective at treating *Haemophilus influenzae*.

7. Doxycycline is a useful antibiotic in COPD patients to treat outpatient upper respiratory tract infections as it has coverage for *Streptococcus pneumoniae and Haemophilus influenzae* infections.

8. Beware of the interaction of metronidazole with coumadin. Clindamycin, amoxicillin, and nafcillin/oxacillin have no significant effects with coumadin. Tylenol in doses exceeding 1500–2000 mg can potentiate the INR.

9. Listeria meningitis should be treated with IV ampicillin. Trimethoprim-sulfamethoxazole is also effective in treating this organism.

10. Patients receiving TPN with lipids or fatty acid emulsions are at risk of fungemia with Candida species and *Malassezia furfur.*

15.53   Year 1—Week 18—Day 1

1. The anti-microsomal antibodies (also known as antithyroid peroxisomal antibodies) will be elevated in Hashimoto's disease (the most common cause of hypothyroidism).

2. Suppression of serum cortisol to less than 5 mg/dl (or suppression of urinary 17-hydroxycorticosteroids to less than 3 mg/dl) with a *high*-dose dexamethasone test (2 mg every 6 h) speaks for the diagnosis of Cushing's *disease* (pituitary is the problem). If there was not suppression of serum cortisol on the *high*-dose dexamethasone test, this would leave adrenal adenoma, adrenal cancer, and ectopic ACTH as possibilities. A high serum ACTH level is seen only with ectopic ACTH (most commonly with small or oat cell cancer of lung). In the patients with low ACTH, the diagnosis of adrenal adenoma and adrenal cancer is distinguished by measuring serum DHEA (or DHEA-S) level or urinary 17-ketosteroids (which are elevated in adrenal cancer).

3. Late-onset congenital adrenal hyperplasia occurs with partial 21-hydroxylase deficiency most commonly and the screening test to differentiate it from polycystic ovarian disease is to measure for an elevated serum 17-hydroxyprogesterone level (seen with CAH). There is another type of late-onset congenital adrenal hyperplasia that involves 11-hydroxylase deficiency (thus serum 11-deoxycortisol will be elevated) and this can be seen in patients presenting with amenorrhea, hirsutism, hypertension, and hypokalemia.

4. Pheochromocytoma (adrenal medulla tumor) is associated with MEN IIA (hyperparathyroidism and medullary carcinoma of thyroid) and MEN IIB (mucosal neuromas and the mentioned thyroid cancer).

5. Eventual definitive treatment of pheochromocytoma is surgery. The patients are given alpha-blockade initially with phenoxybenzamine and then are given an additional beta-blocker (or just switched to labetalol) to control tachycardia prior to surgery.

6. The best serum screening test for acromegaly (which can present with carpal tunnel and hyperphosphatemia) is an insulin-like growth factor 1 (IGF-1) level.

7. The best screening test for Cushing's disease is generally felt to be the 24-h urine free cortisol measurement.

8. Hypoparathyroidism can result from the autoimmune polyglandular syndromes (autosomal recessive as opposed to MEN syndromes which are autosomal dominant) and is seen with low calcium and low PTH level with normal alkaline phosphatase and high phosphorus levels. Osteomalacia generally causes both low calcium and phosphorus with high PTH and alkaline phosphatase levels.

9. There is a condition known as familial dysalbuminemic hyperthyroxinemia in which there is a family history of elevated total T4 levels with normal free t4 levels. No treatment is needed in these patients.

10. Familial hypocalciuric hypercalcemia (FHH) is marked by family history of hypercalcemia and is diagnosed by a measurement of urine calcium to urine creatinine with the ratio generally less than 0.01 (can also be described as calcium reabsorption greater than 99% as opposed to primary hyperparathyroidism in which it is less than 99%). FHH is due to excessive secretion of parathyroid hormone. Intact PTH levels may be mildly elevated, but no treatment is generally required.

15.54　Year 1—Week 18—Day 2

1. Theophylline is notorious for causing drug-induced multifocal atrial tachycardia, even at therapeutic levels.

2. Trapped lung syndrome leads to transudative pleural effusions. Malignant involvement of pleural lining leads to exudative pleural effusions.

3. Aneurysms from syphilis most commonly occur in the ascending aorta.

4. Anatomical areas where chondrocalcinosis can occur include the symphysis pubis and triangular ligament of the wrist. Chondrocalcinosis can be an asymptomatic finding or be seen in association with pseudogout.

5. Generally, doses of prednisone start at 60 mg daily when treating a patient with bullous pemphigoid.

6. Vancomycin is the most notorious antibiotic to cause exacerbation of linear bullous IgA disease.

7. Patients with lupus panniculitis or lupus profundus will respond to hydroxychloroquine.

8. Hypertension is common in patients with adult polycystic kidney disease. Only about 10% of patients will develop berry aneurysms.

9. Homocystinuria leads to dilation of the aorta and pulmonary arteries and is also associated with lens subluxation and osteoporosis.

10. Osteomalacia is adult vitamin D deficiency and can present with significant bone pain and pseudofractures on X-rays.

15.55 Year 1—Week 18—Day 3

1. Propylthiouracil (PTU) stops conversion of T4 to T3. Note that methimazole does not do the same.
2. In patients with pituitary resection, do not follow TSH level as it will be undetectable. Follow free T4 levels.
3. The lab test to follow in patient being corrected from severe hyperthyroidism is the free and total T4 level. The TSH will take much longer to reflect what is really going on.
4. The multiple endocrine neoplasia (MEN) syndromes are inherited in autosomal dominant fashion but the autoimmune polyglandular syndromes are inherited in autosomal recessive fashion.
5. Current standard of care for Bell's palsy is to start treatment with acyclovir and steroids.
6. *Schistosomiasis* can cause pipe-stem fibrosis of the liver.
7. Wilson's disease can present with "sunflower" cataracts.
8. Cystine stones can be radiolucent or radioopaque depending on the sulfur content of the stones.
9. Uric acid stones are always radiolucent. Treat with allopurinol.
10. Never use probenecid in patients with history of uric acid nephrolithiasis.

15.56 Year 1—Week 19—Day 1

1. Patients with severe *Leptospirosis* infections should be treated with IV penicillin.
2. Patients with *Actinomycosis* infections can present with fistula formation and should be treated with penicillin.
3. Patients with *Nocardia asteroids* infections can present with brain abscess, disseminated skin nodules, and pulmonary infiltrates. Treatment is with sulfamethoxazole-trimethoprim first line for up to 6 months to a year, with secondline therapy being minocycline.
4. Patients with listeria infections should be treated with IV ampicillin. Sulfamethoxazole-trimethoprim could be used if a patient had severe penicillin allergy. Cephalosporins will not work.
5. In patients with HACEK endocarditis infections, ceftriaxone is the drug of choice. The most common organisms seen from the HACEK group are *Citrobacter, Eikenella corrodens, and Kingella* species.
6. Patients with permanent lines (ports) found to have *Corynebacterium jeikeium* infections should have those lines removed.
7. Patients with *Candida krusei* will not respond to fluconazole and should be treated with voriconazole or amphotericin B.
8. Patients with streaking cellulitis due to streptococcus could be treated with IV penicillin at high doses and IV clindamycin to bind the toxin.
9. Patients with septic pulmonary emboli on lung X-ray with internal jugular thrombophlebitis should be treated with penicillin and are most likely to have *Fusobacterium necrophorum*.
10. Malassezia furfur causes a "spaghetti and meatballs" appearance on KOH and is treated with topical ketoconazole or systemic therapy if severe.

15.57 Year 1—Week 19—Day 2

1. Inflammatory breast cancer (*peau d'orange* appearance) is treated with neoadjuvant chemotherapy first, then surgery, then radiation therapy to affected bed along with more chemotherapy.
2. Rectal adenocarcinoma is generally treated with neoadjuvant chemotherapy and radiation therapy and then surgical resection.
3. Most anal cancers are squamous cell in histology.
4. A patient who contracts squamous cell cancer of anus or rectum should be tested for HIV disease.
5. Likewise, a patient with HIV disease who complains of rectal pain should have a flexible sigmoidoscopy because of increased incidence of squamous cell cancer of rectum with this disease.

6. Germ cell tumors are comprised of seminomas and non-seminomas. Seminomas are AFP negative (they can be HCG positive at times).
7. Seminomas are radiosensitive, similar to CNS dysgerminomas.
8. Any state of chronic liver disease that leads to cirrhosis could lead to hepatocellular carcinoma.
9. The most common lung cancer to cause hypercalcemia is squamous cell cancer through a PTH-related peptide mechanism.
10. The most common lung cancer to cause gynecomastia is large cell carcinoma.

15.58 Year 1—Week 19—Day 3

1. Patients with invasive head and neck carcinoma usually receive neoadjuvant chemotherapy with cisplatin and radiotherapy before being considered for surgical resection.
2. Adrenal cancer is a very rare phenomenon. Most common cause of a malignancy involving the adrenal gland is metastatic lung cancer.
3. 10% of pheochromocytomas are bilateral, and 10% are malignant.
4. Risk factors for squamous cell cancer of the esophagus include lye ingestion, Plummer-Vinson syndrome (iron deficiency anemia and esophageal webs/cysts), tylosis, and alcohol/smoking abuse.
5. Squamous cell cancer of skin usually arises from an actinic keratosis.
6. The metastatic potential of squamous cell cancer of the skin is greatest when it is from the lower lip or from the ears.
7. Two skin conditions associated with HIV disease are eosinophilic folliculitis and seborrheic dermatitis.
8. Besides HIV disease, think of Parkinson's disease in patients with seborrheic dermatitis affecting them at a very young age (as in the 20s–40s).

9. Embryonal cell carcinoma of the testes is treated after orchiectomy with chemotherapy involving bleomycin, etoposide, and cisplatin.
10. Bleomycin can cause pulmonary fibrosis, Raynaud's phenomenon, and sclerodactyly.

15.59 Year 1—Week 20—Day 1

1. The classical treatment regimen for myeloma was melphalan and steroids. The old treatment regimen for ALL (acute lymphoblastic leukemia) was vincristine and steroids. L-Asparaginase is a chemotherapy medication that has also been found to be effective for ALL treatment with one of its feared side effects being drug-induced pancreatitis.
2. Mefloquine is the drug of choice for treatment of patients traveling to most parts of the world where malaria is prevalent. Doxycycline can be used in several instances as well.
3. The two treatment regimens for babesiosis, which causes hemolytic anemia in afflicted patients include azithromycin with atovaquone or clindamycin with quinine, with both regimens given for 5–7 days (short treatment).
4. *Burkholderia pseudomallei* is an organism that can cause cough and respiratory distress with ability to form lung abscess. It was noted in tsunami victims. Treatment is imipenem with sulfa-based drug.
5. Among the complications of *Mycoplasma* to look out for are bullous myringitis, transverse myelitis, erythema multiforme, and cold agglutinin hemolytic anemia.
6. Among the soft tissue infections one needs to look out for are *viridans streptococci, staphylococcus epidermidis, Eikenella corrodens, Bacteroides species, Corynebacterium*, and even *Peptostreptococc*us.
7. Dog bite infections include *Pasteurella species, Fusobacterium, Staphylococcus aureus, and Capnocytophaga canimorsus.*
8. *Capnocytophaga canimorsus* is the organism that can cause DIC and sepsis with purpura

and skin necrosis in patients with history of asplenia.

9. Ceftriaxone is the drug of choice for treatment of patients with HACEK organism endocarditis.

10. Ceftriaxone is also the drug of choice for patients with advanced carditis and neurological symptoms with Lyme disease.

15.60   Year 1—Week 20—Day 2

1. First-line treatment of Conn's syndrome (primary hyperaldosteronism) is spironolactone. A side effect is breast pain/gynecomastia. Amiloride is second-line treatment.

2. The most common cause of macrocytosis in the general population is chronic use of alcohol.

3. Poxvirus is the cause of molluscum contagiosum, which can also be seen in immunocompetent patients. The classic description of the lesion is a central umbilicated papule.

4. Erysipelas is a cellulitis with sharply demarcated borders with a violaceous hue discoloration and group A streptococci is the most common cause. Treat with IV penicillin initially (only need 7–10 days of treatment).

5. Erysipeloid is a mimicker of erysipelas, except it is caused by *Erysipelothrix rhusiopathiae*, and this organism affects meat handlers and fish handlers. Treatment is with intravenous penicillin.

6. Clindamycin should be part of the treatment plan in treating patients with gas gangrene by *Clostridium perfringens* and necrotizing fasciitis by group A streptococci.

7. With a cellulitis with severe pain and fever, suspect group A streptococcal necrotizing fasciitis.

8. Venous stasis is the most common factor leading to recurrent episodes of cellulitis.

9. Necrotizing fasciitis caused by group A streptococci can begin in deep muscles and not show any cutaneous manifestations until much later in the disease course.

10. Hydroxychloroquine is the treatment of choice for subacute cutaneous lupus erythematosus similar to the other cutaneous manifestations of the diseases in the lupus spectrum. Patients on this medication need eye exams one to two times a year by an ophthalmologist.

15.61   Year 1—Week 20—Day 3

1. Neurocysticercosis can cause both parenchymal based and ventricular based lesions in the brain. The most common scenario is for an isolated lesion. Treatment is with albendazole.

2. The murmur of mild aortic stenosis usually peaks early in systole but it is still a harsh murmur with medium pitch heard best at the second right intercostal space.

3. With a large ASD, one can expect a mid-diastolic murmur at the lower left sternal border with an S2 which is widely split and fixed.

4. The most common cause of isolated mitral regurgitation in the USA now is mitral valve prolapse.

5. Multiple sclerosis, CVA, and sepsis are among the common scenarios where one may encounter hypothermia.

6. The risk of asystole and ventricular fibrillation, as well as the likelihood of seeing Osborn waves on an EKG, increases as the core body temperature drops below 25 degrees Celsius (77 degrees Fahrenheit).

7. Primidone can be used for essential tremor after failure of beta-blocker.

8. A common side effect of glatiramer acetate which is used for multiple sclerosis is transient flushing and chest pain after site injection.

9. A very common cause of mental status changes in patients with multiple sclerosis is urinary tract infection (which may not show overt signs of dysuria or fever in patients with multiple sclerosis).

10. Common locations for hypertensive-induced bleeds in the brain include the pons, the pulvinar nucleus of the thalamus, the putamen, and the posterior fossa area.

15.62 Year 1—Week 21—Day 1

1. Doxycycline and topical clindamycin are acceptable choices for mild hidradenitis suppurativa (apocrine gland involvement) but moderate to severe disease states will require TNF-alpha receptor inhibitor adalimumab.
2. Transferrin saturation levels above 45% should raise suspicion of hemochromatosis. The definitive test is liver biopsy showing appropriate hepatic iron index. Patients with this disease can have second and third MCP arthritis and increased incidence of pseudogout. Phlebotomy helps with the cardiac disease and the hyperpigmentation but usually does not relieve the arthritis or hypogonadism. The number one cause of death is heart failure with the second being liver failure.
3. The first step in management in a patient with upper GI bleed is to give normal saline through two large bore peripheral IV sites. If the patient has signs of liver disease (spider angiomas, splenomegaly, asterixis, palmar erythema), then IV octreotide should be started as well.
4. Pancreatitis and splenic vein thrombosis are causes of isolated gastric varices. Liver disease patients with gastric varices in addition to esophageal varices generally do poorly and should be considered for TIPS (transhepatic portosystemic shunt) to prevent rebleeding from gastric varices if they are appropriate candidates.
5. Primary biliary cirrhosis is associated with antimitochondrial (M2 portion highest) antibodies in over 90% of cases. Patients with early disease respond to ursodeoxycholic acid. There is a preponderance for females. About 50% of patients present with itching and fatigue.
6. Primary sclerosing cholangitis is a disease with male predilection that is associated with ulcerative colitis. Diagnosis is made at ERCP with beading and dilation of the biliary system ("chain of lakes"). There are no effective oral treatments and patients should be considered for liver transplant unless they have cholangiocarcinoma (which can be diagnosed with brushings on ERCP or on biopsy of any strictures seen).
7. Autoimmune hepatitis is marked by impressive transaminitis in young patients (especially females) with elevated globulin fractions and occasionally very positive ANA titers. Patients with the most common type of this disease have positive anti-smooth muscle antibodies (type 2 is anti-liver-kidney-microsomal antibodies). Treatment is with corticosteroids.
8. Acetaminophen toxicity is treated with N-acetylcysteine for 17 doses which acts in place of depleted glutathione (depleted by the metabolites of acetaminophen rather than the parent drug). The pathology is centrilobular necrosis. Worst clinical predictors are prolongation of the PT (prothrombin time) and elevation of total bilirubin.
9. Acute fatty liver in pregnancy can present with encephalopathy or coagulopathy. It is marked by a minimal transaminitis with impressive elevations of total bilirubin and prothrombin time. It occurs in the third trimester and there is microvesicular fat accumulation in hepatocytes. Treatment is immediate delivery. Recurrence in a following pregnancy is rare.
10. Intrahepatic cholestasis of pregnancy is associated with elevated alkaline phosphatase and total bilirubin in the third trimester and is the second most common cause of jaundice in pregnancy after viral hepatitis. Although benign for the mother, it is associated with increased fetal death. Recurrence occurs with other pregnancies or when oral contraceptives are used.

15.63 Year 1—Week 21—Day 2

1. Among the complications of massive blood transfusions are factor wash-out (which leads to continued bleeding and is best treated with

FFP) and hypocalcemia/metabolic alkalosis (which results from the large amount of citrate that tags along with the blood transfusions).

2. TSH replacement for a young woman with no known coronary artery disease should start at near target goal of replacement (1.6 micrograms/kg body weight).

3. Be aware that 5% of all thyrotoxic states may present initially as an isolated T3 thyrotoxicosis. Also be aware that T3 is available commercially so that you should also check T3 levels in patients you suspect to be ingesting thyroid hormone factitiously (common scenario is someone who has been trying to lose weight).

4. The screening test for acromegaly is IGF-1 (somatomedin C).

5. IGF-2 is a hormone that is released in a paraneoplastic fashion usually by sarcomas and leads to hypoglycemia.

6. When you have a patient with Cushing's syndrome, an ACTH level is helpful. It will be *low* if the cause is from the adrenal gland. It will be high if it is from the pituitary or ectopic source (most commonly, it is really high with ectopic source).

7. Small cell lung cancer is the most common carcinoma to cause ectopic ACTH syndrome. These patients generally present with hypertension and hypokalemia (although usually not as profound as the hypokalemia of Conn's syndrome).

8. The two situations where a pituitary adenoma is not treated with surgery initially are: (1) a prolactinoma and (2) a non-functioning adenoma in the setting of severe hypothyroidism.

9. Pleural effusions and pericardial effusions can occur in the setting of severe hypothyroidism.

10. Low voltage on EKG can be seen in patients with hypothyroidism even if no pericardial effusion is present.

15.64   Year 1—Week 21—Day 3

1. Metoclopramide can cause drug-induced Parkinsonism and can even lead to methemoglobinemia.

2. Think of pontine infarct in patients with pin-point pupils and locked-in syndrome.

3. A patient with cerebellar hemorrhage needs urgent neurosurgical consult to evaluate for drainage to prevent cerebellar herniation and to prevent mass effect on the pons.

4. Patients will fall to the same side of a cerebellar hemorrhage or infarct. Vertigo and ataxia are common presenting symptoms as well.

5. A patient with truncal ataxia but intact finger to nose and heel to shin testing should be thought of having alcohol-induced midline cerebellar damage (vermis damage).

6. All patients with pityriasis rosea should be checked for syphilis if they have promiscuous sexual history as it is a mimicker of this condition.

7. Both seborrheic dermatitis and eosinophilic folliculitis are skin conditions seen in HIV disease.

8. The most common cause of Guillain-Barre syndrome worldwide is *Campylobacter jejuni* infections.

9. Vitamin A toxicity, tetracyclines, and steroids are causes of pseudotumor cerebri.

10. Thalamic strokes can be pure sensory, pure motor, mixed sensory-motor, and can present with clumsy hand-dysarthria syndrome. Patients with post-thalamic stroke syndrome have chronic hemisensory pain that can be devastating (known as the Dejerine-Roussy syndrome).

15.65   Year 1—Week 22—Day 1

1. Patients who receive fludarabine are at risk of acquiring *Pneumocystis jirovecii* infection and Listeria infection (through T-cell mediated defect that arises after treatment). This was classically seen in CLL patients who received the medications.

2. Mitoxantrone is used in secondary progressive multiple sclerosis. There is a risk factor for cumulative cardiotoxicity if receiving the drug over an extended period of time (thus check ejection fraction before treatment).

3. Iron may bind Synthroid and cause you to elevate Synthroid dose when not necessary. Space out the medication times by several hours to avoid this problem.

4. Thiazide diuretics (hydrochlorothiazide and chlorthalidone), niacin, pyrazinamide, and cyclosporine can cause drug-induced gout.

5. Patients with diffuse large B-cell lymphoma can undergo tumor lysis syndrome even without chemotherapy treatment. These patients generally get renal failure from uric acid nephropathy.

6. In patients neutropenic for greater than 10 days, think of typhlitis (treatment is metronidazole) if they present with right lower quadrant abdominal pain (although also rule out appendicitis).

7. Patients with both rheumatoid arthritis and Sjogren's syndrome are at increased risk of developing lymphoma (usually diffuse large B-cell lymphoma, which is a non-Hodgkin's lymphoma).

8. The EKG finding of hypercalcemia is a shortened QT interval such that there appears to be no ST-segment.

9. The alkaline phosphatase and the GGT level should be impressively elevated in patients with infiltrative disease of the liver.

10. Death from Addisonian crisis generally arises from a fatal arrythmia due to hyperkalemia or hypoglycemic cerebral crisis.

15.66 Year 1—Week 22—Day 2

1. Aminoglycosides can cause hearing loss by causing cochlear cell dysfunction and loss.

2. Thyroid hormone requirements are expected to increase as a pregnancy moves from trimester to trimester.

3. All patients with chronic liver disease who have negative hepatitis A and hepatitis B serologies need to be vaccinated for these two viruses.

4. If a patient has received the hepatitis A vaccine more than 1 month before exposure to hepatitis A, there is no need to give passive hepatitis A immunoglobulin in most cases.

5. The pharmacological treatment of granulomatosis with polyangiitis is usually a combination of cyclophosphamide and steroids. Plasmapheresis may be an option in patients with rapidly progressive glomerulonephritis findings.

6. The initial treatment of polymyositis and dermatomyositis is IV steroids. These patients then are weaned off steroids after addition of azathioprine.

7. Azathioprine can cause drug-induced pancreatitis.

8. The first-line treatment of osteoarthritis is acetaminophen and not NSAID therapy. WBC count in the joint fluid if obtained should be less than 3000 WBC/ml in patients with osteoarthritis if that disease is the cause of the effusion.

9. The treatment of temporal arteritis is 1 mg/kg of oral steroids initially, with gradual weaning occurring. A late complication of temporal arteritis is aortic dissection.

10. Pseudogout most commonly affects the knee joint. One may see chondrocalcinosis in the joint space in these patients. The patient has rhomboid, weakly positive birefringent crystals in joint fluid.

15.67 Year 1—Week 22—Day 3

1. Among the diseases that can cause an elevated MCV with anemia are hypothyroidism, megaloblastic anemia, and myelodysplastic syndrome.

2. Among the states that can cause an elevated MCV without anemia are use of dilantin, use of hydroxyurea, use of alcohol, and location of Wyoming (the Wyoming is a much needed humor break!).

3. Most frequently asked combination regimen for a patient with ALL would probably include vincristine and prednisone.
4. The LDH level is a very important test as far as prognosis and treatment decisions in patients with ALL.
5. Patients with hairy cell leukemia usually present with pancytopenia and splenomegaly, and they can have a dry bone marrow tap.
6. Anemia of chronic disease usually causes a normocytic anemia, but it can cause a microcytic anemia (macrocytic anemia should not be seen).
7. Congenital sideroblastic anemia causes a microcytic anemia. Acquired sideroblastic anemia, usually seen in chronic alcohol users, is a macrocytic anemia.
8. Hemoglobin E disease causes a microcytic anemia. Be aware that one cannot follow hemoglobin A1C levels in these patients as they have a hemoglobinopathy (leading to unreliable test results) and thus a serum fructosamine would have to be obtained to document glucose control (similar to sickle cell disease patients).
9. Do not initiate allopurinol acutely in gout attack. Colchicine is recommended in twice daily dose for up to several months once allopurinol is started.
10. Colchicine can cause a myositis, usually taking at least a year after once starts the medication. It is seen usually in patients with chronic renal insufficiency who received too high a dose of the medication given the compromised renal function.

15.68 Year 1—Week 23—Day 1

1. Hypothyroidism can present with hoarseness among other non-specific complaints.
2. It is generally safe to give angiotensin receptor blockers in patients who had angioedema from an ace-inhibitor. The mechanisms of angioedema that both medications can cause are unique from each other.
3. *Ehrlichia* infections are marked by WBC inclusions and patients have thrombocytope-

nia, LFT abnormalities, and splenomegaly. Treatment is doxycycline.
4. Ceftriaxone is required in Lyme disease treatment when there is advancing meningoencephalitis symptoms or advanced carditis (manifested by prolonged PR interval).
5. Babesiosis presents with RBC inclusions and a hemolytic anemia. Treatment is either atovaquone and azithromycin or clindamycin and quinine.
6. The first-line treatment of trigeminal neuralgia is carbamazepine.
7. The first-line treatment of absence seizures is ethosuximide. Second-line treatment is valproic acid.
8. Left-sided varicoceles in patients with weight loss should trigger workup for renal cell carcinoma.
9. If a solid mass is seen in a kidney on imaging with clear chest x-ray and no liver metastasis, the next step in management is referral to urology for a nephrectomy.
10. The treatment for myelodysplastic syndrome patients below age 50 is generally bone marrow transplant.

15.69 Year 1—Week 23—Day 2

1. The most common cause of heel pain in the general population is plantar fasciitis.
2. The most common cause of knee pain in the general population is patellofemoral syndrome.
3. The most common cause of lateral hip or thigh pain in the general population is iliotibial band syndrome.
4. The most common neuroleptic drug linked to open neural tube defects in pregnancy is valproic acid.
5. The most common cause for a "dry tap" on bone marrow is myelofibrosis.
6. The most common cause of jaundice in the general population is Gilbert's syndrome.
7. The most common type of AML (acute myelogenous leukemia) to cause gingival hyperplasia is AML M4 type.

8. The most common cause of retinal detachment in the general population is severe myopia.
9. The most common cause of intrinsic renal failure is acute tubular necrosis (muddy brown granular casts on urinalysis).
10. The most common antibody seen in primary biliary cirrhosis is the antimitochondrial antibody assay.

15.70 Year 1—Week 23—Day 3

1. Neurosarcoidosis would be asked in association with other findings of sarcoidosis, such as hilar lymphadenopathy, pulmonary symptoms, uveitis, and cardiac conduction block abnormalities.
2. Pituitary adenomas should not cause posterior pituitary problems.
3. Lymphocytic hypophysitis is a state that usually affects young females, sometimes after pregnancy, that is associated with posterior pituitary problems.
4. Propranolol has been noted to cause loss of mental sharpness or intellect among many patients (it crosses into the CSF barrier). In patients with essential tremor and this complaint, use primidone instead.
5. Beta-blockers as a class may be associated with nightmares.
6. Tricyclic antidepressants may be associated with decreased effective action of central acting hypertensive agents such as reserpine and clonidine.
7. The classic side effect of reserpine is depression. This medication is rarely used in present times for hypertension.
8. The worst prognostic factor in a tricyclic antidepressant overdose is QRS width prolongation.
9. Patients with TCA poisoning should be managed with alkalinization with the pH of the arterial blood gas followed to titrate effect.

10. Dextromethorphan can interact with SSRI agents and lead to increased risk of serotonin syndrome.

15.71 Year 1—Week 24—Day 1

1. Patients with AML who are receiving all-trans-retinoic acid (ATRA) are at risk of retinoic acid syndrome. This involves fever, dyspnea, weight gain, pulmonary infiltrates, pleural/pericardial effusions, leukocytosis, and hypotension and can affect up to 25% of patients on the medication.
2. Treatment of retinoic acid syndrome involves withdrawal of medication for a short while. Patients may be challenged with the medication again after that short withdrawal period. There is no need for specific therapy with NSAID's or steroids.
3. After a short time off the medication in this syndrome, the medication usually can be restarted once the symptoms abate.
4. Polyarteritis nodosa (PAN) spares the lung from involvement classically. These patients can often present with "foot drop" on as their mononeuritis multiplex presentation, although foot drop can occur with any vasculitis. Check for hepatitis B serology on these patients.
5. The treatment of granulomatosis with polyangiitis is most often cyclophosphamide plus steroids.
6. The major side effect of hydroxychloroquine is retinal toxicity. It is first-line agent for all skin and joint manifestations of lupus.
7. Penicillin allergy is *not* a contraindication to use D-penicillamine. D-penicillamine can mimic several diseases, including myasthenia gravis, Goodpasture syndrome, lupus, and polymyositis. It can also cause a nephrotic syndrome.
8. Among the X-ray characteristics of osteoarthritis are subchondral bone sclerosis, asymmetric joint narrowing, osteophyte formation,

and subchondral cyst formation. First-line treatment is acetaminophen.

9. Adult Still's disease is associated with extremely high ferritin levels (sometimes into the tens of thousands), arthritis usually of wrists, shoulders, hips, and knees, transient salmon colored rash at the time of the high fever, and a negative rheumatoid factor.

10. HIV disease can cause a syndrome that mimics Sjogren's syndrome. The disease is called DILS (diffuse infiltrative lymphocytosis syndrome) and has a different clonal population of T-cells which infiltrate the parotid gland. Also, the anti-Ro and anti-La (also known as SS-A and SS-B, respectively) will be negative in DILS.

15.72   Year 1—Week 24—Day 2

1. Low-dose aspirin promotes hyperuricemia by blocking tubular secretion of urate. High-dose aspirin is uricosuric and thus lowers uric acid level by blocking tubular reabsorption of uric acid.

2. Digital infarcts is the most common appearance of rheumatoid vasculitis, which usually occurs in the face of rheumatoid nodules and rheumatoid lung disease.

3. Patients with rheumatoid lung disease usually present with worsening dyspnea (over several months) rather than cough. Methotrexate-induced lung disease usually occurs over a much shorter time period. When in doubt, stop methotrexate and gauge patient clinical response.

4. Methotrexate is associated with alopecia and with oral ulcers. The nausea associated with the medication is helped by administration of folic acid.

5. Familial Mediterranean Fever usually causes short-lived attacks of peritonitis and pleurisy (less than 3 days) and is associated with AA amyloidosis. Colchicine may be helpful in management of the disease.

6. Patients with polymyositis and interstitial lung disease will commonly have anti-histidyl TRNA synthetase antibodies (anti-Jo 1 antibodies). They can also have keratitis of the hands known as "mechanic's hands."

7. Inclusion body myositis responds extremely poorly to any medications. The EMG may show neuropathic features besides the expected myopathy. There can be distal weakness as well present unlike dermatomyositis and polymyositis.

8. *E. coli* is *not* associated with any reactive arthritis syndrome. Yersinia, Shigella, Salmonella, and Campylobacter can cause reactive arthritis. *Ureaplasma urealyticum* and *Chlamydia trachomatis* can cause a reactive arthritis syndrome. Use antibiotics only for the GU-based infections (use doxycycline).

9. Gonorrhea is associated with a migratory arthritis that can be easily treated with IV ceftriaxone (usual course is at least 1 week of treatment).

10. Speaking of STDs, a couple of quick teaching points are as follows: (a) trichomonas does not cause upper genital tract disease; thus, it is not a causative agent of PID and (b) clindamycin and gentamicin is an appropriate combination regiment to treat PID in patients who have severe penicillin allergy and cannot tolerate doxycycline (due to GI intolerance).

15.73   Year 1—Week 24—Day 3

1. Rituximab is a monoclonal antibody against CD-20 which is used in ITP, non-Hodgkin's lymphoma, and CLL.

2. Fludarabine is used for aggressive CLL. A side effect is an increased propensity for *Pneumocystis jirovecii* pneumonia.

3. Check a PPD (or a serum gamma interferon assay) in patients being considered for TNF-alpha receptor blocker therapy (etanercept or

infliximab) as tuberculosis could reactivate during treatment.

4. Interstitial lung disease of scleroderma and polymyositis is treated with cyclophosphamide.

5. Rheumatoid arthritis can cause a variety of problems including scleritis, episcleritis, and scleromalacia perforans.

6. Constrictive pericarditis is associated with an early third heart sound (pericardial knock). It is associated with rheumatoid arthritis, tuberculosis, and fungal diseases (such as coccidiomycosis).

7. Colchicine can cause a myopathy, especially when given at high doses in patients with renal insufficiency. IV or oral colchicine is contraindicated in all patients with advanced renal insufficiency.

8. Oral hairy leukoplakia is characterized by white "fronds" on the lateral edge of tongue that are not removed by scraping with tongue blade. It is a result of synergism of EBV and HIV.

9. Patients with positive antiphospholipid antibodies should be treated only if they have a past medical history of clot or stroke.

10. Cyclophosphamide is the treatment of choice for patients with lupus cerebritis. These patients generally present with seizures and a SPECT nuclear medicine scan may be helpful in diagnosis.

15.74   Year 1—Week 25—Day 1

1. LDH level should be obtained on all patients with acute lymphoblastic leukemia (ALL) as it is prognostic and some decisions about treatment are made based on it.

2. ALL is associated with a high involvement of CNS problems, such that intrathecal chemotherapy is made part of the regimen.

3. The pain associated with sacroiliitis is brought about by flexion, external rotation, and abduction of the hip on the affected side.

4. The pain of trochanteric bursitis worsens with abduction and with lying on the side of

the affected area. Direct pressure over the lateral side of the hip reproduces the pain.

5. Chlorambucil is used to treat the vascular complications of Behcet's disease (which include pulmonary artery aneurysms, arterial clots, and venous clots).

6. Patients with Behcet's disease get visual problems from posterior uveitis.

7. Heart rate control is essential in patients with mitral stenosis as patients with tachycardia will go into pulmonary edema.

8. Beta-blockers are the first line of treatment of patients with prolonged QT syndrome and hypertrophic cardiomyopathy.

9. Side effects of amiodarone include hypothyroidism, hyperthyroidism, interstitial lung disease, LFT abnormalities, bluish discoloration of the skin, and corneal toxicity.

10. Filgrastim can cause musculoskeletal and bone-induced pain (medullary bone pain).

15.75   Year 1—Week 25—Day 2

1. Parasitemia with *Plasmodium falciparum* of greater than 15% should trigger RBC exchange transfusion therapy.

2. Sickle cell disease indications for RBC exchange transfusion include priapism, acute chest syndrome, and stroke syndrome.

3. Steroids should be used in treating patients with neurosarcoidosis and heart disease with conduction blocks.

4. Angioid streaks can be seen in patients with pseudoxanthoma elasticum. These streaks are disruptions in Bruch's membrane and they can appear as if they represent retinal disease (which they do not).

5. Sjogren's syndrome can present with distal RTA and increased risk of lymphoma and pseudolymphoma.

6. There is an increased risk of lymphoma in patients with rheumatoid arthritis independent of the medication risk that might also be present.

7. Serotonin syndrome can present with trismus, teeth chattering, myoclonus, and fever.

8. Low uric acid levels are seen in patients with SIADH and Wilson's disease.

9. Any young patient with liver disease who has a hemolytic anemia should be worked up for Wilson's disease.

10. Allopurinol can lead to a granulomatous hepatitis as well as a hypersensitivity syndrome.

15.76   Year 1—Week 25—Day 3

1. Lithium, reserpine, fentanyl, and clonidine are among the drugs that can cause bradycardia.

2. Severe lithium poisoning requires immediate hemodialysis.

3. Increased intracranial pressure will lead to a bradycardia that carries the company of hypertension.

4. Efavirenz is the medication most linked to vivid dreams and nightmares among the HIV treatment medications.

5. There is an acute retroviral syndrome for which antiretroviral therapy is indicated. The syndrome presents very much like mononucleosis, except it usually has a rash that spares the palms and soles.

6. The fluoroquinolone class is associated with spontaneous tendon rupture, glycemic control problems, and mental status changes in the elderly.

7. Use steroids in treatment of patients with *Pneumocystis jirovecci* if the PAO2 is less than 70 mm HG or the AA gradient is greater than 35.

8. Cullen's sign is periumbilical hemorrhage that can be seen with cases of hemorrhagic pancreatitis.

9. The sign of Leser-Trelat involves the sudden appearance over a few months of numerous seborrheic keratosis or telangiectasias mostly over the trunk in patients with underlying gastrointestinal carcinoma.

10. Sweet's syndrome consists of painful nodules and plaques commonly associated with fever with AML a lurking possibility in the next few years (biopsy shows a neutrophilic dermatitis).

15.77   Year 1—Week 26—Day 1

1. Heparin and low molecular weight heparin can lead to osteoporosis by increasing osteoclast-activating factor. It is advised that all pregnant women who receive heparin be placed on vitamin D and calcium.

2. Heparin can lead to hyperkalemia by interfering with the mineralocorticoid receptor in the adrenal gland.

3. Heparin can cause a "white clot syndrome" in the spectrum of heparin-induced thrombocytopenia which includes formation of arterial clots.

4. Treatment of a clot formed in the setting of heparin-induced thrombocytopenia can involve lepirudin or hirudin if there is no renal insufficiency (use argatroban in those cases with renal function compromise). It is safe to continue coumadin in these patients.

5. A neoplasm must involve 90% of both adrenal glands in order for there to be adrenal insufficiency due to the neoplastic process.

6. In males with osteoporosis, be sure to rule out hypogonadism as a cause.

7. Primary hypogonadism will be marked by low testosterone level and an elevated LH level.

8. Patients with Klinefelter's syndrome are at increased risk of testicular and breast cancer (the latter due to gynecomastia).

9. There is dysautonomia associated with Guillain-Barre syndrome such that blood pressure can fluctuate as much as is seen with spinal cord injury patients.

10. The Miller-Fisher variant of Guillain-Barre syndrome involves a descending paralysis with ataxia and ophthalmoplegia.

15.78   Year 1—Week 26—Day 2

1. Gold is associated with a nephrotic syndrome and an exfoliative dermatitis which requires discontinuation of the drug.

2. D-penicillamine can also cause a nephrotic syndrome but likes to be asked on standard-

ized testing as causing a "myasthenia gravis-like" syndrome.

3. Hydroxychloroquine can cause retinal toxicity and the worsening of psoriatic rash. It is first line for skin manifestations of lupus.

4. Methotrexate can cause small nodule formation, interstitial lung disease, and liver function abnormalities (as well as folate deficiency).

5. Azathioprine can be used as a steroid-sparing agent in many rheumatological diseases such as temporal arteritis or polymyalgia rheumatica.

6. Etanercept and infliximab (TNF-alpha receptor blocker drugs) can reactivate tuberculosis and can worsen existing infections to include worsening into sepsis state.

7. Leflunomide is associated with diarrhea and with liver function test abnormalities. It is a pyrimidine nucleotide inhibitor.

8. Sulfasalazine can cause male infertility (due to azoospermia and oligospermia). It is used mostly in inflammatory bowel disease.

9. Colchicine can be used very effectively in cases of chronic pericarditis and lessens the risk of amyloidosis development in patients with Familial Mediterranean Fever. As mentioned earlier, it can cause a serious state of myositis if given in patients with advanced renal insufficiency.

10. Allopurinol can cause a hypersensitivity syndrome. This can be avoided by testing patients for HLA B 58 allele subtype.

15.79 Year 1—Week 26—Day 3

1. In patients with gout, 24-h uric acid collections should be obtained. If a patient has less than 800 mg per 24 h, they are considered under-excretors and theoretically could be treated with probenecid instead of allopurinol.

2. Contraindications to probenecid include uric acid nephrolithiasis and renal insufficiency. Also, the patient has to be willing to drink 1.5–2 L a day of water (would not work for interns).

3. Rheumatoid arthritis causes marginal joint erosions with periarticular osteoporosis on X-rays of the hands.

4. Lupus does not cause erosions on X-rays but it is still considered an inflammatory arthritis.

5. Gout causes cystic, "punched-out" bone lesions with overhanging edges of bone on X-rays with periarticular sclerosis.

6. The syndesmophytes or bony bridges between the vertebral bodies are marginal in ankylosing spondylitis and non-marginal in reactive arthritis.

7. A finding on X-ray of the knee that might be seen in a patient with pseudogout is calcification in the joint space (chondrocalcinosis).

8. Dapsone can be used for multitude of things such as leprosy, Penumocystis jirovecci prophylaxis, brown recluse spider bites if within 48 hours of episode, and dermatitis herpetiformis.

9. Dermatitis herpetiformis is the rash associated with celiac sprue which appears usually over the extensor surface of the knee.

10. Porphyria cutanea tarda has a high association with underlying hepatitis C disease.

15.80 Year 1—Week 27—Day 1

1. Number needed to treat is 1/absolute risk reduction. Thus, if the absolute risk reduction is 25%, then 1/0.25 is 4, and thus four patients would need to be treated to make a difference. This would be a very good "number needed to treat" and thus would favor treatment being initiated in a patient with the intervention.

2. The positive predictive value is based on the prevalence of the disease.

3. Serum sickness is most associated with acute hepatitis B (not hepatitis C and not HIV disease).

4. Primidone is the second-line treatment for essential tremor.

5. Right heart failure is the most likely cause of finding ascites with a SAAG (serum albumin to ascites gradient) greater than or equal to

1.1 and a total protein content greater than 2.5 mg/dl in ascitic fluid.

6. Verapamil is extremely useful for prophylaxis of migraines with visual auras.

7. Lamotrigine is the preferred agent for treating atonic generalized seizures which are marked by sudden syncope ("drop attacks").

8. Lithium can be used for the prophylaxis of cluster headaches. Acute treatment of a cluster headache is with 100% oxygen.

9. Indomethacin is the preferred treatment of chronic paroxysmal hemicrania, which affects females much more commonly than males, and which has short-lived attacks that can strike multiple times a day (as opposed to cluster headaches which can last hours and strike rarely more than a couple of times a day and which favors males in incidence).

10. The most common type of incontinence in the general population is detrusor instability (urge incontinence).

15.81 Year 1—Week 27—Day 2

1. Hypercapnea generally develops after FEV1 value drops below 1 L in patients with COPD.

2. Oxygen is the only proven intervention that prolongs the survival of patients with COPD.

3. Smoking will dramatically worsen the emphysema of patients with alpha-1-antitrypsin disease.

4. Doxycycline covers *Streptococcus pneumonia* well and atypical organisms such as Chlamydia and Mycoplasma. Pancreatitis is among its side effects.

5. Long-acting beta-agonists (formoterol and salmeterol) should be considered in patients with COPD who are not optimal and are already on ipratropium and inhaled steroids.

6. Ectopic ACTH syndrome can be seen with small cell lung cancer and should be suspected in patients with a lung mass and new onset hypertension and hypokalemia (not induced by medication).

7. Carcinoid syndrome can cause ectopic ACTH production.

8. Hypertrophic pulmonary osteoarthropathy is a paraneoplastic process of non-small cell lung cancer that can cause tibial periostitis and new onset clubbing.

9. Squamous cell cancer causes hypercalcemia by PTH-related peptide production.

10. Goal of oxygenation in a patient with COPD is a PAO_2 of 55–60 mm Hg. The $PACO_2$ may elevate slightly to get to this O_2 level but not enough to cause clinical concern.

15.82 Year 1—Week 27—Day 3

1. *Fusarium* is a fungus with acute angle branching hyphae (similar to Aspergillus) which tends to have a very aggressive course. Treatment involves double coverage of antifungal agents.

2. *Aspergillus* can cause aggressive pulmonary disease particularly in those patients who have been neutropenic for over 10 days.

3. Another consideration in patients who are neutropenic for over a week and develop lower right quadrant pain is typhlitis. Treatment is with metronidazole.

4. *Aeromonas* is a freshwater bacteria that can cause an aggressive cellulitis in patients with liver disease. It can be seen after alligator bites or after piranha bites.

5. *Vibrio vulnificus* is a saltwater gram-negative organism that can cause aggressive cellulitis in liver disease patients. It is marked by bullous lesions. Treatment is doxycycline and a third-generation cephalosporin if inpatient.

6. The shawl sign of dermatomyositis is an erythema that involves the anterior neck and shoulders. It is associated with a better outcome than those without this sign. Antibody MI-2 is usually present.

7. Patients with myositis (poly or dermato) who have interstitial lung disease will usually have positive anti-Jo 1 titers (histidyl TRNA synthetase).

8. Ursodeoxycholic acid can be used for patients with primary biliary cirrhosis. It has

also been used in patients planning rapid weight loss in hopes to avoiding gallstone formation.

9. Cutaneous larval migrans is most often caused by *Ancylostoma braziliense* in the western world.

10. The complement levels in patients with renal failure due to Goodpasture's syndrome are usually normal.

15.83 Year 1—Week 28—Day 1

1. *Rhodococcus equi* can cause cavitary lung disease in patients with HIV disease who work on horse farms.

2. The three most common causes of periorbital edema are nephrotic syndrome, Trichinosis, and hypothyroidism.

3. Massive hemoptysis is usually felt to be >600 ml/24 h.

4. Bronchopulmonary aspergillosis is treated with steroids and itraconazole.

5. "Hook" osteophytes are seen in hemochromatosis and usually involve the metacarpophalangeal joints (second and third MCP most commonly).

6. Arthritis of the first carpometacarpal joint is osteoarthritis.

7. Coarctation of the aorta can cause rib notching (due to formation of collateral vasculature).

8. Nasal ipratropium is very effective for gustatory rhinitis.

9. Cefazolin should be stopped within 24 h after a surgery if being used for skin prophylaxis.

10. *Entamoeba histolytica* infections can mimic inflammatory bowel disease. Treatment is with metronidazole and paromomycin (to eliminate spores).

15.84 Year 1—Week 28—Day 2

1. Pancreatitis due to high triglycerides is usually caused by elevated chylomicrons which interfere with the amylase assay and give a normal or near-normal value with elevated lipase.

2. Besides hypertriglyceridemia, other causes of pancreatitis include hypercalcemia, alcohol, gallstones (the most common), pancreas divisum (an anatomic variant that is found in 7% of the population in which the main pancreatic duct drains completely into the duct of Santorini and the minor papilla), and drug-induced causes (furosemide, estrogen, valproic acid, tetracycline, pentamidine, salicylates, sulfas, azathioprine, L-asparaginase, thiazides, ddI/ddC medications used for HIV).

3. The procedure which is the next step in management for a patient with cholangitis already on antibiotics (on the boards the desired choice will be ampicillin, gentamicin, and metronidazole) is ERCP with sphincterotomy.

4. Acetaminophen is the most common cause of acute liver failure in the USA. A patient with acute fulminant hepatic failure should be transferred to a center with expertise in liver transplantation.

5. Hemangiomas can be detected with tagged, pooled RBC nuclear scan. Only large hemangiomas (usually larger size than 10 cm) will require surgical excision.

6. The most common causes of lower GI bleeding are diverticulosis and angiodysplasias.

7. Irritable bowel syndrome requires 3 months of abdominal pain that is relieved with defecation and is associated with a change in either the frequency or consistency of the stool, and two or more of the following for at least 25% of the days. (1) Disturbed defecation (3+/day or 3 or less per week), (2) altered form of stool, (3) altered stool passage, (4) passage of mucus, or (5) bloating or feeling of abdominal distension.

8. Treatment of irritable bowel syndrome includes fiber supplementation with psyllium if constipated, loperamide if having diarrhea, exercise, lactose restriction, fluids, and anticholinergic medications if having spasms.

9. The D-xylose test checks for malabsorption involving the jejunum (small bowel). The test is abnormal if after 2 h there is less than 20 mg/dl in serum or less than 5 g in 5 h in urine.

10. A qualitative screen for fat malabsorption is the fecal fat stain (Sudan Black). The diagnostic test is a 72-h stool collection showing a fat output of greater than 7% of intake (between 60 and 100 g).

15.85 Year 1—Week 28—Day 3

1. Sinus pulmonary tract infections, GI tract infections (with Giardia as well), and otitis media are hallmarks of IGA deficiency.

2. IGA deficiency is associated with ataxia-telangiectasia syndrome, celiac sprue, inflammatory bowel disease, and autoimmune hepatitis.

3. Drugs such as Dilantin and D-penicillamine (and less commonly hydroxychloroquine) have been able to induce IGA deficiency.

4. Patients with IgA deficiency are at risk of developing anaphylaxis when given fresh frozen plasma or blood transfusions.

5. Among the lesser-known diseases that give a Wood's lamp fluorescence pattern are Microsporum tinea capitis, Pseudomonas super-infection in burn patients, vitiligo (appears ivory-white which helps to distinguish from tinea versicolor), and herpetic eye infections.

6. The urine of patients with ethylene glycol poisoning will fluoresce under Wood's lamp.

7. Erythrasma infections will fluoresce coral red under a Wood's lamp.

8. Methanol poisoning can lead to papillitis (acute visual loss).

9. Isopropyl alcohol causes an osmolar gap but generally not an anion gap metabolic acidosis.

10. Treat sporotrichosis and histoplasmosis with itraconazole as first-line agent for most manifestations except acute meningitis state.

15.86 Year 1—Week 29—Day 1

1. Patients with HIV disease can have any presentation of tuberculosis, including diffuse interstitial infiltrates and the miliary version of the disease (millet-seed lesions throughout the lung).

2. The most common fast-growing atypical mycobacteria species are the following: Chelonae, fortuitum, and abscessus.

3. *Mycobacterium gordonae* is a common contaminant as it can be found in freshwater.

4. Nocardia can cause brain abscess disease as well as lung disease. IV amikacin is used by many physicians along with sulfamethoxazole-trimethoprim if a brain abscess is present.

5. Whipple's disease patients can present with hyperpigmentation throughout their body.

6. Anterior mediastinal widening can be caused by "*terrible*" lymphoma, *thymoma*, *teratoma*, or substernal *thyroid* gland (the four "t" terms).

7. Posterior mediastinal widening is usually due to neurogenic or esophageal cysts processes but can be caused by histoplasmosis.

8. Q-Fever is caused by *Coxiella burnetii* and can cause endocarditis and liver failure.

9. Rifampin is used in treatment of severe Legionella lung infections along with azithromycin.

10. The treatment of Lemierre's syndrome is with penicillin. If a patient has significant penicillin allergy, then use clindamycin in those individuals for treatment.

15.87 Year 1—Week 29—Day 2

1. Patients with long-standing rheumatoid arthritis (RA) and hoarseness should be evaluated for cricoarytenoid joint involvement.
2. Hoarseness can occur in Ortner's syndrome, where the enlarged left atrium due to mitral stenosis impinges on the left recurrent laryngeal nerve.
3. Hoarseness has been noted in epidemiological studies with *Chlamydia pneumoniae* infections.
4. Hypothyroidism can present with subtle signs such as rhinitis and hoarseness.
5. Goodpasture's disease is rarely seen in patients above age 50.
6. Aortic dissection can occur years after one is given the diagnosis of temporal arteritis.
7. A young patient who is found to have black, bloody synovial fluid should be suspected of having pigmented villonodular synovitis. Treatment is with synovectomy.
8. Polyarteritis nodosa classically spares the lung. Microscopic polyangiitis, which can have a positive P-ANCA test, can involve the lung and the kidneys.
9. Ethambutol can cause drug-induced gout, but pyrazinamide is the most common medication in tuberculosis treatment with this side effect.
10. A 24-h uric acid collection may be asked to be done as the next step in management of a patient with gout. This is to see if a patient is an over-producer or under-excretor. 90% of patients are under-excretors and thus candidates for treatment with probenecid if they can drink 2 L of water per day. Allopurinol is preferred agent if patient has history of urate nephrolithiasis.

15.88 Year 1—Week 29—Day 3

1. Golfer's elbow is also known as medial epicondylitis. It is an overuse injury to the tendinous origin of the flexor pronator muscle mass.
2. Golfer's elbow is evident on exam by tenderness at the medial epicondyle and pain with resisted wrist flexion and forearm pronation.
3. Cubital tunnel syndrome refers to ulnar nerve neuropathy due to usually direct trauma to the ulnar nerve in the cubital tunnel.
4. Surgical treatment of cubital tunnel surgery is needed if there is motor weakness, a positive electromyogram, or if conservative treatment fails.
5. Tennis elbow is lateral epicondylitis. Pathology is usually small tears of the extensor carpi radialis brevis muscle that extends from the lateral epicondyle.
6. Radial tunnel syndrome involves radial nerve entrapment, frequently involving the posterior interosseus branch of the radial nerve at the proximal edge of the supinator muscle.
7. Biceps tendinitis develops in athletes who require repetitive elbow flexion and supination.
8. There may be tenderness in the antecubital fossa in patients with biceps tendinitis.
9. Rotator cuff problems should be suspected in patients with decreased internal rotation when the shoulder is abducted.
10. The proximal tibia is the most common location for stress fracture of the leg.

15.89 Year 1—Week 30—Day 1

1. Iliotibial band syndrome most commonly manifests with lateral knee pain.
2. Diffuse idiopathic skeletal hyperostosis (DISH) is seen with flowing calcifications down at least four anterior vertebral bodies.
3. There is no morning stiffness associated with DISH.
4. DISH does have an association with diabetes mellitus.
5. Athletes do get increased left ventricular mass usually by enlargement of myocardial muscle fiber size.
6. Overtraining in athletes may lead to an increase in basal heart rate and chronic fatigue.

7. Wrestlers can get a herpes infection complex known as herpes gladiatorum.
8. Pain in the anterior groin area with flexion, abduction, and external rotation points to sacroiliac joint disease.
9. Trochanteric bursitis manifests as tenderness over the lateral hip on palpation.
10. The pain of trochanteric bursitis is worse when one lies on the affected side, and it worsens on abduction of the affected side.

15.90   Year 1—Week 30—Day 2

1. Prominent U-wave in lead III can be seen with low potassium, class Ia antiarrhythmic use, and CNS disease with long QT intervals.
2. Broad, prominent T-waves over the anterior leads can be seen in hyperacute MI.
3. T-wave alternans predicts a high possibility of arrythmia in the post-MI setting.
4. Signal averaged EKGs are used to check for the possibility of ventricular arrythmias.
5. Lown-Ganong-Levine syndrome involves a short PR interval, no delta waves, and a propensity to go into rapid atrial fibrillation.
6. Deeply symmetrical T-waves over most leads, but especially all the anterior leads, can be seen with CNS events (such as stroke).
7. Aortic valve endocarditis can cause ring valve abscess which can manifest on EKG as a prolonging PR interval due to invasion into conduction system.
8. QRS widening is an ominous sign in patients with TCA poisoning.
9. Macrocytosis is most commonly due to alcohol abuse in the general population.
10. Methadone is the only opioid that reproducibly has been shown to prolong the QT interval.

15.91   Year 1—Week 30—Day 3

1. Spherocytes are seen in hereditary spherocytosis and autoimmune hemolytic anemia. Those conditions are marked by a rise in MCHC.

2. The osmotic fragility test helps diagnose hereditary spherocytosis.
3. A direct Coombs test is positive in patients with autoimmune hemolytic anemia.
4. Paroxysmal nocturnal hemoglobinuria involves thrombosis of unusual vessels such as the mesenteric and portal veins. It is diagnosed nowadays by flow cytometry defects in CD55 and CD59 of the red blood cells.
5. Hairy cell leukemia is treated with 2-CDA and is associated with recurrent Legionella pneumonia infections.
6. TTP is marked by normal PT and PTT values, and it is treated by plasmapheresis. IVIG is second-line therapy.
7. HIV status should be checked in all patients with ITP and TTP.
8. If a patient with ITP does not respond to steroid therapy, splenectomy is usually the next step in management.
9. Beta-thalassemia trait is marked by an increased hemoglobin A2 fraction.
10. The MCV value will rise in most cases of myelodysplasia. White blood cells in this disorder will be hypogranular and hyposegmented.

15.92   Year 1—Week 31—Day 1

1. Yellow nail syndrome is marked by bronchiectasis, sinusitis, pleural effusions that can be chylous in nature, and, of course, yellow nails on physical exam.
2. *Serratia marcescens* is a gram-negative rod that can cause pneumonia and can produce a reddish pigment that appears as if it was bloody sputum.
3. Pheochromocytoma of the bladder should be considered in patients with palpitations and piercing headaches just before, during, and after micturition.
4. Acute vertigo occurring immediately after pressing on the tragus portion of the ear should raise suspicion for perilymphatic fistula.

5. Lithium, beta-blockers, and antimalarials are the most common medications to flare the rash of psoriasis.

6. Basal cell carcinoma is estimated to metastasize at a rate of 1 in 10,000.

7. For every 1000 patients with actinic keratosis, one out of those 1000 will convert to squamous cell carcinoma of the skin in most series (0.1 percent).

8. Disopyramide cannot be used in patients with history of acute angle closure glaucoma due to its anticholinergic properties.

9. Propafenone is the only anti-arrhythmic with the side effect of taste disturbance. This drug cannot be used in patients with structural heart disease.

10. The three types of atrial septal defects are ostium primum, ostium secundum, and sinus venosus.

15.93 Year 1—Week 31—Day 2

1. Verner-Morrison syndrome is another name for VIPoma, one of the functional tumors that can cause diarrhea.

2. In a patient with beta-thalassemia trait who has a normal hemoglobin A2 fraction (after previously being elevated), suspect iron deficiency anemia has ensued.

3. It is expected that the MCV will rise in patients being treated with hydroxyurea.

4. Tularemia is transmitted by the Dermacentor ticks and by *Amblyomma americanum* (the Lone star Tick).

5. Amantadine has uses in Parkinson's disease (for tremor) and in multiple sclerosis (for chronic fatigue syndrome).

6. Ehrlichia infections can be marked by WBC inclusions known as morulae. The treatment of this infection is with doxycycline.

7. The meglitinides are the only other class of hypoglycemic agents, meaning the only other medications to stimulate endogenous insulin secretion besides the sulfonylureas.

8. MEN syndromes are inherited in autosomal dominant fashion. Hypoglandular autoim-

mune syndromes are inherited in autosomal recessive fashion.

9. Beta-blockers are the first-line therapy for patients with hypertrophic cardiomyopathy and for patients with prolonged QT syndrome.

10. Niacin is felt to be the only drug that reliably lowers the lipoprotein (a) level.

15.94 Year 1—Week 31—Day 3

1. Turcot syndrome is felt to be the only colon polyp syndrome that is inherited in autosomal recessive fashion. It is marked by occurrence of brain tumors as well.

2. Gardner's syndrome, associated with jaw and skull osteomas, can be also seen in association with carcinoma of the ampulla of Vater.

3. Meckel's diverticulum can include ectopic pancreatic and gastric tissue. It is when the tumor contains ectopic gastric tissue that bleeding usually occurs. It is manifested by bright red blood per rectum rather than melena.

4. Antimitochondrial antibodies are found in over 90% of patients with primary biliary cirrhosis. First-line treatment is ursodeoxycholic acid.

5. Leflunomide is the only DMARD (disease modifying anti-rheumatic drug) to be a pyrimidine nucleotide inhibitor. It is used for rheumatoid arthritis, sometimes in conjunction with methotrexate. LFT abnormalities are the most common side effect.

6. Pigmented villonodular synovitis should be suspected in young patients with joint fluid that is dark red to black in color. Synovectomy is the treatment of choice.

7. The lemniscal pathways of the central nervous system are involved in light touch, vibration, and proprioception.

8. Riluzole is an anti-glutamate agent that has been used in treatment algorithms of patients with amyotrophic lateral sclerosis.

9. Entacapone and tolcapone are COMT inhibitors (catechol-O-methyl transferase inhibitors) that are used in conjunction (not

monotherapy) usually with carbidopa-levodopa in treating Parkinson's disease.

10. Lamotrigine is a very useful medication in treating atonic seizures (drop attacks prominent).

15.95   Year 1—Week 32—Day 1

1. HSV encephalitis causes changes in MRI usually at the temporal lobes or inferior frontal lobes.
2. The test of choice to diagnose HSV encephalitis is PCR for DNA of HSV. The first test may be initially negative so a second test may need to be ordered.
3. Treatment of HSV encephalitis is with 10 mg/kg of IV acyclovir every 8 h.
4. WPW is associated with Ebstein's anomaly where the right ventricle appears nearly as small as the right atrium due to abnormal displacement of the tricuspid valve.
5. Definitive treatment of WPW is radiofrequency ablation. Procainamide is the answer on the test if the patient presents acutely in rapid atrial fibrillation with this condition.
6. The first step in complete heart block management is to stop all AV-nodal blocking agents, such as beta-blockers or digoxin.
7. The best treatment for progressive multifocal leukoencephalopathy is to treat the underlying HIV disease with antiretrovirals.
8. Atovaquone can be used to cover PCP and toxoplasmosis prophylaxis in patients with sulfa allergy.
9. If a patient with a sulfa allergy develops acute toxoplasmosis, then one could use pyrimethamine and clindamycin for treatment.
10. Intracerebral metastasis is much more common than leptomeningeal carcinomatosis in patients with solid tumors.

15.96   Year 1—Week 32—Day 2

1. Ataxia is the most common initial presentation of leptomeningeal carcinomatosis.
2. Paradoxical split of the S2 most commonly correlates to a left bundle branch block on EKG.

3. Persistent split of the S2 heart sound most commonly correlates to a right bundle branch block on EKG.
4. A fixed split of S2 heart sound most commonly correlates to the presence of an atrial septal defect.
5. Patients with ostium secundum ASD do not need endocarditis prophylaxis when undergoing invasive procedures.
6. A step-up in oxygen saturation from the right atrium to the right ventricle of at least 5% is needed before entertaining the diagnosis of VSD.
7. A patient with a pleural fluid glucose less than 40 mg/dl in the setting of a complicated parapneumonic effusion needs a chest tube for drainage of the effusion.
8. Lupus patients have the "shrinking lung" syndrome that can strike which is a loss of lung volume due to inflammation involving the inspiratory muscles of respiration.
9. Lupus patients can also develop diffuse alveolar hemorrhage with increased DLCO on PFTs. Hemoptysis is seen 75% of the time in these patients. Treat with cyclophosphamide.
10. Graves' disease can lead to exophthalmos, lid retraction, conjunctival irritation, and periorbital swelling.

15.97   Year 1—Week 32—Day 3

1. Four drug therapy for tuberculosis treatment needs to be employed in all areas which run a multidrug resistance rate of greater than 4%.
2. A pleural fluid mesothelial cell count of greater than 5% along with a pH of pleural fluid greater than 7.4 speaks strongly against tuberculous origin of pleural effusion.
3. Tuberculous pleural effusions are rarely hemorrhagic and are rarely large in size.
4. Doxycycline is a useful antibiotic for outpatient community-acquired pneumonia treatment.
5. Amphotericin-B is the drug of choice in treating severe to life-threatening fungal infections.

6. Fusarium is a fungus with acute angle branching hyphae that can be resistant to antifungal treatment. Using aggressive surgical debridement when called for is essential.
7. Ticarcillin-clavulanate and sulfa-based drugs are acceptable treatments of *Stenotrophomonas* infections.
8. *Stenotrophomonas* infections are universally resistant to imipenem.
9. Sarcoidosis might manifest acutely with uveitis (usually posterior), parotid gland enlargement, and fever, known as Heerfordt's syndrome.
10. The fast-growing atypical mycobacteria include *M. fortuitum, M. chelonae, and M. abscessus.*

15.98   Year 1—Week 33—Day 1

1. D-penicillamine and amiodarone are among the drug-induced causes of bronchiolitis obliterans with organizing pneumonia (BOOP).
2. PCP can cause pneumothorax due to ability to form bronchopleural fistulas.
3. Ethambutol can cause optic neuritis. Pyrazinamide can cause drug-induced gout.
4. Hydroxychloroquine can cause both retinal and corneal toxicity. The drug must be discontinued if retinal toxicity is noted (usually seen as bullseye lesions near the macula).
5. The number needed to treat is the value of the number one divided by the absolute risk reduction).
6. Do not use rifampin in HIV patients taking protease inhibitors as it will increase the P450 pathway in the liver and deliver less than ideal protease inhibitor levels.
7. Pouchitis as a possible complication from underlying ulcerative colitis is treated with metronidazole.
8. Azathioprine and L-asparaginase can cause pancreatitis.
9. Twitching of the eyelids while on looks upward in gaze occurs in patients with myasthenia gravis.

10. Avoid aminoglycosides in patients with myasthenia gravis as they can cause worsening of manifestations of the disease.

15.99   Year 1—Week 33—Day 2

1. The most common culprit for emphysematous cholecystitis and pyelonephritis is *Escherichia coli.*
2. Diabetes mellitus increases the risk of acquiring tuberculosis by at least ten-fold.
3. Fusobacterium can cause diabetic periodontitis. Surgery may be needed early as part of treatment.
4. Diabetes mellitus patients may have aggressive infections due to increased hypoxia of tissue, decreased phagocytosis, and decreased wound healing.
5. Steroids are used as an adjunct in treating tuberculous meningitis.
6. Bezold's abscess is found at the tip of the petrous bone in patients who have malignant otitis externa.
7. Patients with clostridial infections should also receive clindamycin to bind toxin (penicillin treats the underlying infection but does not do anything as far as the toxin).
8. Avoid performing intravenous pyelogram testing in patients with diabetes mellitus suspected of having papillary necrosis.
9. Papillary necrosis presents with flank pain, hematuria, peritoneal signs, and usually 3 days into therapy of UTI treatment.
10. A patient with cranial nerve palsy and underlying diabetes mellitus should be investigated for Mucor infection, especially if there is sinusitis present as well.

15.100 Year 1—Week 33—Day 3

1. Patients with rheumatological disease should be discontinued from their biological treatment agent (such as TNF-alpha receptor inhibitor) at least one cycle before the planned operation to promote best wound healing possible. Medications such as meth-

otrexate and hydroxychloroquine can be continued through the surgical operation.

2. Use epinephrine early in patients suspected of anaphylaxis.

3. There is a late phase of anaphylaxis that might occur as late as 8–12 h after the initial episode. Steroids are beneficial really only for the late phase of anaphylaxis.

4. Serum tryptase levels will be elevated in patients with systemic mastocytosis and with anaphylaxis. This may be helpful in distinguishing patients with urticaria and angioedema from true anaphylaxis.

5. Celiac sprue can present at any age. The best antibody to detect this disease is tissue transglutaminase.

6. Suspect Wilson's disease in young patients with liver disease and unexplained hemolysis.

7. D-penicillamine is used acutely in the treatment of Wilson's disease. Trientine and zinc are treatments that can be used for chronic copper chelation.

8. Vitamin E deficiency can lead to areflexia.

9. A couple of neat diagnoses to consider in patients with recurrent aseptic meningitis are Behcet's syndrome, Mollaret's meningitis (felt to be caused by HSV), and Vogt-Koyanagi-Harada syndrome (associated with uveitis and CN 8 damage).

10. In a lupus patient with aseptic meningitis, look through medications to make sure patient does not have NSAIDs in the drug profile.

15.101 Year 1—Week 34—Day 1

1. Always measure the negative inspiratory force and FVC value in patients with Guillain-Barre syndrome as they may have diaphragmatic involvement and might need protective intubation.

2. Plasmapheresis is the treatment of choice for patients with renal failure and respiratory failure in Goodpasture's syndrome.

3. Creutzfeldt-Jakob disease can be diagnosed using the 14-3-3 protein of the CSF.

4. Transverse myelitis can be seen in patients with multiple sclerosis, SLE, and post-vaccination, especially hepatitis B.

5. Post-MMR vaccination, one can see acute disseminated encephalomyelitis.

6. Hypercalcemia is mediated by PTH-related peptide when it is driven by squamous cell cancer.

7. Hypercalcemia of breast cancer and multiple myeloma will respond to steroids.

8. Carbamazepine is the anti-epileptic most prone to causing hyponatremia.

9. The most common medication to cause hyponatremia are thiazide diuretics (HCTZ and chlorthalidone).

10. There is a hemolytic anemia associated with CLL and it is important to recognize by getting appropriate tests (Coombs test, LDH, haptoglobin) as this anemia is treated by steroids rather than treating the CLL with fludarabine.

15.102 Year 1—Week 34—Day 2

1. Antibiotics, anticonvulsants (usually carbamazepine), and NSAIDs are the three most common causes of toxic epidermal necrolysis states.

2. The fungi with acute angle branching hyphae that cause disease in humans are Fusarium and Aspergillus.

3. Discoid lupus and sarcoidosis should be considered in a patient with scarring alopecia.

4. Anti-Saccharomyces cerevisiae antibodies (ASCA) can be seen in patients with Crohn's disease.

5. Probenecid is contraindicated in patients with history of uric acid nephrolithiasis.

6. Acetaminophen in doses exceeding 1500 mg daily may cause potentiation of the INR if a patient is on coumadin.

7. Nasal ipratropium is effective in treating cases of gustatory rhinitis.

8. Urticarial vasculitis should be suspected in all patients with pain from their sites rather

than the usual pruritis symptoms of most urticaria states.

9. Daptomycin is the first lipopeptide antibiotic to be released on the market. It covers gram-positive organisms only, including VRE and MRSA.

10. Nitrofurantoin requires a creatinine clearance in a patient of above 40–50 cc/min to work as this is the kidney function needed to be able to reach high enough concentration of the drug in urine.

15.103 Year 1—Week 34—Day 3

1. Think of *Schistosome* dermatitis in patients with severe itching and a papular rash shortly after swimming in a freshwater lake in the Midwest.

2. Treatment of most U.S. based Schistosome dermatitis is with topical/oral antihistamines and corticosteroids. Anti-helminthic treatment is rarely needed.

3. *Giardia lamblia* and malaria infections do not cause eosinophilia.

4. Ivermectin can be used in treating *Schistosomiasis* and Norwegian scabies, with this variant of scabies being seen in patients with HIV disease.

5. Hyperpigmentation changes can occur in patients with hyperthyroidism.

6. Pretibial myxedema is most commonly seen in patients with hyperthyroidism.

7. IVIG has been used in treating some patients with Stevens-Johnson's syndrome.

8. Nasal packing for epistaxis can lead to staphylococcal toxin shock syndrome.

9. Erythroplakia is much more likely to lead to progression to squamous cell carcinoma than is leukoplakia.

10. Kikuchi-Fujimoto disease is a necrotizing lymphadenitis syndrome that presents with lesions mimicking a vasculitis and commonly causes posterior cervical lymphadenopathy. It may be linked to lupus as well.

15.104 Year 1—Week 35—Day 1

1. Patients with hairy cell leukemia have abnormal lymphocytes with projections (hair-appearing) from their membranes. The only other situation where cells may mimic those of hairy cell leukemia are the cells of splenic marginal zone lymphoma.

2. Suspect constrictive pericarditis in patients with significant dyspnea on exertion yet normal ejection fraction and no valvular heart disease.

3. Patients with WPW (Wolff–Parkinson–White) syndrome having symptomatic episodes need radiofrequency ablation.

4. Consider WPW heavily in the differential of a young patient with atrial fibrillation with a very rapid ventricular rate.

5. The most common supraventricular tachycardia seen in the general population is an AV-nodal reentrant tachycardia.

6. Nitrofurantoin can cause a pulmonary toxicity marked by interstitial pneumonitis.

7. Amoxicillin-clavulanate can potentiate the INR in patients taking warfarin. Patients with amoxicillin alone do not seem to have this effect.

8. Serotonin selective uptake inhibitors (SSRI) can be tapered after one single major depressive disorder if side effects after the patient has noted improvement in major depression symptoms for at least 4–9 months on average. Such tapering may be needed for erectile dysfunction or hyponatremia as complications of therapy.

9. A Horner's syndrome may be noted in patients with lateral medullary infarction (as part of the Wallenberg's syndrome).

10. Gerstmann syndrome is marked by acalculia, finger anomia, left-right confusion, and dysgraphia.

15.105 Year 1—Week 35—Day 2

1. Patients placed on high-dose sulfamethoxazole-trimethoprim therapy for a prolonged period of time are at risk of developing folic acid deficiency.

2. Blastomycosis is marked by broad-based budding fungi and can cause significant mucocutaneous disease as well as isolated plaque lesions.

3. Histoplasmosis can cause WBC inclusion bodies and a posterior fibrosing mediastinitis.

4. Molluscum contagiosum appears as a pearly papule with an umbilicated center. It is caused by poxvirus.

5. Among the infectious causes of erythema nodosum are streptococcus, Yersinia, tuberculosis, and coccidiomycosis.

6. Among the non-infectious causes of erythema nodosum are the use of oral contraceptive pills, Behcet's syndrome, and sarcoidosis.

7. Nocardia asteroids will respond to minocycline and amikacin, besides the usual medication given for this condition which is trimethoprim-sulfamethoxazole.

8. Imipenem will not be effective against *Nocardia braziliensis*, which is one of the most common causes of nodular lymphangitis in this country.

9. *Nocardia asteroides* can cause brain abscess formation as well as disseminated subcutaneous nodules.

10. *Nocardia* is a partially acid-fast organism, so a positive AFB stain should not automatically push you into tuberculosis treatment without looking at all other possibilities.

15.106 Year 1—Week 35—Day 3

1. Patients who have been revascularized within the last 5 years (by either CABG or stent with angioplasty) and have no cardiac symptoms are generally safe to go to the OR for surgery in most situations.

2. Autoimmune hepatitis may not have antibodies present upon testing. The most common two that are found are anti-smooth muscle antibody and anti-liver-kidney-microsomal antibody.

3. The most common supraventricular tachycardia is AV-nodal reentrant tachycardia.

4. About 20% of patients with temporal arteritis will have signs and symptoms of polymyalgia rheumatica. 11% of patients with temporal arteritis will have a normal ESR.

5. Mononeuritis multiplex is most commonly seen with polyarteritis nodosum of all the rheumatological diseases.

6. 30% of patients with polyarteritis nodosum will have antibodies against hepatitis B.

7. Cryoglobulinemia can be seen with both hepatitis B and hepatitis C. Serum sickness is seen only with acute hepatitis B.

8. The DLCO is essential in differentiating the origin of restrictive lung diseases. A DLCO value that is low speaks for parenchymal lung disease as the cause of the restrictive lung disease.

9. Kyphoscoliosis, morbid obesity, and neurological diseases (such as ALS) are among the causes of restrictive lung diseases not due to parenchymal lung disease.

10. Grapefruit juice is notorious for raising cyclosporine levels.

15.107 Year 1—Week 36—Day 1

1. Prolymphocytic B-cell leukemias are characterized by rapid disease progression and generally are unresponsive to therapy, although there are some good results with rituximab at times.

2. Most patients with hairy cell leukemia present with pancytopenia and splenomegaly.

3. The projections from the cell of hairy cell leukemia can resemble those seen in splenic marginal zone lymphoma. The best way to distinguish the two are by flow cytometry and annexin A immunostaining which is quite commonly seen in hairy cell leukemia.

4. T-cell prolymphocytic leukemia generally presents at about age 63 (median) and presents with splenomegaly, LAD, occasional skin infiltrative features, and pleural effusions (in about 15% of patients).

5. There is a strong relationship between the T-cell large granular cell leukemia and Felty's syndrome of rheumatoid arthritis.
6. The tap of a patient with hairy cell leukemia can be dry similar to patients with myelofibrosis.
7. HTLV-1 was the first retrovirus discovered capable of causing cancer in humans.
8. Patients with T-cell leukemia are at risk of developing Candida, PCP, aspergillus, CMV, and even Strongyloides infections. The malignant lymphocytes may have lobulated nuclei, sometimes giving them the appearance of "flower cells."
9. Paroxysmal nocturnal hemoglobinuria is best diagnosed with flow cytometry showing defects in CD-55 and CD-59 which involve the red cell membrane.
10. The most common clinical manifestation of patients with paroxysmal nocturnal hemoglobinuria is thrombosis.

15.108 Year 1—Week 36—Day 2

1. Think of Zollinger-Ellison syndrome (ZES) in a patient with ulcers in the second and third part of the duodenum with coexisting hypercalcemia and diarrhea.
2. Most common cause of an elevated gastrin level in the general population is not ZES but rather use of a proton pump inhibitor.
3. The first step in evaluating a patient for possible Zencker's diverticulum is a barium swallow rather than an EGD.
4. Gilbert's syndrome is the most common cause of an elevated bilirubin level in the general population.
5. 7% of patients in the general population are estimated to have pancreas divisum yet only a few of those patients will ever develop clinical pancreatitis
6. Candida esophagitis is marked by a "shaggy" esophagus on barium swallow.
7. Patients with calcification of the gallbladder (porcelain gallbladder) need removal of gallbladder due to high risk of gallbladder cancer.

8. HIV disease can cause colitis, esophagitis, and cholangiopathy.
9. Hypercalcemia develops in Paget's disease only when those patients are immobilized for a significant amount of time.
10. Osteomalacia can cause diffuse bone pain in the elderly. It is marked by low vitamin D levels, calcium levels, and phosphorus levels.

15.109 Year 1—Week 36—Day 3

1. Vancomycin can worsen linear bullous IGA dermatitis.
2. Linear bullous IGA dermatitis can be treated with dapsone.
3. Filgrastim administration can induce Sweet's syndrome as well as an inflammatory arthritis.
4. Filgrastim is usually only given after a patient has one previous episode of neutropenic fever.
5. Treatment of recurrent idiopathic pericarditis can involve use of colchicine as steroid-sparing agent.
6. The most important aspect of management of mitral stenosis is heart rate control (beta-blockers are first-line therapy).
7. The most common reason for heart failure in a pregnant patient is peripartum cardiomyopathy.
8. Never rechallenge a patient or try to desensitize a patient who has had a hypersensitivity reaction to a medication.
9. Glycoprotein 2b-3a inhibitors (such as tirofiban and abciximab) should be used in patients with positive troponin I labs and ST-segment depression on the EKG.
10. Chronic hypertension is the most common cause of left ventricular hypertrophy in a patient.

15.110 Year 1—Week 37—Day 1

1. Patients who develop pre-eclampsia have been shown to have a higher incidence of metabolic syndrome later in life.
2. The risk of venous thrombosis is increased seven to ten-fold in pregnancy and is the highest right after delivery.
3. In pregnancy, T-cells go from T-helper 1 dominance to T-helper 2 dominance, thus diseases that rely on TH-1 dominance, such as rheumatoid arthritis, multiple sclerosis, and thyroiditis improve and diseases such as SLE which rely on TH-2 predominance worsen.
4. Diseases with Th-1 dominance, though, can re-appear quickly after pregnancy such as post-partum thyroiditis, especially if the women have a high titer of anti-microsomal antibodies.
5. Intrahepatic cholestasis of pregnancy is associated with a higher risk of preterm birth and higher incidence of cholelithiasis.
6. Guillain-Barre syndrome has a Miller-Fisher variant where the paralysis is descending rather than ascending (most common direction) and that variant is associated with ataxia and ophthalmoplegia as early symptoms in the course of disease.
7. Ovarian torsion is most likely to present in women with ovarian cysts but can occur in normal ovaries in about 20% of cases.
8. The key to ovarian torsion is that nausea and vomiting start with the onset of pain, as opposed to appendicitis where nausea and vomiting start well after pain starts.
9. One can occasionally see evidence of an abdominal aortic aneurysm (AAA) on plain abdominal X-ray as the aorta wall can appear calcified.
10. The incidence of AAA is estimated at 14% in patients above age 65 and five times more likely to occur in men than women.

15.111 Year 1—Week 37—Day 2

1. Sudden death in patients with prolonged QT syndrome can be triggered by states of emotion or exercise.
2. Patients with prolonged QT syndrome with symptoms refractory to beta-blockers could be considered for left-sided cardiac sympathetic denervation, AICD placement, or pacemakers depending on the clinical situation.
3. There is a link between IGA deficiency and inflammatory bowel syndrome.
4. IVIG infusion does not seem to be a problem for patients with serum IGA levels of at least 7 mg/dl as far as possible anaphylactic reactions.
5. Patients with CLL have increased risk of infection with encapsulated organisms.
6. Recurrent pneumonias in patients with common variable immunodeficiency may lead to the development of bronchiectasis.
7. There may be benefit to IVIG infusion in patients with CLL who have low serum IGG levels and who have history of recurrent significant infections.
8. Besides *Giardia* infection, there is an increased risk for *Campylobacter jejuni* and *Yersinia* infections in patients with IGA deficiency.
9. Dilantin can lower IGA levels within 3–4 months of starting therapy and lead to complete deficiency in about 5% of patients (this is reversible by stopping the medication).
10. There is a marked risk of lymphoma in patients who have common variable immunodeficiency.

15.112 Year 1—Week 37—Day 3

1. Most peripancreatic fluid collections will resolve spontaneously within 6 weeks. Drainage should be done if infection is suspected or if obstructive symptoms develop due to mass effect.

2. Alcohol is the most common cause of chronic pancreatitis. It is associated with calcifications of the pancreas.

3. Among the antibodies found in celiac sprue are the anti-endomysial, antireticulin, and antigliadin antibodies. Patients with celiac sprue have small bowel biopsies showing blunting or atrophy of villous structures with hypertrophy of the crypts. IGA is found in immunofluorescence. Gluten-free diet is the treatment. Celiac sprue is associated with lymphoma, and sometimes iron deficiency anemia will be the first and only clinical manifestation. The skin disease associated with this condition is dermatitis herpetiformis. If antibodies remain positive, then suspect non-compliance with dietary regimen.

4. Mesalamine (5-ASA) is considered first-line therapy for patients with mild to moderate active ulcerative colitis. Patients who have acute flares should be treated with intravenous corticosteroids.

5. Infliximab is superior to 6-mercaptopurine and metronidazole combination therapy for treatment of fistulas in Crohn's disease. Infliximab works against tumor necrosis factor-alpha.

6. Patients with tropical sprue have similar lesions to celiac sprue except the former has a lymphocytic infiltrate rather than a monocytic infiltrate. Treatment of tropical sprue can be carried out with tetracycline 250 mg four times daily and folic acid 5 mg daily therapy. Suspect if recent trip to the Caribbean or India. Most patients present with mild eosinophilia and a megaloblastic anemia. They can have fat globules in stool.

7. *Helicobacter pylori* is associated with a low-grade non-Hodgkins lymphoma called MALToma, in which nearly 80% will regress just with antibiotics and might be diagnosed by biopsing an area of redundant mucosal folds.

8. There has historically been no role for treatment of *Helicobacter pylori* in patients with non-ulcer dyspepsia.

9. Patients who have been vaccinated for hepatitis B will not show a positive anti- HBc IgM or IgG (no core antibodies). The Hbe Ag (e-antigen) usually reflects active viral replication and is positive in most cases of acute hepatitis B. Sometimes, just the core IGM antibody will be positive in acute cases (window period).

10. Patients with right heart failure will have ascites that has a serum/ascites albumin gradient (calculated by subtraction) greater than 1.1 (as seen in portal hypertension, myxedema, and Budd-Chiari syndrome) with total protein greater than 2.5 (like in tuberculous peritonitis, peritoneal carcinomatosis, pancreatitis, and nephrotic syndrome).

15.113 Year 1—Week 38—Day 1

TN—True negative, TP—True positive, FN—False negative, FP—False positive.

1. Selection bias is eliminated as long as the randomization of subjects does not allow systematic unbalanced allocation of study subjects with predictive factors for cancer mortality into one of the study groups. This selection bias can be eliminated by "intention to treat" analysis, rather than according to whether the subjects received the screening or not.

2. Trials performed using volunteers are called efficacy studies. Trials performed on population-based subjects are called effectiveness studies.

3. A cohort study would have study subjects categorized based on the exposure or lack of exposure of a risk factor (smoking in pregnancy) and then followed to determine if a particular outcome (low birth weight babies) results. A clinical trial is a prospective study in which an intervention is applied. In a case control study (which is always retrospective), you would select patients that are normal and those that have a unfavorable outcome (low birth weight) and then compare the frequency of a variable (maternal smoking) in both groups. Cross-sectional

studies look at exposure and outcome at the same point in time.

4. A statistically significant test ($p < 0.05$) rejects the null hypothesis (the null hypothesis states that no differences of effect will be found). Thus, $p < 0.05$ indicates that a difference was found and that there is less than 5% probability that it occurred by chance. Trends in studies usually point to the need for larger, more involved study of a specific association.

5. Sensitivity reflects the performance of a test in patients who have the disease [(TP/(TP + FN)]. Thus, sensitivity looks for "positive in disease." Specificity reflects the performance of a test in patients who do not have the disease [(TN/(TN + FP)]. Thus, specificity looks for "negative in health."

6. Predictive value of a test is dependent on the prevalence of a disease. The positive predictive value of a test is best described as "of those who have a test positive, how many will actually have the disease?" or [TP/(TP + FP)]. The negative predictive value is best described as "of those who have a test negative, how many actually do not have the disease" or [TN/(TN + FN)].

7. "Intention to treat" is a method of analysis that involves analyzing data based on initial randomization into treated and untreated groups, regardless of subsequent outcomes such as poor compliance, crossovers, or migration. Thus, it is essential to answering the question " Does the decision to treat a certain population improve their outcome?"

8. The relative risk can be calculated by dividing the incidence of a disease in exposed individuals by the incidence of the disease in unexposed individuals.

9. Among the drugs notorious for anticholinergic side effects in the elderly are amitriptyline, doxepin, diphenhydramine, chlorpheniramine, dicyclomine, oxybutynin, and methocarbamol.

10. The first intervention of a patient with Parkinson's disease who is having lots of falls is not to add amantadine but rather to give the patient a four-wheeled walker.

15.114 Year 1—Week 38—Day 2

1. The hamate bone is the most common carpal bone fractured by golfers.

2. Gonorrhea is associated with tenosynovitis, most commonly at the wrist mimicking the primary disease state of De Quervain's tenosynovitis.

3. Pseudogout should be highly considered as the cause of wrist pain in older adults. Osteoarthritis of the first carpometacarpal joint can also cause this symptom.

4. The most common rash associated with disseminated gonorrhea is a hemorrhagic pustule on a erythematous base. Treatment of disseminated gonorrhea is ceftriaxone IV for 7–14 days.

5. As cephalosporins go further up in "generation," they have better gram-negative coverage and lose gram-positive coverage compared to first-generation cephalosporins.

6. Cephalosporins and fluoroquinolones are amongst the most common causes of *C. difficile* colitis.

7. Cefazolin should not be continued for more than 24 h post-operatively if it was used for skin prophylaxis.

8. Doxycycline has been used in the treatment of acne rosacea. It has also been used in the treatment of reactive arthritis that is presumed to have been acquired from post-Chlamydia infection.

9. *Ureaplasma urealyticum* and *Mycoplasma hominis* are other causative organisms of nongonococcal urethritis.

10. Multiple sclerosis is most common between the ages of 15 and 45 and is nearly unheard of after the age of 70. Vasculitis diseases such as temporal arteritis and CNS angiitis are misdiagnosed often as multiple sclerosis in patients above age 70 years old.

15.115 Year 1—Week 38—Day 3

1. Pseudogout is associated with hemochromatosis, hypomagnesemia, hypophosphatemia, hypothyroidism, and familial hypocalciuric hypercalcemia.
2. One can see calcification of the triangular ligament of the wrist in patients with pseudogout.
3. Colchicine is helpful in reducing the number of recurrent attacks in patients with pseudogout. Allopurinol has no role in treating this disease.
4. Plan for synovial biopsy when one has a monoarticular process that continues to recur and cannot be explained by autoimmune or crystal-based phenomenon.
5. Patients with aortic stenosis need repair at the point they become symptomatic with either one of syncope, heart failure, or angina.
6. Anecdotal evidence links aortic stenosis with GI bleeding (through arteriovenous malformations of the GI tract). This is known as Heyde's syndrome and is felt to be a type 2a von Willebrand's factor disease.
7. Free wall rupture usually occurs 1–4 days post-myocardial infarction. It tends to occur with the first MI of patients due to lack of collateral circulation and tends to form where infracted tissue meets normal tissue.
8. VSD and papillary muscle rupture are possible complications 1–4 days post-MI. They both can show systolic murmurs. A Swan-Ganz catheter would show a step-up in oxygen saturation between the right atrium and the right ventricle in VSD.
9. Mechanical complications such as listed number 7 and number 8 of this day are felt to affect about 0.1% of post-MI patients.
10. Even with surgical therapy, the mortality associated with free wall rupture post-MI approaches 50%.

15.116 Year 1—Week 39—Day 1

1. Patients who have been neutropenic for 10–14 days and develop right lower quadrant pain are at risk of having typhlitis.
2. Initial treatment of typhlitis includes starting metronidazole and obtaining CT scan of abdomen and general surgical consultation.
3. Patients with cirrhosis are at risk of *Yersinia enterocolitica* infection which can cause a mesenteric adenitis that resembles appendicitis.
4. *Enterobius vermicularis* (the pinworm) would be the parasite most likely if a worm is found as the culprit of a patient with appendicitis.
5. Treatment options in seborrheic dermatitis include low-dose topical steroids (5% or less hydrocortisone), 2% ketoconazole topical preparations and topical zinc preparations. The zinc preparation must be left on skin for at least 5 min for best therapeutic effect.
6. AL amyloid is seen in patients with primary amyloidosis and those patients with multiple myeloma.
7. Beta-2-microglobulin amyloid is the amyloid fibril that can afflict hemodialysis patients (at least 5 years of hemodialysis usually) with carpal tunnel syndrome.
8. Patients with isolated elevated alkaline phosphatase levels and normal bone scans should be suspected of having infiltrative processes of the liver, such as amyloidosis.
9. Patients with splenic and renal infarcts on CT scan of abdomen with no explanation should be considered for endocarditis workups.
10. Marginal zone lymphomas can occur in the splenic area of patients.

15.117 Year 1—Week 39—Day 2

1. The paraneoplastic process of hypercalcemia is usually due to PTH-related peptide in solid tumors such as squamous cell lung cancer. About one-third of non-Hodgkin's lympho-

mas can have hypercalcemia mediated by calcitriol.

2. The anti-Yo antibody is helpful in detecting subacute cerebellar degeneration in patients with breast and ovarian cancer and less useful for detecting this entity in patients with small cell lung cancer.

3. The anti-Hu (anti-neuronal antibody 2) is used to detect limbic encephalomyelitis which may afflict patients with Hodgkin's disease, small cell lung cancer, and testicular cancer.

4. Calcitonin may be used in the first 24 h to treat extreme elevations of serum calcium but its effect is nowhere near as potent as IV hydration with normal saline and concomitant furosemide.

5. Patients with normal pressure hydrocephalus may present with lower extremity Parkinsonism.

6. Polymyalgia rheumatica can present initially as a seronegative symmetrical polyarthritis before its more usual presentation of hip and shoulder stiffness.

7. Enthesopathy is inflammation at insertion point of tendon or ligament into bone, it can be seen in such diseases as ankylosing spondylitis, reactive arthritis, psoriasis, and arthritis associated with inflammatory bowel disease.

8. There has been epidemiological evidence linking hidradenitis suppurativa and spondyloarthropathies.

9. Samter's syndrome is the triad of bronchial asthma, nasal polyposis, and intolerance to aspirin.

10. Patients with silicosis are at high risk of developing tuberculosis.

15.118 Year 1—Week 39—Day 3

1. Progesterone is associated with a vasculitis and angioedema syndrome.

2. Celiac sprue has a link between IGA deficiency and diabetes mellitus type 1.

3. Prednisone may be used in patients who are refractory to the gluten-free diet in patients with celiac sprue.

4. Dapsone is used to ameliorate the pruritis of dermatitis herpetiformis which may be seen in patients with celiac sprue.

5. If multiple liver and renal infarcts are seen, one should consider and embolic source and order a transesophageal echocardiogram to look for marantic or infectious endocarditis.

6. Treatment of HACEK endocarditis with IV ceftriaxone. If you suspect this entity, you must tell the lab to hold blood cultures for up to 14 days.

7. Early post-operative prosthetic valve endocarditis should be treated with vancomycin, rifampin, and gentamicin.

8. Most pleural effusions associated with tuberculosis are non-bloody.

9. Pulmonary emboli can cause large pulmonary effusions, which can be either transudative or exudative in nature.

10. Hypothyroidism is associated with either exudative or transudative pleural effusions. The pleural effusion may have a moderately high triglyceride level as well.

15.119 Year 1—Week 40—Day 1

1. Capacity is determined by a physician (does not need to be a psychiatrist). Competency is determined by a court. A demented patient can have the capacity to make advance directive choices if he demonstrates an understanding of the choices presented to him.

2. Patients under age 18 may be able to make decisions about their health care legally in some states if they are pregnant.

3. Jehovah's witness patients should be asked if they wish to receive blood products in life-threatening situations. If not, that wish cannot be overturned.

4. In a patient who is fasting as part of his religion, if he demonstrates no depression and understands his decision to fast, an ethics consult is not needed if the patient is hospitalized and wishes to continue to fast.

5. You may override a patient's autonomy if he poses a risk to the community, such as a patient with tuberculosis who refuses treatment.

6. A document with a signature to proceed with a procedure is not in and of itself considered informed consent. The procedure must be explained to the patient to the standard of the doctor's profession and risks and benefits explained in the patient's language to include the alternative of no treatment.

7. The most reliable end point in assessing the screening efficacy in a randomized trial involving oncology is the cause-specific cancer mortality.

8. Generalizability is a confounding effect that is not addressed by randomization in a definitive cancer-screening trial of volunteer study subjects with cancer mortality end points. The phenomenon introduced by the volunteer subjects is known as the healthy volunteer effect.

9. When a spectrum (such as the indolence of prostate cancer) of a disease is not considered in the randomization of patients, then the study is susceptible to the confounding effect of length bias. Overdiagnosis is an extreme form of length bias.

10. Randomized, controlled trials with cancer mortality end points are the best way to avoid lead-time bias, because they measure mortality in both screened and non-screened patients from the same point of time, namely when they enter the study rather than when they were diagnosed with the cancer.

15.120 Year 1—Week 40—Day 2

1. Plasmapheresis is the preferred first-line therapy for patients with TTP. IVIG can be used if plasmapheresis is not possible.

2. Spherocytes are seen in peripheral smear in patients with hereditary spherocytosis and autoimmune hemolytic anemia.

3. Piperacillin-tazobactam is the preferred agent of choice in patients with diabetic foot ulcers. Recall for testing purposes though that ticarcillin-clavulanic acid does cover Pseudomonas.

4. Ticarcillin-clavulanic acid and sulfa drugs can be used for treating Stenotrophomonas pneumonias (remember that this organism is resistant to imipenem).

5. The second most common cause for ectopic ACTH syndrome after small cell lung cancer is carcinoid tumors.

6. *Candida krusei* will generally not respond to fluconazole.

7. Membranous nephropathy is the most common cause of idiopathic nephrotic syndrome in Caucasian patients.

8. Focal segmental glomerulosclerosis is the most common cause of idiopathic nephrotic syndrome in African American patients.

9. Do an age-appropriate search for solid tumors in all patients with membranous nephropathy.

10. Renal vein thrombosis occurs in highest incidence in nephrotic syndrome patients in those who are found to have membranous nephropathy.

15.121 Year 1—Week 40—Day 3

1. Among the medications that can cause gingival hyperplasia are the dihydropyridine calcium channel blockers, cyclosporine, and dilantin.

2. Carbamazepine is the neuroleptic most linked to hyponatremia through an SIADH-like mechanism.

3. Fluoroquinolones have been associated with mental status changes in the elderly and with sudden tendon ruptures.

4. Among the medications that can increase acid reflux are theophylline, nitrates, and calcium channel blockers.

5. Alpha-blockers can induce rhinitis in patients similar to estrogen.

6. The initial treatment of patients with Raynaud's phenomenon is calcium channel blockers. Alpha-blockers are second line.

7. Dihydropyridine calcium channel blockers can cause proteinuria and lower extremity edema.

8. There is a drug interaction between theophylline and fluoroquinolones, especially ciprofloxacin (can cause dangerous theophylline levels).

9. Heparin, including low molecular weight forms, can induce osteoporosis within a few months by increasing osteoclast-activating factor.

10. Amiodarone and minocycline are the two most common drugs that can cause bluish discoloration of the skin.

15.122 Year 1—Week 41—Day 1

1. The most common cause of retinal detachment in the general population is severe myopia.

2. Latanoprost, which works through the prostaglandin receptor, can lead to severe myalgias. It is used for glaucoma.

3. Subconjunctival hemorrhages resolve on their own and usually are caused by states such as frequent constipation or coughing (where a Valsalva maneuver might occur).

4. Per medical literature and for tests, conjunctivitis is not associated with eye pain as opposed to iritis, episcleritis, scleritis, and glaucoma.

5. The leading cause of the "red eye" is viral conjunctivitis.

6. Rheumatoid arthritis patients can have a whole host of complications with the eye, including episcleritis, scleritis, and scleromalacia perforans.

7. Iritis/uveitis is associated with a constricted pupil on physical exam.

8. Optic neuritis and trigeminal neuralgia are associated with multiple sclerosis.

9. Amantadine can help the chronic fatigue syndrome of multiple sclerosis.

10. Patients with multiple sclerosis can complain of blurry vision after a hot shower as heat decreases nerve conduction, especially along demyelinated nerves.

15.123 Year 1—Week 41—Day 2

1. Activated protein C resistance is seen in patients with factor V Leiden mutation. The actual pathophysiology is that of increased resistance (although beware that many labs will report that as a low ratio).

2. Prothrombin 20210 mutation (a zip code for thrombosis one might opine) is one of the most common inherited mutations among Caucasians leading to increased thrombotic risk.

3. Dilute Russell Viper Venom test is one of the panel tests for lupus anticoagulant.

4. Acute DVT can drop levels of protein C, protein S, and antithrombin III levels acutely (which then return to normal after the active state resolves).

5. Idiopathic hypercalciuria patients will have kidney stones. Prevention of these kidney stones can occur with use of thiazide diuretics.

6. PTH can be subtly elevated in patients with familial benign hypocalciuric hypercalcemia.

7. Hypothyroidism can lead to an increased prolactin level (due to increased TRH).

8. In patients taking beta-blockers for HTN, one should still give epinephrine first before considering glucagon in the setting of anaphylaxis.

9. Diabetes patients can have a low sex hormone binding globulin level which leads to low testosterone levels.

10. *Candida* infections and *Malassezia furfur* are the two fungal organisms to most worry about in patients with fungemia who are receiving TPN therapy with lipid supplementation.

15.124 Year 1—Week 41—Day 3

1. AZT-associated myopathy in HIV disease is lower than previously seen in the past due to lower dosing of the medication in current regimens.

2. Nucleoside reverse transcriptase inhibitors are associated with acute ascending neuropa-

thy and possible lactic acidosis. In this setting, the patient must be taken off the medication immediately.

3. Efavirenz is associated with CNS side effects such as insomnia and delirium.

4. Abacavir can lead to an acute hypersensitivity reaction marked by fevers, LAD, morbilliform rash, hepatitis, abdominal pain, and shortness of breath.

5. Paroxysmal nocturnal hemoglobinuria (PNH) is associated with defects in the RBC membrane at CD-55 and CD-59 and can lead to thrombosis of major vessels and of hemolytic anemia.

6. Thombotic thrombocytopenic purpura (TTP) is caused by antibodies to the metalloproteases of the von Willebrand factor (which do not allow the large multimers of VWF to be broken down).

7. HIV-associated myelopathy (vacuolar) may mimic B-12 deficiency.

8. Distal symmetrical polyneuropathy is probably the most common neurological manifestation of HIV disease and is highly associated as well with HIV antiretroviral drugs, such as DDI, DDC, and D4T.

9. Foscarnet can be used to treat CMV disease. It is associated with renal insufficiency and hypophosphatemia.

10. Cranial nerve palsy may be the presenting sign of tuberculosis. Treatment of CNS manifestations of tuberculosis includes corticosteroids in addition to antibiotics against tuberculosis.

15.125 Year 1—Week 42—Day 1

1. Epiphrenic esophageal diverticulum can be quite large such that it can mimic a lung abscess or a mass. Use a barium swallow to exclude this as a possibility.

2. CMV disease can cause an inflammatory demyelinating polyneuropathy in patients with advanced HIV disease (such that it can mimic Guillain-Barre syndrome).

3. Acute treatment of toxoplasmosis is with sulfa medication and pyrimethamine (use clindamycin instead of sulfa if there is an allergy to sulfa). Toxoplasmosis can involve the basal ganglia.

4. If a patient had a CD4 count above 200 for at least 6 months, then prophylaxis against Pneumocystis and toxoplasmosis can be discontinued.

5. Cryptococcal meningitis might lead to increased intracranial pressure more so than any other meningitis. Initial treatment is with amphotericin B (not the liposomal complex) and 5-flucytosine.

6. Hemiparesis, ataxia, seizures, cranial nerve palsies, and mental status changes can occur in patients with progressive multifocal leukoencephalopathy.

7. Atrial myxomas can cause distal emboli to brain and to the lower extremities.

8. The treatment for the vascular complications of Behcet's syndrome is chlorambucil.

9. Eruptive xanthomas can be seen with familial hypertriglyceridemia. Most patients with pancreatitis with this disorder have triglyceride levels above 1000 mg/dl.

10. Herpes gestationis is a blistering disorder of pregnancy marked by large bullae usually located around the umbilicus. The treatment is corticosteroids as no other immunosuppressive agent is safe to give during the pregnancy.

15.126 Year 1—Week 42—Day 2

1. Patients with hereditary spherocytosis are at risk of gallstones and many undergo cholecystectomies at a young age.

2. The osmotic fragility test is the way to test for hereditary spherocytosis.

3. White blood cell count and platelet count elevation usually accompanies elevated hemoglobin level in patients with polycythemia vera.

4. Of all the myeloproliferative disorders, essential thrombocytosis would be the most

likely to present with lack of splenomegaly (although splenomegaly is present in roughly half of patients with this disorder).

5. The first step in management in an active smoker with CAD and COPD is smoking cessation.

6. Be cognizant that gout may strike patients with myeloproliferative disorders (due to constant cell turnover).

7. Gastric carcinoids are associated with pernicious anemia.

8. Prolactinomas should have prolactin levels in excess of 200 mg/dl if they are above 1 cm in size.

9. Pheochromocytoma patients with hypercalcemia should be screened for hyperparathyroidism.

10. Males with UTIs should receive generally a minimum of 7 days duration of antibiotic therapy in most treatment cases.

15.127   Year 1—Week 42—Day 3

1. Patients with high titer rheumatoid factors who have rheumatoid arthritis are at risk for vasculitis, rheumatoid nodules, and rheumatoid lung disease.

2. Endocarditis can cause a positive rheumatoid factor titer.

3. Roth spot lesions can be seen with endocarditis and similar lesions can also be seen in patients with AML.

4. Behcet's disease is a rheumatological disorder marked by arthritis, pathergy, pulmonary artery aneurysms, genital ulcers, painful oral ulcers, and venous/arterial clots.

5. Pathergy refers to the phenomenon where one develops pustules at areas of trauma, such as venipuncture sites.

6. Sarcoidosis can present with acute parotid gland enlargement and with acute uveitis accompanied by fever (Heerfordt's disease).

7. Sarcoidosis can also present with ankle arthritis, erythema nodosum, and bilateral hilar lymphadenopathy (Lofgren's syndrome).

8. Consider tuberculosis unlikely as the cause of a pleural effusion if the mesothelial cell count exceeds 5% or if the pH of the pleural fluid exceeds 7.40 value.

9. Mesotheliomas spread commonly by direct growth rather than by hematogenous or lymphangitic spread.

10. Patients with asbestos exposure will usually have mid-lung zone pleural plaques and even calcified diaphragmatic plaques.

15.128   Year 1—Week 43—Day 1

1. Li-Fraumeni syndrome involves multiple carcinomas of the breast, brain, adrenal gland, sarcomas, laryngeal cancers, and leukemias and is due to tumor suppressor gene deletion on chromosome 17.

2. Gardner's syndrome can involve the ampulla of Vater with carcinoma, and it can also present with osteomas of the jaw and skull along with soft tissue tumors such as epidermal inclusion cysts.

3. Peutz-Jeghers syndrome patients (freckling of lips and oral mucosae as a feature) can present not only with hamartomas of the small bowel (most common) but also with colon adenocarcinoma.

4. Fluoroquinolones are associated with spontaneous tendon rupture in the elderly.

5. Bilateral plantar fasciitis and recurrent Achilles tendonitis in a young patient should trigger a workup for ankylosing spondylitis.

6. Dilantin and phenobarbital can raise the alkaline phosphatase level in the serum.

7. Acanthosis nigricans is a hallmark of insulin resistance.

8. Hemorrhage can occur into a long-standing pituitary adenoma and may cause retroorbital headache pain if it extends into the cavernous sinus. These patients are at risk for adrenal insufficiency and should receive immediate hydrocortisone IV and have an emergent neurosurgical evaluation.

9. A patient with myxedema coma must be given steroids first before thyroid replacement as Addison's disease can be associated

with hypothyroidism (as seen in polyglandular autoimmune type 2 syndrome).

10. Suppression of serum cortisol by a high-dose dexamethasone test rules out the pituitary gland as the cause of Cushing's syndrome.

15.129 Year 1—Week 43—Day 2

1. Nystagmus can be seen in patients with normal levels of dilantin (phenytoin). Nystagmus does not imply a toxicity state with this medication in all cases.
2. Atrial myxoma is the most common primary cardiac tumor.
3. Cytogenetics is the most important predictor of AML survival.
4. Minocycline can cause drug-induced lupus.
5. Sulfasalazine can help patients with arthritis from colitis.
6. Clozapine is helpful for psychosis in Huntington's patients.
7. Isosthenuria or the inability to concentrate or dilute urine occurs in acute tubular necrosis.
8. Beta-lactams can cause drug-induced hemolytic anemia.
9. Acute fatty liver and pre-eclampsia can cause schistocytes to be noted in peripheral smear testing of patients.
10. Evan's syndrome features idiopathic thrombocytopenia purpura combined with autoimmune hemolytic anemia.

15.130 Year 1—Week 43—Day 3

1. Cerebral infarction is the most common CNS manifestation of bacterial endocarditis.
2. 75% of cerebral infarcts in the setting of endocarditis involve the middle cerebral artery and its branches.
3. In general, valve replacement surgery is usually delayed for 10–14 days (if possible) after a cerebral infarction has occurred in the setting of endocarditis.

4. Ceftriaxone is the medication of choice in treating endocarditis caused by the HACEK group of organisms.
5. Cerebral angiography is indicated for patients with endocarditis who have evidence of a mycotic aneurysm (by clinical symptoms), a cranial nerve deficit, or subarachnoid hemorrhage.
6. Intussusception in adults is usually due to a solid lesion (such as a polyp or tumor) and thus evaluation for malignancy is always indicated.
7. Sigmoid volvulus most commonly occurs in the elderly population and it usually is not due to any anatomical lesion.
8. Small bowel volvulus is usually due to history of prior surgery causing the presence of adhesions.
9. Emphysematous cholecystitis is a surgical emergency.
10. Patients with porcelain gallbladders should have surgical removal as there is a significant chance of gallbladder adenocarcinoma.

15.131 Year 1—Week 44—Day 1

1. Patients with Churg-Strauss vasculitis will have adult-onset asthma, mononeuritis multiplex, and eosinophilia.
2. Patients with chronic eosinophilic pneumonia have no peripheral eosinophilia (the eosinophils are found on bronchoalveolar lavage) and the chest film looks exactly opposite of what you would see in congestive heart failure with sparing of the central areas and predominantly peripheral infiltrates.
3. There are cases of Churg-Strauss vasculitis reported as one starts a leukotriene-inhibitor and quickly tapers systemic steroid therapy.
4. Byssinosis is an interstitial lung disease brought about by exposure to cotton textile materials and presents with Monday chest tightness.

5. Berylliosis is a granulomatous disease that can cause hilar lymphadenopathy and upper lobe infiltration.
6. Asbestosis prefers the lower lobes for fibrosis, as opposed to silicosis which affects the upper lobes.
7. Lymphangioleiomyomatosis can lead to cystic lung disease in women.
8. Lymphangioleiomyomatosis can also lead to spontaneous pneumothorax and chylous pleural effusions.
9. Patients with hypothyroidism can present with pericardial effusion.
10. Patients with lupus can have lung manifestations to include interstitial pneumonitis, pleural effusions and "shrinking lung" syndrome.

15.132 Year 1—Week 44—Day 2

1. Creutzfeldt-Jacob disease patients have rapid mental decline and have startle myoclonus.
2. If a transplant patient is allergic to sulfa-based drugs, those patients will be desensitized to allow use of the medication.
3. All adrenal masses must be ruled out for pheochromocytoma before surgical removal ensues.
4. Adult polycystic kidney disease patients have a high incidence of hepatic cysts by age 50 (over half the patients will have this finding by that age).
5. Progressive cerebellar degeneration by mid-life is a hallmark of a prion disease known as Gerstmann-Straussler-Scheinker disease.
6. Kuru and fatal familial insomnia syndrome are two other prion diseases.
7. Workers in the aerospace industry are at risk of berylliosis which presents with hilar LAD and reticulonodular opacities.
8. Breast cancer is the most likely solid tumor malignancy to not present with weight loss.
9. Patients with the aspirin triad cannot be given any NSAIDs ideally for pain treatment (sal-

salate is the safest of COX-1 inhibitors if one must be used).
10. Patients with Lewy body disease present with impressive visual hallucinations early on in their dementia course.

15.133 Year 1—Week 44—Day 3

1. Granulomatosis with polyangiitis might present with hearing loss early in its course.
2. Syphilis can cause paroxysmal cold hemoglobinuria and the test of choice in this situation is Donath-Landsteiner antibodies.
3. The Miller-Fisher test of normal pressure hydrocephalus is to remove 30 ML of CSF and then see if there is gait improvement.
4. The Miller-Fisher variant of Guillain-Barre syndrome is ataxia, ophthalmoplegia, and ascending weakness.
5. A pontine infarct occurs in patients with hypertension and might leave the patient with small pinpoint pupils.
6. Cerebral amyloidosis should be thought about in patients with recurrent lobar hemorrhages in areas not classically affected by hypertension. MRI spin echograms are now used to look for footprints of amyloid, thus bypassing brain biopsy for diagnosis.
7. Dapsone is helpful for the pruritis associated with dermatitis herpetiformis.
8. Topical tretinoin is the advised step in treating a patient with acne with exclusively comedonal features.
9. Measure an IGF-2 level in patients suspected of having recurrent leiomyosarcoma who are presenting with hypoglycemia.
10. COPD is the comorbid disease most associated with atypical mycobacteria infections.

15.134 Year 1—Week 45—Day 1

1. Digibind is only to be used in digoxin toxicity when a patient faces a life-threatening arrythmia.

2. Digoxin levels are not reliable for nearly 2 weeks after a patient receives Digibind therapy.
3. Bidirectional ventricular bigeminy is a classic arrythmia seen in patients who have digoxin toxicity.
4. Aspirin irreversibly inhibits cyclooxygenase and causes platelet dysfunction in this manner.
5. Patients with markedly low platelet counts will have abnormal platelet function assay testing simply from the low number of platelets.
6. In general, do not place chest tubes for drainage in patients with chylothorax or hepatic hydrothorax.
7. Among the causes of chylothorax are Castleman's disease, histiocytosis X, and lymphangioleiomyomatosis.
8. Renal cell cancer patients can have a paraneoplastic process known as Stauffer's syndrome whereby they have transaminitis with no liver lesions noted.
9. DVT in nephrotic syndrome patients commonly occurs due to loss of antithrombin III in the urine.
10. Histoplasmosis will present with posterior mediastinitis and WBC inclusions, as well as a possible rash that resembles molluscum contagiosum.

15.135 Year 1—Week 45—Day 2

1. Metronidazole and piperacillin-tazobactam are agents that can be used to treat typhlitis which is also known as adult necrotizing enterocolitis.
2. *Clostridium septicum* and other gram-negative organisms need to be considered in patients with typhlitis.
3. Typhlitis has a greater than 50% chance of recurrence in patients with previous episode.

4. Xanthelasma is a feature that can be seen in patients with primary biliary cirrhosis.
5. The gold standard radiologic test to diagnose splenomegaly is a liver-spleen scan.
6. The gold standard test to diagnose gastroparesis is a nuclear medicine gastric scintigraphy scan.
7. Translocation of chromosomes 12, 21 and hyperdiploid state greater than 50 but less than 65 are favorable findings in patients with ALL.
8. In patients with diffuse alveolar damage, survivors of this state seem to have resolution of the fibrosis within 6 months.
9. Adult necrotizing enterocolitis is known commonly as typhlitis and can develop in patients with neutropenia usually greater than a week in duration.
10. Albendazole is used in long-term therapy in treating patients with *Echinococcus* infections (praziquantel is used only in the short term).

15.136 Year 1—Week 45—Day 3

1. Microscopic polyangiitis has pulmonary involvement and generally a very poor prognosis.
2. Post-capillary venulitis is the most common type of vasculitis.
3. Henoch-Schonlein purpura is an IG-A driven process that can cause hematuria, rash, and abdominal pain.
4. Mixed cryoglobulinemia is seen in patients with hepatitis B and hepatitis C, and it will have a positive rheumatoid factor seen.
5. Hypersensitivity vasculitis does not cause pain, whereas erythema nodosum (septal panniculitis) does cause pain.
6. Steroids are indicated in sarcoid if there is cardiac or neurological involvement, severe systemic disease (such as with uveitis and parotitis), hypercalcemia, lupus pernio, and nephrocalcinosis.

7. Urticarial vasculitis is associated with C1Q precipitin which is also associated with history of lung disease and cigarette smoking.

8. C-ANCA may be negative in patients presenting with only limited granulomatosis with polyangiitis (for example, only isolated sinusitis or laryngeal inflammation).

9. Methotrexate has been used as a steroid-sparing agent in patients with large vessel vasculitis.

10. Polyarteritis nodosum and Churg-Strauss vasculitis both could have P-ANCA positive directed toward myeloperoxidase.

15.137 Year 1—Week 46—Day 1

1. Indications for Digibind in digoxin toxicity are progressive bradyarrhythmias unresponsive to atropine and an overall serum digoxin level above 12–15 mg/dl.

2. Digoxin levels are best drawn 6–8 h after administration of last dose for best accurate levels.

3. The first symptoms of digoxin toxicity seem to be GI in nature (abdominal pain, nausea) rather than the yellow halo visual effects.

4. Lymphocytotoxic antibodies can be seen in TRALI (transfusion-related acute lung injury).

5. C3 and C5a levels may drop acutely in patients with TRALI.

6. Acute lupus myocarditis is treated with high-dose steroids (1 g daily initially). T-wave inversions may be the only finding on EKG.

7. Abnormal waveforms in the PTT may be seen in patients with sepsis.

8. Bacteria are at times noticed engulfed in macrophages and monocytes in patients with bacteremia.

9. Diastolic dysfunction CHF is most commonly due to long-standing hypertension.

10. Methyldopa may give a false positive Coombs test, and ironically it may also cause a true hemolytic anemia. Clinical correlation is recommended, as always.

15.138 Year 1—Week 46—Day 2

1. Hydralazine is recommended to be added to methyldopa when an adjunctive therapy is needed to control hypertension in a pregnant woman.

2. False negative skin testing may occur for 4–6 weeks after a severe local reaction or anaphylaxis from insect sting.

3. Glucagon drips may be needed when treating epinephrine-unresponsive anaphylaxis in patients on beta-blocker therapy.

4. Among the problems encountered in pregnancy include rhinitis and epulis (gingival hyperplasia due to hormones).

5. Most patients with severe local reaction to insect sting will not have anaphylaxis with next exposure to insect sting.

6. Follow sedimentation rate and C-reactive protein levels in patients you are treating for osteomyelitis.

7. The left parietal lobe near the angular gyrus is the most common location of the lesion causing Gerstmann syndrome.

8. Lateral medullary infarction involves the proximal inferior cerebellar artery at its most proximal occlusion site.

9. The medial medullary syndrome is due to infarction of the anterior spinal artery most commonly due to occlusion of the paramedian branches. It can also occur with occlusion of the vertebral artery or basilar artery.

10. Gabapentin is a very useful treatment for glossopharyngeal nerve dysfunction in relieving pain associated with this syndrome.

15.139 Year 1—Week 46—Day 3

1. Periosteal elevation on plain films can be seen late in the course of osteomyelitis in adults as opposed to children where it is seen early in the course of disease.

2. Mycoplasma can cause transverse myelitis, bullous myringitis, and cold agglutinin hemolytic anemia.
3. Chlamydia pneumonia infections are classically associated with hoarseness.
4. Patients with *Chlamydia psittaci* infections usually are quite ill on presentation.
5. Diffuse large B-cell lymphoma is the most common non-Hodgkin's lymphoma type to afflict adults.
6. Guttate psoriasis is worsened by acute streptococcal infections.
7. Pustular psoriasis usually worsens as a patient is being weaned from systemic steroids.
8. Small lymphocytic lymphoma is related to chronic lymphocytic leukemia (CLL). CD-23 is usually positive in these patients.
9. Erythroderma is seen in patients with psoriasis, cutaneous T-cell lymphoma when associated with Sezary syndrome, and pityriasis rubra pilaris.
10. Mantle cell lymphoma is CD5 positive and can be moderately aggressive in disease presentation with an expected 3-to-5-year median survival.

15.140 Year 1—Week 47—Day 1

1. Small frequent meals strategy is the first-line treatment of gastroparesis patients.
2. There is a risk of ischemic bowel in patients taking certain medications for gastroparesis.
3. Motility agents are used in patients with irritable bowel syndrome with constipation as predominant symptom.
4. Erythromycin will increase the risk of myositis in any HMG-Coa reductase inhibitor that works through the cytochrome P450-3A4 system.
5. Gardner's syndrome is associated with an increased risk of ampulla of Vater cancer that causes silvery colored stools.
6. Leser-Trelat sign is the rapid development of seborrheic keratosis over the back of an individual in a short period of time and is associated with GI malignancy.

7. Gastrin level is the screening test for Zollinger-Ellison (ZES) syndrome. Patients with gastrin levels between 200 and 1000 mg/dl can be stressed with a secretin stimulation test, and if the gastrin level paradoxically rises, then one should strongly suspect ZES.
8. Somatostatinomas are associated with gallstones, diarrhea, and diabetes mellitus.
9. Sulfonylurea ingestion will be associated with elevated C-peptide levels, whereas insulin exogenous administration will not be associated with elevated C-peptide levels.
10. Scarring alopecia and follicular plugging of the helix and antihelix areas of the ears are classic signs of discoid lupus.

15.141 Year 1—Week 47—Day 2

1. Dapsone can cause methemoglobinemia. Cimetidine is used in addition to methylene blue in these patients.
2. Vitamin C can help in refractory cases of methemoglobinemia.
3. Vitamin C and cranberry juice can help acidify the urine in patients with struvite infections.
4. Hemochromatosis should be thought in patients with osteoarthritis in unusual places.
5. Anatomical snuff-box pain without trauma in adults should have one thinking about De Quervain's tenosynovitis and carpometacarpal osteoarthritis.
6. Pseudogout loves to attack the wrists and knees bilaterally.
7. Hemochromatosis, hypomagnesemia, and hyperparathyroidism are among the states that can lead to pseudogout.
8. Among the fun learning cases of diseases that cause hypercalcemia are Addison's disease, Zollinger-Ellison syndrome, and familial benign hypocalciuric hypercalcemia.
9. Anterior thigh pain with concomitant paresthesia should have someone concerned about meralgia paresthetica, which is entrapment of the lateral femoral cutaneous nerve as it passes under the inguinal ligament.

10. Among the causes of sacroiliac (SI) joint pain besides ankylosing spondylitis are reactive arthritis and psoriasis.

15.142 Year 1—Week 47—Day 3

1. Polymyalgia rheumatica and scleroderma can both cause a symmetrical inflammatory arthritis.
2. Sine wave pattern QRS morphology can be seen in patients with severe hyperkalemia.
3. Sodium polystyrene sulfate decreases total body potassium stores.
4. High doses of sulfa-based medications such as used in treating *Pneumocystis jirovecii* infections can lead to hyperkalemia.
5. Broad, tall T-waves with normal potassium levels noted in a patient should raise concern for hyperacute MI.
6. Hypomagnesemia will worsen atrial arrhythmias.
7. Atovaquone can be used for patients for *P. jirovecci* prophylaxis who cannot tolerate sulfa drugs or dapsone.
8. Pentamidine can also be used for P. jirovecci prophylaxis in the situation described in Pearl #7. Side effects of this medication include drug-induced pancreatitis as well as hypo- or hyperglycemia.
9. Adrenal insufficiency, vitiligo, and hypothyroidism are all part of the polyglandular autoimmune syndrome, type 2.
10. Diffuse esophageal spasm can cause chest pain that responds to nitrates and causes a "corkscrew pattern" to barium swallow if obtained while the patient is symptomatic.

15.143 Year 1—Week 48—Day 1

1. Fomepizole can be used to treat methanol and ethylene glycol poisonings by its actions on alcohol dehydrogenase.
2. Patients with methanol poisoning can present with blindness from optic atrophy.
3. The key to recognizing poisonings from methanol and ethylene glycol will be an osmolar gap in the setting of a metabolic acidosis. These patients need to be started on fomepizole or ethanol drips urgently and may even need hemodialysis if they are critically ill.
4. Folic acid is added to the treatment of methanol poisoning.
5. Oxalate crystals may be seen in patients with ethylene glycol poisoning.
6. Patients with small cell lung cancer and lymphoma should be treated regardless of performance status with chemotherapy due to the high chemo-sensitive nature of these diseases.
7. Tamoxifen will worsen hot flashes, possibly lead to ocular toxicity, and increase the risk of DVT.
8. Sulfa and tetracycline are the two antibiotics most linked to fixed drug eruption.
9. Patients with EBV mononucleosis demonstrate a morbilliform exanthem when given ampicillin.
10. CMV is the likely cause for a mononucleosis-like picture in a patient with negative EBV testing.

15.144 Year 1—Week 48—Day 2

1. CLL is the most common hematological disorder associated with angioedema in the elderly.
2. Although ARBs may cause angioedema, it is through a different mechanism than ACE-inhibitors, thus it is felt to be safe to give an ARB to patients with previous angioedema from ACE-inhibitor.
3. Pulmonary alveolar proteinosis is treated with bronchoalveolar lavage bilaterally. This procedure will require anesthesiology assistance.
4. The anti-Jo antibody is positive in patients with polymyositis and interstitial lung disease.
5. The anti-Ro antibody may be seen positive in patients with subacute cutaneous lupus erythematosus.

6. Patients with pernicious anemia have an increased incidence of gastric carcinoid polyps.
7. Menetrier's disease is a state of extreme hypertrophy of the rugal folds of the stomach and it is associated with a higher risk of gastric adenocarcinoma.
8. Turcot's syndrome is felt to be the only one of the colon polyp syndromes which is inherited in autosomal recessive fashion.
9. Li-Fraumeni syndrome is associated with deletion of the tumor suppressor gene on chromosome 17 and thus one sees carcinomas of the larynx, leukemias, sarcomas, adrenal carcinomas, breast carcinoma, and brain carcinomas with this disorder.
10. Kallman's syndrome is hypogonadotropic hypogonadism associated with anosmia. Expect low LH and low testosterone levels.

15.145 Year 1—Week 48—Day 3

1. The initial treatment for all functional adenomas except prolactinoma is generally surgical removal.
2. Sauna takers lung is a hypersensitivity pneumonitis associated with *Aureobasidium* species.
3. Silo filler's lung is marked by acute shortness of breath upon exposure to nitrogen dioxide.
4. Dengue fever has a hemorrhagic variant that can lead to death when aggressive. Biggest risk factor for getting such variant is previous infection with any strain of dengue fever.
5. Monoamine oxidase inhibitors (MAO-I) are useful for the treatment of atypical depression (marked by hyperphagia, excess sleep, and other features).
6. Trimethaphan is a ganglionic-receptor blocker that has been used in the treatment of hypertension in patients with aortic dissection.
7. Screening tests are part of secondary prevention. Primary prevention would be vaccination services for instance.

8. Likelihood ratios are more likely to be used in cohort studies, whereas odds ratios are more likely to be used in case control studies.
9. A phrase to accurately describe specificity would be the following. "Of those people who don't have a disease, how many people would have a negative screening test."
10. The characteristics of a screening test are the following: (a) able to be applied to a large population, (b) cost-effective, (c) relatively painless, and (d) available to most of the population.

15.146 Year 1—Week 49—Day 1

1. Beta-blockers and diuretic therapy might increase VMA, metanephrine, and catecholamine levels so beware of getting these tests in patients on current dosing with these medications. Clonidine tends to decrease those levels and thus could be used while working up for pheochromocytoma.
2. Serum serotonin level and the urine 24-h HIAA level will be elevated in patients with carcinoid syndrome.
3. *Coxiella burnetii* is the causative agent for Q-fever which can present with pneumonia, endocarditis, or liver failure. Treat with doxycycline.
4. Jaccoud's arthritis, which is a nondeforming arthritis but which is marked by ulnar subluxation of the digits, is seen nowadays occasionally with SLE but was first described with rheumatic fever.
5. Even though the arthritis of lupus is nonerosive, it is an inflammatory arthritis.
6. Leflunomide is a pyrimidine inhibitor which has been used in the treatment of rheumatoid arthritis with side effects including LFT abnormalities and diarrhea.
7. *Streptococcus bovis* and *Clostridium septicum* bacteremia can be seen with endocarditis in the setting of colon carcinoma.
8. Porcelain gallbladder patients are at risk for gallbladder carcinoma and should have cholecystectomy.

9. NSAID use is one of the most common causes for lithium toxicity in the general population.
10. Hemodialysis is the treatment of choice for patients with severe lithium toxicity.

15.147 Year 1—Week 49—Day 2

1. Daptomycin, which exclusively covers gram-positive organisms, can cause a myositis so periodic CPK monitoring while on therapy is recommended.
2. Patients with Clostridium septicemia should be looked at for an underlying source, such as an occult abscess, colon carcinoma, or soft tissue infection.
3. The treatment of tropical sprue involves high-dose doxycycline until the megaloblastic anemia resolves and until symptoms of malabsorption abate (usually about 3–6 months). Folic acid replacement is needed at high dose of doxycycline.
4. Severe carditis and severe neurological symptoms of Lyme disease are treated with IV ceftriaxone.
5. Midodrine can cause hypertension when patients lie supine. Midodrine is used in patients with orthostatic hypotension who do not respond to mineralocorticoid therapy.
6. Iron studies must be checked in patients while they are undergoing erythropoietin therapy.
7. Patients with sickle cell anemia of the SS type should not have splenomegaly (as they infarct splenic tissue). Patients with sickle cell disease, SC variant (meaning sickle-hemoglobin C), can have splenomegaly.
8. Target cells are seen on peripheral smear in patients with beta-thalassemia trait and hemoglobin C disease.
9. Schistosoma haematobium infections can cause squamous cell carcinoma of the bladder.
10. Use red cell exchange transfusion in patients with sickle cell disease if priapism, chest pain syndrome, or CNS symptoms are present.

15.148 Year 1—Week 49—Day 3

1. Diabetes mellitus, liver disease, and renal insufficiency are all risk factors for development of Legionella infections.
2. Listeria infections are found in greater number in patients with leukemias, in pregnancy, and with liver disease. Treat Listeria with ampicillin as cephalosporins do not work. Use trimethoprim-sulfamethoxazole if penicillin allergic.
3. Steroid therapy will not work in patients with cold agglutinin disease.
4. Warm agglutinins can be seen in patients with HIV disease, SLE, inflammatory bowel disease, and in patients with Evan's syndrome (hemolytic anemia with spherocytes noted and with idiopathic thrombocytopenia purpura).
5. Mycoplasma and certain lymphoproliferative disorders can cause cold agglutinin disease.
6. Trimethylaminuria is an amino acid disorder that can be seen in young adults. Patients with this disorder smell like rotting fish.
7. Patients with isovaleric acidemia as an amino acid disorder will complain of excessive sweaty feet.
8. Danazol is an anabolic steroid that could be used in the treatment of warm autoimmune hemolytic anemias. It is also used in treating hereditary angioedema.
9. Splenectomy does not help in treating patients with cold agglutinin disease.
10. Splenectomy is helpful in managing patients with refractory cases of warm agglutinin disease and has even been tried in patients with recurrent thrombotic thrombocytopenia purpura (TTP).

15.149 Year 1—Week 50—Day 1

1. Smoking and asbestos exposure increases the risk for bronchogenic carcinoma exponentially.

2. Smoking does not increase the risk for malignant mesothelioma even in patients with heavy asbestos exposure.
3. A Horner's syndrome can be seen in patients with Wallenberg's syndrome (lateral medullary infarction) as well as in patients with Pancoast tumors (bronchogenic carcinomas) destroying the cervical sympathetic plexus.
4. Bronchioalveolar carcinoma can mimic pneumonia both clinically and radiographically.
5. Carcinoid syndrome is the second most common cause of ectopic ACTH syndrome.
6. von Hippel–Lindau syndrome is associated with pheochromocytoma and renal cell carcinoma.
7. Chronic hydronephrosis/vesicoureteral reflux can cause nephrotic syndrome with the predominant histology being focal segmental glomerulosclerosis.
8. There is a marked rise in the incidence of tuberculosis in patients who have silicosis.
9. A PPD needs to be checked on all patients before beginning therapy with TNF-alpha receptor blockers.
10. Back pain may be the initial presenting sign of patients with rhabdomyolysis. If your young patient with new onset low back pain has a social history that includes cocaine or IVDA, I would check a CPK level as part of his workup.

15.150 Year 1—Week 50—Day 2

1. Dysfunctional uterine bleeding in young females should raise the suspicion of von Willebrand's factor deficiency.
2. Type 2b von Willebrand's disease patients may present with thrombocytopenia.
3. First-line treatment of prolonged QT syndrome is beta-blocker therapy.
4. Prolonged ST-segment can be seen in patients with hypocalcemia, whereas a shortened segment is seen in hypercalcemia.
5. Hypocalcemia in the setting of previous thyroid surgery should raise the suspicion of damage or injury to the parathyroid glands.

6. Thiazide diuretics are used to treat calcium-based kidney stones as they lead to decrease calcium excretion.
7. Dilantin levels need to be corrected in the setting of a low albumin state.
8. Calcium replacement in the setting of hypokalemia and digoxin toxicity could actually worsen the digoxin toxicity; thus, all patients should be on monitored floor if calcium is planned to be given in this setting.
9. Gitelman's syndrome and Bartter's syndrome patients have normal blood pressure levels.
10. Amiloride is the first-line treatment of Lidle's syndrome, which mimics hyperaldosteronism except there are no detectable aldosterone levels in these patients.

15.151 Year 1—Week 50—Day 3

1. Clues to appendicitis on CT scan include fat stranding near the cecum and a bright density near the cecum which commonly represents an appendicolith.
2. Previous lymphangiograms can leave enlarged lymph nodes in patients for life. Previously treated lymphoma can look the same on CT scan as well.
3. Patients with bullous COPD disease are at risk for spontaneous pneumothorax.
4. It is prudent to check alpha-1-antitrypsin levels in patients with underlying COPD who are less than 50 years of age.
5. Acne rosacea is worsened the most by exposure to hot liquids as it causes a flushing reaction.
6. Sebaceous gland hyperplasia may be seen in the setting of acne rosacea.
7. Perioral dermatitis is a skin condition that mimics acne rosacea but is predominant in the skin near the oral area as its name implies. Treatment is best with doxycycline but this condition can flare during pregnancy at which time topical metronidazole may be the best option.
8. Delayed relaxation phase is a hallmark sign of hypothyroidism. Severe long-standing

hypothyroidism can also lead to hypertrophy of proximal musculature.

9. Pretibial myxedema is most commonly seen in the setting of hyperthyroidism.

10. If a patient notices ptosis and hoarseness that worsens as the day wears on, but improves after an overnight sleep, suspect myasthenia gravis.

15.152 Year 1—Week 51—Day 1

1. *Erysipelothrix rhusiopathiae* is the organism that causes erysipeloid and this condition will not respond to vancomycin therapy effectively.

2. Splenomegaly can be detected at times on a plain film of the abdomen.

3. Loss of a psoas shadow on a plain abdominal film should raise the suspicion of psoas abscess.

4. Persistent unilateral serous otitis media in a patient with smoking history should raise suspicion of a squamous cell carcinoma in the nasopharynx.

5. Collapse of a vertebral disc with compromised disc space on plain films of the back should raise suspicion for vertebral body osteomyelitis.

6. Chronic drug users who are "skin poppers" are at risk for amyloidosis.

7. Up to 10% of acute subarachnoid hemorrhage will be missed on a CT scan of the head.

8. Deep inverted T-waves can be seen in the setting of subarachnoid hemorrhage.

9. Cryptococcal infections can lead to chronic CSF pressure elevation as these organisms and their subsequent scarring/inflammation lead to blockage of CSF reabsorption in the arachnoid granulation area.

10. Cryptococcus can present as a primary infection of the lung with large lesions mimicking primary lung cancer or metastatic disease to lung.

15.153 Year 1—Week 51—Day 2

1. Late latent syphilis is generally treated with three rounds of benzathine penicillin G (each shot separated by 1 week's time).

2. The acromioclavicular joint is the most common joint injured in acute shoulder injuries.

3. Amantadine is helpful for the chronic fatigue syndrome of multiple sclerosis.

4. Lesions in the CNS in the setting of multiple sclerosis should occur in different parts of the CNS and at least 3 months apart if the disease is truly present (thus the term of a disease of "time and space").

5. An increased CSF IgG index and the presence of oligoclonal bands are not specific for multiple sclerosis.

6. Modafinil is a narcolepsy drug that has been used to treat patients with multiple sclerosis who do not respond to amantadine and have chronic fatigue syndrome.

7. Tolterodine has been used in patients with urge incontinence but should not be used in patients with glaucoma in past medical history.

8. Mitoxantrone has been used in the treatment of relapsing-remitting multiple sclerosis.

9. Human papillomavirus testing should be done if liquid-based cytology is being used in Pap Smear testing as it helps best guide decision making when trying to interpret Pap Smear results.

10. Women with high grade squamous intraepithelial neoplasia and grade 1 cervical intraepithelial neoplasia (CIN) have a 35% risk of developing grade 2–3 CIN.

15.154 Year 1—Week 51—Day 3

1. Most scientific recommendation bodies advocate for PSA testing for screening only if the patient's life expectancy exceeds 10 years and patient agrees to testing in shared decision making.

2. A prostate size greater than 40 g or a PSA level greater than 3 is usually recommended

to be present before using finasteride for treatment of BPH.

3. It will take 3–4 months for finasteride to begin to provide relief for symptoms of benign prostatic hyperplasia (BPH).

4. Nimodipine should be given for 21 days after subarachnoid hemorrhage in patients with this condition.

5. Recurrent *Neisseria meningitidis* infections should raise the suspicion of late complement deficiency (C5–9).

6. Tularemia and leishmaniasis are among the infections that can present with a sporotrichoid pattern infection.

7. Patients with *Ehrlichia* infections should have rapid defervescence once started on doxycycline, usually within 24–48 h.

8. It is essential in acute stroke patients to keep the temperature in the normal range and to keep blood sugar levels above 80 mg/dl.

9. Patients with premature ovarian failure will have elevated FSH values.

10. Hemochromatosis can cause infertility by both infiltrating the testes or by its effect on the pituitary gland.

15.155 Year 1—Week 52—Day 1

1. Nitrate therapy combined with hydralazine can provide additional benefit in treating patients with congestive heart failure (CHF).

2. Hydralazine can cause a reflex tachycardia and should always be avoided in patients with acute aortic dissection.

3. Procainamide and hydralazine are the two most common medications to cause drug-induced lupus. This is marked by positive anti-histone antibodies but remember the first step in workup is to get an ANA test.

4. Colchicine can cause bone marrow suppression, particularly in patients with underlying renal disease.

5. Anti-Jo-1 positive myositis states are marked by an increased risk for the development of interstitial fibrosis.

6. Most patients with esophageal cancer are staged with endoscopic ultrasound if feasibly possible.

7. Endoscopic ultrasound is as effective as CT and MRI in staging pancreatic cancer patients.

8. Chronic pancreatitis is a risk factor for subsequent development of pancreatic cancer.

9. Patients with essential thrombocytosis will get immediate relief from a state of burning and redness of the digits with aspirin.

10. Isolated gastric varices can be seen in cases of acute pancreatitis if thrombosis of the splenic vein occurs.

15.156 Year 1—Week 52—Day 2

1. Consider doing a subtotal IGG class enumeration in patients with normal immunoglobulin levels who get recurrent infections such as sinusitis and pneumonia. IGG2 is the most common subclass deficiency.

2. Recurrent otitis media in the adult should trigger a workup for a humoral deficiency.

3. T-cell and B-cell enumeration is helpful as well in working up patients with recurrent sinusitis and pneumonia.

4. To check to see if an immunoglobulin deficiency is significant, get pre-vaccination titers of pneumovax, tetanus, and diphtheria, and then give vaccine and get post-vaccination titer levels 4 weeks later to see if there is a significant response.

5. Among the causes of Guillain-Barre syndrome are *Campylobacter jejuni* infections and mycoplasma infections.

6. Mycoplasma infection can also lead to bullous myringitis, transverse myelitis, and erythema multiforme.

7. The most common cause of erythema multiforme in the general population is HSV 1 infection.

8. Think of an upper GI bleed in patients with a large discrepancy between BUN and creatinine with no clinical evidence of dehydration.

9. *Rhodococcus equi*, Nocardia, Tuberculosis, and *Staphylococcus aureus* are among the causes of cavitary lung disease.

10. Coccidiomycosis causes thin-walled cavitary lung disease in patients with exposure in the Southwest USA.

15.157 Year 1—Week 52—Day 3

1. Fluconazole and itraconazole will increase cyclosporine levels.
2. After discontinuation of systemic steroids, it is not unusual to see a flare of pustular psoriasis.
3. Middle aged to elderly men can get keratoacanthomas of the scrotum known as Fordyce spots. No treatment is needed.
4. There is an association between multiple dermatofibromas and systemic lupus erythematosus.
5. Granuloma annulare is a skin condition marked by annular grouped papules that usually appears in weight bearing areas (such as joints) and is seen with increased incidence in diabetes mellitus.
6. Hutchison's sign of melanoma involves the pigment of melanoma from the paronychial part spreading onto the nailfold.
7. Minocycline is the oral antibiotic most often used in patients who need treatment for acne.
8. Morphea is the term to use for localized scleroderma usually involving skin and subcutaneous tissue.
9. Necrobiosis lipoidica diabeticorum is a skin lesion found in the anterior shin of diabetics that does not respond to improved glycemic control (must use intralesional steroids for treatment).
10. Acanthosis nigricans is associated with acromegaly, diabetes mellitus, Cushing's syndrome, thyroid disorders, and polycystic ovarian disease.

Further Reading

Adrogue HJ, Madias NE. Hypernatremia. N Engl J Med. 2000;342(20):1493–9. https://doi.org/10.1056/NEJM200005183422006.

Anderson KE, Bloomer JR, Bonkovsky HL, Kushner JP, Pierach CA, Pimstone NR, Desnick RJ. Recommendations for the diagnosis and treatment of the acute porphyrias. Ann Intern Med. 2005;142(6):439–50. https://doi.org/10.7326/0003-4819-142-6-200503150-00010.

Aurigemma GP, Gaasch WH. Clinical practice. Diastolic heart failure. N Engl J Med. 2004;351(11):1097–105. https://doi.org/10.1056/NEJMcp022709.

Bornstein SR. Predisposing factors for adrenal insufficiency. N Engl J Med. 2009;360(22):2328–39. https://doi.org/10.1056/NEJMra0804635.

Bosch X, Poch E, Grau JM. Rhabdomyolysis and acute kidney injury. N Engl J Med. 2009;361(1):62–72. https://doi.org/10.1056/NEJMra0801327.

Boulton AJ, Kirsner RS, Vileikyte L. Clinical practice. Neuropathic diabetic foot ulcers. N Engl J Med. 2004;351(1):48–55. https://doi.org/10.1056/NEJMcp032966.

Braverman AC. Aortic dissection: prompt diagnosis and emergency treatment are critical. Cleve Clin J Med. 2011;78(10):685–96. https://doi.org/10.3949/ccjm.78a.11053.

Brodsky RA. Narrative review: paroxysmal nocturnal hemoglobinuria: the physiology of complement-related hemolytic anemia. Ann Intern Med. 2008;148(8):587–95. https://doi.org/10.7326/0003-4819-148-8-200804150-00003.

Brugge WR, Lauwers GY, Sahani D, Fernandez-del Castillo C, Warshaw AL. Cystic neoplasms of the pancreas. N Engl J Med. 2004;351(12):1218–26. https://doi.org/10.1056/NEJMra031623.

Camilleri M. Clinical practice. Diabetic gastroparesis. N Engl J Med. 2007;356(8):820–9. https://doi.org/10.1056/NEJMcp062614.

Danese S, Fiocchi C. Ulcerative colitis. N Engl J Med. 2011;365(18):1713–25. https://doi.org/10.1056/NEJMra1102942.

Delacretaz E. Clinical practice. Supraventricular tachycardia. N Engl J Med. 2006;354(10):1039–51. https://doi.org/10.1056/NEJMcp051145.

DeLoughery TG. Microcytic anemia. N Engl J Med. 2014;371(26):2537. https://doi.org/10.1056/NEJMc1413161.

Freeman WK, Gibbons RJ. Perioperative cardiovascular assessment of patients undergoing noncardiac surgery. Mayo Clin Proc. 2009;84(1):79–90. https://doi.org/10.1016/S0025-6196(11)60812-4.

Frohman EM, Wingerchuk DM. Clinical practice. Transverse myelitis. N Engl J Med. 2010;363(6):564–72. https://doi.org/10.1056/NEJMcp1001112.

George JN. Clinical practice. Thrombotic thrombocytopenic purpura. N Engl J Med. 2006;354(18):1927–35. https://doi.org/10.1056/NEJMcp053024.

Gines P, Schrier RW. Renal failure in cirrhosis. N Engl J Med. 2009;361(13):1279–90. https://doi.org/10.1056/NEJMra0809139.

Gollapudi RR, Teirstein PS, Stevenson DD, Simon RA. Aspirin sensitivity: implications for patients with coronary artery disease. JAMA. 2004;292(24):3017–23. https://doi.org/10.1001/jama.292.24.3017.

Grubb BP. Clinical practice. Neurocardiogenic syncope. N Engl J Med. 2005;352(10):1004–10. https://doi.org/10.1056/NEJMcp042601.

Gruchalla RS, Pirmohamed M. Clinical practice. Antibiotic allergy. N Engl J Med. 2006;354(6):601–9. https://doi.org/10.1056/NEJMcp043986.

Hotez PJ, Brooker S, Bethony JM, Bottazzi ME, Loukas A, Xiao S. Hookworm infection. N Engl J Med. 2004;351(8):799–807. https://doi.org/10.1056/NEJMra032492.

Irwin RS, Madison JM. The diagnosis and treatment of cough. N Engl J Med. 2000;343(23):1715–21. https://doi.org/10.1056/NEJM200012073432308.

Jacob JT, Mehta AK, Leonard MK. Acute forms of tuberculosis in adults. Am J Med. 2009;122(1):12–7. https://doi.org/10.1016/j.amjmed.2008.09.018.

Joshi N, Caputo GM, Weitekamp MR, Karchmer AW. Infections in patients with diabetes mellitus. N Engl J Med. 1999;341(25):1906–12. https://doi.org/10.1056/NEJM199912163412507.

Kaszala K, Huizar JF, Ellenbogen KA. Contemporary pacemakers: what the primary care physician needs to know. Mayo Clin Proc. 2008;83(10):1170–86. https://doi.org/10.4065/83.10.1170.

Kelkar PS, Li JT. Cephalosporin allergy. N Engl J Med. 2001;345(11):804–9. https://doi.org/10.1056/NEJMra993637.

Lazarus SC. Clinical practice. Emergency treatment of asthma. N Engl J Med. 2010;363(8):755–64. https://doi.org/10.1056/NEJMcp1003469.

Levine JS, Ahnen DJ. Clinical practice. Adenomatous polyps of the colon. N Engl J Med. 2006;355(24):2551–7. https://doi.org/10.1056/NEJMcp063038.

Lieberman DA. Clinical practice. Screening for colorectal cancer. N Engl J Med. 2009;361(12):1179–87. https://doi.org/10.1056/NEJMcp0902176.

Lien YH, Shapiro JI. Hyponatremia: clinical diagnosis and management. Am J Med. 2007;120(8):653–8. https://doi.org/10.1016/j.amjmed.2006.09.031.

Lucey MR, Mathurin P, Morgan TR. Alcoholic hepatitis. N Engl J Med. 2009;360(26):2758–69. https://doi.org/10.1056/NEJMra0805786.

Luzuriaga K, Sullivan JL. Infectious mononucleosis. N Engl J Med. 2010;362(21):1993–2000. https://doi.org/10.1056/NEJMcp1001116.

Mannucci PM. Treatment of von Willebrand's disease. N Engl J Med. 2004;351(7):683–94. https://doi.org/10.1056/NEJMra040403.

Marcocci C, Cetani F. Clinical practice. Primary hyperparathyroidism. N Engl J Med. 2011;365(25):2389–97. https://doi.org/10.1056/NEJMcp1106636.

McColl KE. Clinical practice. Helicobacter pylori infection. N Engl J Med. 2010;362(17):1597–604. https://doi.org/10.1056/NEJMcp1001110.

Mizgerd JP. Acute lower respiratory tract infection. N Engl J Med. 2008;358(7):716–27. https://doi.org/10.1056/NEJMra074111.

Musher DM, Musher BL. Contagious acute gastrointestinal infections. N Engl J Med. 2004;351(23):2417–27. https://doi.org/10.1056/NEJMra041837.

Park MA, Li JT. Diagnosis and management of penicillin allergy. Mayo Clin Proc. 2005;80(3):405–10. https://doi.org/10.4065/80.3.405.

Reddy KR, Schiff ER. Approach to a liver mass. Semin Liver Dis. 1993;13(4):423–35. https://doi.org/10.1055/s-2007-1007370.

Sahn SA, Heffner JE. Spontaneous pneumothorax. N Engl J Med. 2000;342(12):868–74. https://doi.org/10.1056/NEJM200003233421207.

Schlechte JA. Clinical practice. Prolactinoma. N Engl J Med. 2003;349(21):2035–41. https://doi.org/10.1056/NEJMcp025334.

Segal BH. Aspergillosis. N Engl J Med. 2009;360(18):1870–84. https://doi.org/10.1056/NEJMra0808853.

Skubitz KM, D'Adamo DR. Sarcoma. Mayo Clin Proc. 2007;82(11):1409–32. https://doi.org/10.4065/82.11.1409.

Spechler SJ. Barrett esophagus and risk of esophageal cancer: a clinical review. JAMA. 2013;310(6):627–36. https://doi.org/10.1001/jama.2013.226450.

Stewart AF. Clinical practice. Hypercalcemia associated with cancer. N Engl J Med. 2005;352(4):373–9. https://doi.org/10.1056/NEJMcp042806.

Tsokos GC. Systemic lupus erythematosus. N Engl J Med. 2011;365(22):2110–21. https://doi.org/10.1056/NEJMra1100359.

van de Beek D, de Gans J. Dexamethasone in adults with community-acquired bacterial meningitis. Drugs. 2006;66(4):415–27. https://doi.org/10.2165/00003495-200666040-00002.

Warner E. Clinical practice. Breast-cancer screening. N Engl J Med. 2011;365(11):1025–32. https://doi.org/10.1056/NEJMcp1101540.

Whyte MP. Clinical practice. Paget's disease of bone. N Engl J Med. 2006;355(6):593–600. https://doi.org/10.1056/NEJMcp060278.

Year 2: Internal Medicine Learning Using the "1,2,3 Methodology"

16

16.1 Introduction

As the "internal medicine" learner heads into year 2 of internal medicine residency, there is a usual equal balance between inpatient and outpatient rotations. Therefore, the pearls that are used in this section are an overall fairly equal blend of inpatient topics and outpatient topics within each specialty, as well as an increasing incidence of pearls involving traditional outpatient specialties such as rheumatology, endocrinology, and benign hematology. There is an intended repetition of some of the pearls topics of year 1 that bear refreshing in the very similar manner that the internal medicine learner using this book would be repeating the same specialty topic from Part I of this book during the same month of the year. This programmed repetition of facts will help increase familiarity with the difficult and challenging material of internal medicine for both clinical success on the wards and in the clinics, as well as in the classroom while taking standardized internal medicine questions.

16.2 Year 2—Week 1—Day 1

1. Patients with portal gastropathy causing recurrent bleeding should be considered for shunt placement therapy.
2. First-line treatment of patients with esophageal varices is beta-blocker therapy. Nitrates have proven to be a nice adjunct in a few studies.
3. Thyroglobulin is a useful tumor marker in patients with papillary and follicular thyroid cancer.
4. Papillary and follicular thyroid cancer like to metastasize to the lungs and bones.
5. Calcitonin is the test to order as a tumor serum marker in patients with medullary cancer of the thyroid.
6. Gonorrhea can cause a tenosynovitis when disseminated as well as hemorrhagic pustules usually found on the dorsum of the hand.
7. Turcot's syndrome is a colon polyp syndrome that is associated with brain tumors and is felt by most authorities to be inherited in an autosomal recessive fashion.
8. Baker's cysts can be seen in patients with rheumatoid arthritis and in patients with osteoarthritis.
9. Alopecia can occur in patients with autoimmune thyroid disease. It has also been associated with valproic acid use and with conditions such as discoid lupus.
10. Less than 50% of patients with serotonin syndrome will have actual rigidity although most will have myoclonus. Myoclonus is not the same as hemiballismus, which is the uncontrollable flinging of the arms that is seen with an infarct of the subthalamic nucleus of Luys.

J. Lezama, *Internal Medicine Learning A to Z and 1, 2, 3*, https://doi.org/10.1007/978-3-031-57546-4_16

16.3   Year 2—Week 1—Day 2

1. Megakaryocytic proliferation is felt to the cause of the fibrosis in chronic idiopathic myelofibrosis.
2. Nailfold capillaroscopy should be done in all patients with Raynaud's phenomenon.
3. Calcium channel blockers are first-line therapy for Raynaud's phenomenon. Alpha-blockers are second-line therapy.
4. Among the causes of male gynecomastia are aldactone therapy, Klinefelter's syndrome, and use of cimetidine.
5. Giardia lamblia infections are markedly increased in patients with IgA deficiency and common variable immunodeficiency.
6. Excessive chewing gum users can develop a chronic diarrhea from excess sorbitol due to the gum.
7. Presence of nasal polyposis in a patient with malabsorption from pancreatic insufficiency should lead one to suspect the diagnosis of cystic fibrosis.
8. Consider protein-losing enteropathy in patients with very low albumin levels who have no demonstratable proteinuria.
9. Patients with pure seminomatous testicular cancers should have AFP negative. 20% of them may have an elevated HCG level.
10. Monostotic Paget's disease most commonly involves the pelvis as the site of disease.

16.4   Year 2—Week 1—Day 3

1. Patients with all types of viral hepatitis (A, B, or C) are at risk of cryoglobulinemia.
2. Patients with essential mixed cryoglobulinemia with hepatitis C will have positive rheumatoid factors.
3. Rheumatoid factor can be seen with many disease states, including infections such as endocarditis.
4. High titers of rheumatoid factor in patients with rheumatoid arthritis are predictive of eventual formation of rheumatoid nodules, rheumatoid lung disease, and vasculitis.

5. Patients with polyarteritis nodosa (PAN) typically have sparing of the lungs in their disease process.
6. Patients with PAN will have positive hepatitis B surface antigen in approximately 35% of cases. The sural nerve is the preferred biopsy site in most cases.
7. Treatment of patients with eosinophilic folliculitis should include testing for underlying HIV disease.
8. Herpes gestationis is a blistering disorder of the skin that is seen during pregnancy.
9. The preferred initial agent to treat hypertension in pregnancy is alpha-methyldopa.
10. Hydralazine can be added as an adjunct hypertensive agent to pregnant women who are not completely responding to alpha-methyldopa.

16.5   Year 2—Week 2—Day 1

1. Hepatitis B is more transmissible in a needle-stick situation than is hepatitis C or HIV.
2. A patient who is a smoker and has a positive low anterior cervical lymph node or a supraclavicular node needs a CXR as the next step in management (before lymph node biopsy).
3. Post-tussive rales heard best in the supraclavicular area with the bell is the classic auscultatory sign with active tuberculosis.
4. Most cases of fever of unknown origin declare themselves in the next 2 years from initial start of symptoms. One strong entity to always consider is Hodgkin's disease, and one should consider CT scan of thorax even when CXR is unremarkable.
5. Consider going to CT scan of chest even with normal CXR if there is recurrence of an elevated thyroglobulin in a patient with history of follicular or papillary thyroid cancer.
6. Systemic fibrinolysis can be seen in patients with acute pancreatitis.
7. Argatroban is a direct thrombin inhibitor that will artificially increase INR to a higher level than expected for a given dose of coumadin. Continue argatroban until INR level is at least 4.0 when using argatroban.

8. Lepirudin and hirudin are options for anticoagulation in patients with HIT.
9. Antibodies are not usually necessary to diagnose HIT (heparin-induced thrombocytopenia) as the platelet count drop is so dramatic that the diagnosis becomes evident easily.
10. Patients with HIT can get arterial clots (known as white clot syndrome).

16.6   Year 2—Week 2—Day 2

1. Parvovirus B19 infection can cause an aplastic crisis in patients with sickle cell disease.
2. Red cell exchange transfusions should be used in sickle cell disease when acute chest pain syndrome, acute neurological syndrome, or priapism is present.
3. Trazadone causes priapism at a rate of about 1 in 5000 patients.
4. Consider hypercapnea (so get ABG) as a cause of mental status changes in a patient with COPD.
5. Patients receiving oxybutynin can have mental status changes due to the anticholinergic properties of the drug.
6. Mirtazapine can also have anticholinergic properties and has been noted to cause weight gain in patients.
7. MAO-inhibitors have still been used in selected cases of atypical depression. One must avoid use of meperidine in these patients.
8. The most common reason for an acute crisis within 30 min of a platelet transfusion is bacterial contamination of products as platelets are stored at room temperature.
9. FFP can cause anaphylaxis so if a patient develops urticaria and wheezing during transfusion, then stop transfusion immediately and give epinephrine.
10. Multiparous women are at risk for febrile non-hemolytic transfusion reactions due to the presence of multiple alloantibodies.

16.7   Year 2—Week 2—Day 3

1. Patients with myelodysplasia will have characteristic findings on peripheral smear such as hypolobulated and hypogranular WBCs and WBCs with pseudo-Pelger-Huet anomaly.
2. Sulfamethoxazole-trimethoprim is an antibiotic that has been associated with drug-induced suppression of bone marrow.
3. Patients with factor 12 deficiency will not bleed. They will have a prolongation of the PTT that will correct with a mixing study.
4. Imatinib mesylate is the first-line treatment of patients with CML.
5. Type O is the universal donor for RBCs. Type AB is the universal donor for FFP.
6. Plasmapheresis is performed with fresh frozen plasma. In fact, if plasmapheresis was unavailable to start treatment of TTP, you could start treatment by giving FFP.
7. Both myelofibrosis and hairy cell leukemia can cause a "dry" tap. The clue will be leukocytosis usually with myelofibrosis, whereas leukopenia with hairy cell leukemia.
8. Treat hairy cell leukemia with 2-chlorodeoxyadenosine (CDA).
9. The prognosis for treated hairy cell leukemia is very good one given effective treatment regimen available.
10. Washed RBCs and platelets should be used for patients with IGA deficiency requiring transfusion.

16.8   Year 2—Week 3—Day 1

1. CMV can be associated with a host of problems in HIV disease including colitis, esophagitis, and even cauda equina syndrome.
2. Foscarnet should be used in CMV patients who are ganciclovir-refractory and is associated with side effects of hypophosphatemia and renal insufficiency.

3. Fleets enema repeated administration could cause hyperphosphatemia.
4. Repeated doses of magnesium citrate for constipation should be avoided in patients with renal failure as they can develop hypermagnesemia.
5. Focal segmental glomerulosclerosis can lead to nephrotic syndrome in patients with Fabry disease, morbid obesity, chronic heroin use, and chronic vesicoureteral reflux.
6. Cryptococcus can mimic lesions of molluscum contagiosum in patients with HIV disease (central umbilicated papules).
7. HIV itself can cause an eosinophilia due to aberration of ratio of T-helper subset 2 cells compared to T-helper subset 1 cells.
8. Suspect *Pneumocystis jirovecii* pneumonia in patients with spontaneous pneumothorax and diffuse infiltrates on chest film.
9. Pentamidine can lead to side effects of hyperglycemia, hypoglycemia, and pancreatitis.
10. Suspect atrial flutter in all patients with a heart rate of 150 until proven otherwise. Sometimes the flutter waves are upright rather than saw-tooth (this is known as atypical atrial flutter).

16.9   Year 2—Week 3—Day 2

1. Acute aortic dissection can lead to a diastolic decrescendo murmur that is best heard over the right sternal border.
2. Aortic regurgitation, mitral valve prolapse, and acute aortic dissection are among the cardiac manifestations of Marfan's syndrome.
3. Disopyramide has strong anticholinergic properties and should be avoided in patients with urinary retention issues and in patients with acute delirium.
4. Atrial tachycardias can be associated with increased nocturia due to release of atrial natriuretic peptide.

5. Patients with amyloidosis of heart theoretically are at increased risk of digoxin toxicity.
6. Always suspect digoxin toxicity in patients with long-standing chronic atrial fibrillation who present acutely ill with regular rhythms on auscultation and EKGs.
7. Brugada syndrome is demonstrated on EKG with a RBB pattern with chronic ST-segment elevation in leads V1, V2, and V3. This syndrome has been associated with risk of sudden death and has even been noted in a case study in a patient using cocaine on a chronic basis.
8. Sneddon syndrome is manifested by livedo reticularis with history of multiple cerebral ischemic insults.
9. Dapsone is the first-line agent for treating leprosy.
10. Dapsone may also be used in hemolytic anemias as an adjunct to prednisone. It has also been used to reduce sphingomyelinase toxin in patients with brown recluse spider bite but the efficacy of this indication is greatest within 48 h of the bite.

16.10   Year 2—Week 3—Day 3

1. Among the causes of nodular lymphangitis are sporotrichosis, *Nocardia braziliensis*, and *Mycobacterium marinum*.
2. Itraconazole is the first-line treatment of patients with Sporotrichosis. Beware of QT interval prolongation.
3. Isoniazid will not be effective in treating Mycobacterium marinum infections (usually need clarithromycin plus rifabutin and may be even ethambutol).
4. Bullous pemphigoid is a condition marked by tense bullae, usually arising in the elderly, with no paraneoplastic association.
5. Pemphigus vulgaris does have paraneoplastic association, particularly to ovarian cancer in females.

6. Among the causes of carpal tunnel syndrome are amyloidosis, hypothyroidism, multiple myeloma, acromegaly, pregnancy, and rheumatoid arthritis.

7. Consider first carpometacarpal osteoarthritis and De Quervain's tenosynovitis in patients presenting with pain at the anatomical snuffbox.

8. Fever must be present before diagnosing a patient with thyroid storm.

9. Hydatidiform mole must be considered in pregnant women presenting with clinical signs of pre-eclampsia in the first trimester of pregnancy.

10. Gilbert syndrome is the most common cause of an unconjugated bilirubin increase in the general population.

16.11   Year 2—Week 4—Day 1

1. Antimitochondrial antibodies will be positive in over 95% of patients with primary biliary cirrhosis.

2. Patients with primary biliary cirrhosis can develop xanthelasma even in the absence of abnormal lipid panels.

3. Ursodeoxycholic acid is the treatment of patients with primary biliary cirrhosis.

4. Budd-Chiari syndrome is associated with acute abdominal pain with the rapid development of ascites. The syndrome is marked by thrombosis of the hepatic vein.

5. Collagenous colitis should be considered in elderly patients with diarrhea and biopsy shows increased lymphocytes in the lamina propria.

6. Beware of toxic megacolon in patients with known *C. difficile* colitis who begin to develop a distended abdomen.

7. First-line treatment of autoimmune hepatitis is corticosteroid therapy.

8. Presence of *Streptococcus bovis* or *Clostridium septicum* endocarditis or bacteremia should lead to a colonoscopy as the next step in management due to high association with colon cancer.

9. Systemic mastocytosis can lead to a leukemia-like state with mast cells in the bone marrow. These patients will have flushing similar to carcinoid tumors.

10. Sandostatin is the preferred treatment of patients with pure carcinoid tumor.

16.12   Year 2—Week 4—Day 2

1. Patients with ascites due to right heart failure will have a total protein greater than 2.5 mg/dl and have a SAAG (serum albumin to ascites gradient) greater than 1.1 value.

2. Among the causes of microangiopathic hemolytic anemia are DIC, HUS, malignant hypertension, HELLP syndrome, and acute fatty liver of pregnancy.

3. The treatment for HELLP syndrome and acute fatty liver of pregnancy is urgent delivery of fetus.

4. A normal C4 level precludes hereditary angioedema as the cause of a patient's angioedema.

5. Danazol is an anabolic steroid that is used in the treatment of hereditary angioedema and has also been used in the treatment of ITP that is refractory to steroids.

6. Patients with multiple myeloma will have negative bone scans.

7. Patients with osteoblastic lesions will have positive bone scans.

8. Among the tumors causing osteoblastic lesions are prostate cancer, renal cancer, breast cancer, thyroid cancer, and lung cancer.

9. The calcitonin level is elevated in patients with medullary cancer of the thyroid. Be wary of the presence of occult pheochromocytoma in these patients.

10. Anaplastic variant of thyroid cancer is the most aggressive of all the thyroid tumors. Lymphoma is a cause of thyroid cancer in the elderly as well.

16.13 Year 2—Week 4—Day 3

1. Among the physiological changes in the elderly are increased half-life of lipophilic drugs (such as benzodiazepines), decreased liver blood flow and decreased reductive/hydroxylation/oxidative/demethylation metabolism ("phase 1 reactions") by the liver, and decreased renal blood flow, tubular function, renal mass, and GFR.
2. Phase 2 liver metabolic reactions of glucuronidation, acetylation, and sulfation remain unchanged in activity in elderly patients.
3. "Fleet" enemas are notorious for sometimes creating a state of hyperphosphatemia.
4. Antacid abuse in an elderly patient with diarrhea, and it is usually associated with the magnesium antacids. There are also certain laxatives that can cause hypermagnesemia with abuse, along with melanosis coli (darkening of the colon) if they contain an anthracene derivative. Fixed drug eruptions are not uncommon in elderly patients using laxatives with phenolphthalein.
5. Antacid abuse with aluminum containing compounds is associated with constipation.
6. Warfarin is a drug that is metabolized by phase 1 metabolism by liver and thus lower doses are generally needed in the elderly.
7. Beta-blockers are notorious for causing nightmares in the elderly population.
8. There is decreased gastric acidity and increased gastric emptying time in the elderly.
9. Use of cimetidine is associated with the development of gynecomastia. Aldactone (spironolactone) can cause both gynecomastia and breast tenderness.
10. Depression in elderly patients can present with psychosis. New-onset schizophrenia is rare in the elderly. Electroconvulsive therapy (ECT) works well in patients with depression with psychotic features.

16.14 Year 2—Week 5—Day 1

1. A patient with acute right-sided upper and lower extremity weakness should have stat MRI looking for epidural abscess or hematoma that may require stat laminectomy and drainage by neurosurgery.
2. Acute rheumatic fever is associated with carditis, arthritis, erythema marginatum, subcutaneous nodules, and fever.
3. Serratia marcescens infections may cause reddish pigmentation of sputum that resembles hemoptysis.
4. Potts puffy tumor describes frontal bone osteomyelitis which may arise as a complication of sinusitis.
5. Friedlander bacillus is another name for *Klebsiella pneumonia*, which has an increased incidence in nursing home patients.
6. Patients with tuberculosis who have aggressive pericarditis need glucocorticoid therapy along with treatment with antibiotics
7. Patients with cranial nerve palsies due to diabetes mellitus will have sparing of pupillary function.
8. Transverse myelitis is usually associated with multiple sclerosis but it can be seen in patients status post-hepatitis B vaccination, lupus, and other selected post-infectious states.
9. Inclusion body myositis presents with distal muscle weakness as well as proximal muscle weakness and responds poorly to anti-inflammatory treatment.
10. Never forget to give thiamine to a patient with nystagmus, gait difficulty, cranial nerve palsy, and disorientation as they may have Wernicke's syndrome.

16.15 Year 2—Week 5—Day 2

1. Patients with normal pressure hydrocephalus may present with lower extremity Parkinsonism signs.
2. Metoclopramide may induce a Parkinson's disease-like state.

3. Pseudotumor cerebri may be caused by vitamin A, corticosteroid therapy, and tetracycline.
4. Tetracycline use may cause drug-induced pancreatitis.
5. Many patients with high triglyceride levels will also have low HDL levels. Diabetic patients requiring insulin may see an improvement in triglyceride levels simply from the initiation of insulin as it is a cofactor for lipoprotein lipase.
6. Bronchitis is the most common cause of hemoptysis in the general population.
7. Bronchiectasis is the second most common cause of hemoptysis in the general population.
8. HIV disease, amyloidosis, and lymphoma are among the few causes of acute renal failure associated with large kidneys on imaging.
9. Enthesopathy is the term used to describe inflammation at the site where a tendon attaches to bone.
10. Plantar fasciitis is best treated with rest and NSAID therapy. It is the most common cause of heel pain in the general population.

16.16 Year 2—Week 5—Day 3

1. The finding of hypertension in a young female patient with vascular bruits should raise the suspicion of Takayasu's arteritis.
2. Takayasu's arteritis and temporal arteritis are large vessel vasculitis that need treatment with prednisone at 1 mg/kg daily.
3. Calcinosis cutis can be seen with scleroderma and CREST syndrome patients.
4. Pulmonary hypertension can be seen in patients with CREST syndrome.
5. The anti-centromere antibody is positive in CREST syndrome, whereas the anti-SCL-70 or anti-topoisomerase antibody is positive in patients with diffuse scleroderma.
6. Bilateral adrenal gland enlargement in a patient with lung cancer should raise the suspicion of metastatic lung cancer disease.
7. Lead poisoning can lead to a microcytic anemia with hyperuricemia and abdominal pain.

8. Patients with necrotizing fasciitis need surgical debridement immediately. If streptococcus is the suspected pathogen, add clindamycin to the treatment regimen to bind the strep toxin.
9. Patients with polycythemia vera will present with itching after taking hot showers. They will have splenomegaly on exam.
10. Aspirin is safe to give to patients with essential thrombocytosis and polycythemia vera as long as there is not an occult iron deficiency anemia that has not been worked up yet.

16.17 Year 2—Week 6—Day 1

1. Hemochromatosis can cause male infertility both through primary hypogonadism and through pituitary dysfunction.
2. Sulfadiazine can cause male infertility, usually through oligospermia.
3. Sperm banking should be considered in patients with testicular cancer who are planning to receive bleomycin, cisplatinum, and etoposide.
4. Bleomycin can cause Raynaud's phenomenon, sclerodactyly, and pulmonary fibrosis.
5. Etoposide could lead to a secondary leukemia, most commonly AML that can be very refractory to treatment.
6. Fludarabine is usually used as single agent therapy for patients with aggressive CLL.
7. There is a hemolytic anemia associated with CLL that can be treated simply with steroids without having to use fludarabine.
8. Wilson's disease needs to be ruled out in all young patients with liver failure, especially if there are neurological or psychiatric comorbid diseases present.
9. Treatment of dilantin hypersensitivity is to acutely stop dilantin and start corticosteroid therapy.
10. Prolactinoma is the only functioning pituitary tumor that does not get treated by surgery (treat with bromocriptine or other dopamine agonist receptor therapy).

16.18 Year 2—Week 6—Day 2

1. Patients with type 2 diabetes mellitus may have anemia due to erythropoietin deficiency even with normal renal function.
2. A celiac sprue panel in patients with iron deficiency anemia and no occult blood loss to explain the state.
3. Ceftriaxone needs to be used in treating Lyme disease when there is severe carditis and when there are severe neurological symptoms (otherwise use doxycycline or amoxicillin if allergic to doxy).
4. West-Nile virus needs to be considered in patients with flu-like illness with weakness pattern resembling poliomyelitis. A high protein value will be obtained in CSF analysis.
5. Recombinant factor VIIa can be used in treating patients with factor 8 inhibitor.
6. Diabetes mellitus patients seem at higher risk of rhabdomyolysis if taking both fibrate therapy and HMG-CoA reductase (statin) therapy than the general population.
7. Caution needs to be used with thyroid replacement in the elderly as over-correction may lead to atrial fibrillation and osteoporosis.
8. The diagnosis of benign follicular adenoma versus follicular carcinoma in the pathology specimens of patients with a follicular thyroid abnormality can be challenging such that further molecular methods should be used to distinguish between the two entities.
9. Among the coronary artery pathological findings in patients with sudden death at a young age are anomalous coronary artery, atherosclerotic CAD, coronary artery hypoplasia, coronary aneurysm, intramyocardial coronary bridge, and coronary dissection.
10. Other causes of cardiac sudden death in young adults include bicuspid aortic stenosis, embolic myocardial infarction, and various cardiomyopathy states.

16.19 Year 2—Week 6—Day 3

1. Acrodermatitis enteropathica is the acral rash associated with zinc deficiency. Consider this in patients with poor nutrition or chronic alcoholism.
2. Non-small cell lung cancer is the neoplasm associated with hypertrophic pulmonary osteoarthropathy.
3. Ectopic ACTH syndrome, subacute cerebellar degeneration, limbic encephalitis, and Lambert-Eaton syndrome are among the paraneoplastic processes associated with small cell lung carcinoma.
4. Nearly 90% of both adrenal glands must be destroyed by tumor before adrenal insufficiency will develop.
5. Consider adrenal hemorrhage as a possible cause of adrenal insufficiency in patients taking coumadin.
6. Hypertriglyceridemia is the most common lipid abnormality in patients with chronic renal failure.
7. Arsenic has been used in refractory cases of AML and its main side effect is QT interval prolongation.
8. Normal septal depolarization is noted on an EKG by a small Q-wave in lead V6 and loss of this Q-wave might imply an old septal infarct.
9. Folinic acid therapy needs to be given to patients in treating methanol toxicity.
10. The urine chloride level is the most reliable test to get in patients with metabolic alkalosis to see if there will be a response to normal saline.

16.20 Year 2—Week 7—Day 1

1. The osmotic fragility test should be ordered in patients suspected to have hereditary spherocytosis.
2. Minimal change disease histology causing nephrotic syndrome in adults can be seen in patients with HIV involvement of the kidney and in those patients with Hodgkin's disease.

3. Only 20% of carcinoid syndrome patients will present initially with isolated cardiac valvular abnormalities.

4. Uncal herniation usually presents with a unilateral dilated pupil. Bilateral small pupils in a patient with hypertension should raise suspicion for a pontine infarct.

5. Paroxysmal nocturnal dyspnea is typically absent in patients with underlying shortness of breath who are afflicted with constrictive pericarditis.

6. Short metacarpals is the classic physical finding in patients with pseudopseudohypoparathyroidism   and pseudohypoparathyroidism.

7. Dilation and segmentation of retinal veins may be seen on fundoscopic exam of patients with Waldenstrom's macroglobulinemia.

8. Delayed relaxation of the left ventricle may be seen in patients with severe hypothyroidism.

9. Aspergillus and Fusarium are fungal diseases that can present on microscopic exam with acute angle branching hyphae. Fusarium can present with acute infection in the toenail spaces in immunocompromised patients.

10. Right atrial infarction and acute pericarditis can lead to a depression of the PR segment.

16.21   Year 2—Week 7—Day 2

1. Sterile pyuria is the most common genitourinary finding in patients having tuberculosis afflicting the GU tract.

2. Pyrazinamide is the most common anti-tuberculous drug to lead to drug-induced gout.

3. Levofloxacin at doses of 1000 mg/day are used for anti-tuberculous activity.

4. A pleural fluid sample that has 5% or more mesothelial cells is unlikely to be caused by tuberculosis. The pH of the sample is also almost always less than 7.4 in patients with tuberculous effusion.

5. Post-CABG patients can develop large effusions after their procedures which are exudative and may take months to resolve.

6. Poxvirus is the causative agent of molluscum contagiosum.

7. Of all the rheumatological diseases, systemic sclerosis is the one most linked to colonic pseudo-obstruction.

8. HLA-DR4 is the most common HLA type associated with severe, destructive rheumatoid arthritis.

9. Griseofulvin can still be used effectively to treat tinea capitis.

10. The JC virus is the cause of progressive multifocal leukoencephalopathy.

16.22   Year 2—Week 7—Day 3

1. Wedge-shaped appearing "infiltrates" on chest X-rays might actually represent lung infarction in the setting of pulmonary emboli.

2. Posterior myocardial infarctions demonstrate with various findings such as tall R-wave in lead V1 or significant ST-segment depression along leads V1–V2.

3. Afterload reduction is crucial in the treatment of aortic insufficiency and mitral regurgitation.

4. Heart rate control is crucial in treating patients with mitral stenosis and when these patients go into tachycardia, they are at risk of pulmonary edema.

5. When patients with aortic stenosis become symptomatic, then they should have surgical valve replacement.

6. Lactic acid levels and LDH levels may be normal in patients with ischemic and necrotic bowel.

7. Suspect mesenteric ischemia when there is focal small bowel dilation on plain X-rays with little or no abnormalities of the large intestine.

8. Patients with new onset left bundle branch block and chest pain should be treated as are those patients with ST-segment elevation as far as doing a careful assessment as far as the need for acute cardiology intervention.

9. Patients on steroids and morphine for pain control may not manifest abdominal pain in the setting of visceral perforation.
10. *Enterobius vermicularis* is the parasite that most commonly affects the appendix in humans in North America and may lead to acute appendicitis.

16.23 Year 2—Week 8—Day 1

1. Theophylline is notorious for leading to atrial arrythmias even in the setting of normal levels.
2. Look out for interaction between the fluoroquinolones and theophylline, with ciprofloxacin the one most indicated in the literature.
3. Ciprofloxacin does not provide useful coverage of *Streptococcus pneumoniae* infections.
4. Nitrofurantoin has been associated with causing pulmonary interstitial fibrosis.
5. Terbutaline has been associated with causing pulmonary edema (known as tocolytic-induced pulmonary edema).
6. All-trans retinoic acid may lead to pulmonary infiltrates which are transient and usually resolve with discontinuing the drug for a short period of time. NSAIDs and steroids have been used for treatment of acute symptoms but literature is not convincing on use of either of them in this setting.
7. Arsenic is one of the treatments if standard therapy fails that can be used for the treatment of acute myelogenous leukemia.
8. Valproic acid is the anti-epileptic agent most associated with drug-induced alopecia among members of its class.
9. Patients with niacin deficiency (pellagra) can get a rash along the V-area of their neck (sunlight driven) known as Casal's necklace.
10. Corkscrew hairs and perifollicular hemorrhages are hallmark signs of scurvy or vitamin C deficiency.

16.24 Year 2—Week 8—Day 2

1. Herpes zoster infections that involve a lesion at the tip of the nose should be investigated further for ophthalmological involvement (the lesion at the tip of the nose is called Hutchison's sign).
2. Steroids and acyclovir are commonly used in treatment of Bell's palsy.
3. Painless 3rd nerve cranial palsy patients should be worked up for diabetes mellitus.
4. Insulin resistance seems to be the mechanism for the disease process of acanthosis nigricans and polycystic ovarian disease.
5. Side effects of lithium include hypercalcemia, nephrogenic diabetes insipidus, and hypercalcemia.
6. A couple of OTC (over the counter) warnings are included in the following: (a) do not use dextromethorphan for cough suppression in patients with SSRI as serotonin syndrome may ensue and (b) beware of using NSAIDs in patients with lithium on board as lithium toxicity may ensue.
7. Consider CT scan or MRI scan of head in patients with nausea and vomiting with negative GI workup and negative metabolic workup.
8. Consider infection, cancer, and iron deficiency anemias as probable causes of patients with continued thrombocytosis as outpatients.
9. Yellow-orange discoloration of the creases of the palm of the hand signifies type 3 hyperlipoproteinemia and the finding is known as Palmar striated xanthomas.
10. The most common cause of hypercalcemia in outpatient population is hyperparathyroidism.

16.25 Year 2—Week 8—Day 3

1. Patients with porphyria cutanea tarda can have Wood's lamp fluorescence of their gums due to deposition of the porphyrins in that location.

2. Consider acute intermittent porphyria in patients with histories of acute abdomen episodes with no organic cause found. One should order 24-h porphyrin studies in these patients.
3. Three disease states to remember as possibly causing transudative pleural effusions include pulmonary embolus, hepatic hydrothorax, and hypothyroidism.
4. Erythema ab igne is a rash that may appear in patients using chronic heating pads.
5. Livedo reticularis rash is seen in patients with antiphospholipid antibody syndrome, other rheumatological diseases like R.A., parvovirus infections, and cholesterol emboli syndrome.
6. Cholesterol emboli syndrome can occur within one week of initiation of coumadin or direct thrombin inhibitor therapy.
7. Dexamethasone should be employed in the treatment regimen of patients with high-altitude cerebral edema.
8. Calcium channel blockers can be used in the treatment of high-altitude pulmonary edema as they help bring down pulmonary artery pressures.
9. High resting pulmonary artery pressures might be associated with tricuspid regurgitation on an echocardiogram and tall R-waves in lead V1 on an EKG.
10. The ELISA D-dimer's greatest value is in its negative predictive value for deep venous thrombosis/pulmonary emboli.

16.26 Year 2—Week 9—Day 1

1. The strongest evidence for gout or pseudogout is to not only see the classic crystals but also to see them embedded in a neutrophil or macrophage.
2. There is no role for using allopurinol in treating patients with pseudogout.
3. There is a "shrinking lung syndrome" of lupus marked by respiratory muscle weakness with PFTs showing normal DLCO with classic restrictive lung indices.
4. The DLCO helps distinguish interstitial pneumonitis of lupus from diffuse alveolar

hemorrhage from lupus as it is elevated in the latter and low in the former.
5. It is tough at times to distinguish between rheumatoid lung involvement and interstitial fibrosis of methotrexate. A reasonable first option is to stop methotrexate and switch to another agent for RA control (such as leflunomide or etanercept) and then see if the lung disease improves.
6. Cefotaxime or ceftriaxone is the first-line treatment of spontaneous bacterial peritonitis.
7. Lead poisoning and myeloproliferative disorders are among the disease states that can lead to gout.
8. *Pasteurella multocida* is the most common cause of cellulitis after a cat bite.
9. Amoxicillin-clavulanate is the first-line therapy after a cat or dog bite in a non-penicillin allergic patient.
10. Alligator and piranha bites predispose patients to Aeromonas cellulitis.

16.27 Year 2—Week 9—Day 2

1. HIV disease and chronic pulmonary emboli should be ruled out in patients with pulmonary hypertension.
2. Multiple coagulation disorders in one patient increase that patient's risk for clots dramatically.
3. Loss of antithrombin III is the reason for increased coagulable risk in patients with nephrotic syndrome.
4. Low molecular weight heparin medications cannot be used in patients with heparin-induced thrombocytopenia.
5. EKG and CXR findings may be completely normal in patients with significant pulmonary emboli.
6. Raynaud's phenomenon is best treated with calcium channel blockers for first-line agent treatment.
7. Turcot syndrome is marked by colon polyps and brain tumors.
8. The most common cause of a Charcot joint of the shoulder is syringomyelia.
9. The most common cause for Charcot joint of the knee is syphilis.

10. Active coumadin use precludes the ability to test for protein C and protein S. Active heparin use precludes the ability to test for antithrombin III and APC resistance (but you can test for the actual underlying Factor V Leiden gene mutation).

16.28　Year 2—Week 9—Day 3

1. Diagnosis of hypereosinophilic syndrome requires a sustained eosinophil count above 1500 cells/microliter for over 6 months.
2. Patients with persistent eosinophilia should have stool exams for ova and parasite and blood cultures. If these are negative, the next steps involve bone marrow exam to exclude a hematological malignancy or myelodysplasia, as well as serum tryptase levels looking for systemic mastocytosis.
3. Chronic myelomonocytic leukemia has been associated with the presence of eosinophilia.
4. Vasculitis states, polyarteritis nodosa, systemic sclerosis, inflammatory bowel disease, and sarcoidosis have all been described with eosinophilia.
5. Thromboembolic disease such as Budd-Chiari syndrome has been described in patients with hypereosinophilic syndrome.
6. Imatinib is the drug of choice for chronic eosinophilic leukemia.
7. Among the target organs of the hypereosinophilic syndrome are skin, heart, lungs, GI system, and the nervous system in which findings range from transverse myelitis, mononeuritis multiplex, sensory or motor neuropathy, and eosinophilic meningitis.
8. HIV disease and Borrelia infections are among the few viral/bacterial causes of persistent eosinophilia.
9. Addison's disease, Hodgkin's lymphoma, and non-Hodgkin's lymphoma can also cause eosinophilia.
10. Toxoplasma, Dientamoeba, and *Isospora belli* are the three most common causes of eosinophilia caused by protozoans (which usually do not cause eosinophilia).

16.29　Year 2—Week 10—Day 1

1. Patients with multiple myeloma generally have normal alkaline phosphatase levels.
2. The alkaline phosphatase level should be followed every 6–12 months in patients with Paget's disease to monitor for osteosarcoma formation.
3. The COX-2 inhibitors ironically are the safest NSAIDs to give to patients with history of aspirin triad (asthma, nasal polyps, aspirin sensitivity).
4. Salsalate is the safest regular NSAID to give to patients with aspirin sensitivity due to low COX-2 activity.
5. NSAIDs can cause both a nephritic and a nephrotic syndrome picture on urinalysis.
6. NSAIDs have even been linked to protein-losing enteropathy where the serum albumin is low with no protein loss in urine.
7. Type 1 autoimmune polyendocrine syndrome can involve the following three entities: chronic mucocutaneous candidiasis, hypoparathyroidism, and autoimmune adrenal insufficiency.
8. Patients with cortisol levels of less than 2 mg/dl in their early morning blood samples have sufficient evidence to make a diagnosis of adrenal insufficiency with no further testing needed.
9. Consider osteoporosis workup in a patient with a wedge deformity vertebral body fracture.
10. Gastric carcinoid lesions can be found in patients with pernicious anemia.

16.30　Year 2—Week 10—Day 2

1. Although primidone can be used in patients with essential tremor not responding to beta-blocker therapy, be careful with side effects of ataxia and vomiting that may occur as you start to titrate therapy.
2. Iron deficiency anemia needs to be explored in patients with restless leg syndrome. Dopamine receptor agonist therapy is replac-

ing benzodiazepine therapy as first-line treatment

3. HSV-1 is felt to be the most likely causative agent of Bell's Palsy.
4. Methotrexate is an effective agent to use in patients with polymyalgia rheumatica who are being weaned off steroid therapy slowly.
5. Ventricular septal defects (VSD) tend to occur in patients who are post-myocardial infarction (MI) and who are elderly, have hypertension, and who are suffering from first MI due to lack of collateral vessels and lack of time for fibrosis to occur.
6. VSDs can be difficult to manage even surgically due to difficulty in suturing ventricular septum in acute stages of process
7. A loud holosystolic murmur radiating across the precordium from the left sternal border should give great suspicion to a VSD in patient with acute coronary syndrome.
8. The systolic murmur of tricuspid regurgitation will be accentuated by inspiration.
9. It is common to see tricuspid regurgitation present in patients with pulmonary hypertension.
10. Babesiosis can be treated with a regimen of azithromycin and atovaquone or with a regimen of clindamycin and quinine.

16.31   Year 2—Week 10—Day 3

1. Sulfasalazine, cyclosporine, and infliximab are treatment options for pyoderma gangrenosum.
2. Streptococcus is the most common infectious agent to cause erythema nodosum. Other infectious causes include Yersinia, coccidiomycosis, and tuberculosis.
3. Aphthous ulcers can be seen in patients with inflammatory bowel disease.
4. Acrodermatitis enteropathica is the rash that is seen with zinc deficiency.
5. Scurvy is seen with perifollicular plugging and corkscrew hair formation. Treatment is ascorbic acid and complications include left ventricular dysfunction leading to heart failure.

6. Dermatitis herpetiformis and lichen planus lesions are pruritic.
7. Tissue transglutaminase is felt to be the most sensitive and most specific antibody to detect celiac sprue.
8. Oral beta-carotene is the treatment of variegate porphyria, which demonstrates features of both porphyria cutanea tarda and acute intermittent porphyria.
9. Urticaria and vasculitis can be seen with hepatitis A.
10. There has been an association in the literature between hepatitis C and lichen planus. The better known dermatological association of hepatitis C is porphyria cutanea tarda, which is caused by lack of activity or by deficiency of uroporphyrinogen decarboxylase.

16.32   Year 2—Week 11—Day 1

1. Both pyrazinamide and ethambutol have been associated with drug-induced gout when being used in the treatment of tuberculosis infections.
2. Silo filler's lung disease causes respiratory distress shortly after exposure to nitrogen dioxide (it is not Farmer's lung which is a restrictive lung disease).
3. Dapsone can lead to methemoglobinemia, so be cautious of patients who complain of hypoxia that are on this medication.
4. Methylene blue can ironically cause methemoglobinemia if given in excess doses.
5. Methylene blue is the preferred treatment of choice in cases of methemoglobinemia where the level is 15% or above.
6. Do not give methylene blue for treatment of methemoglobinemia if the patient has underlying G6PD deficiency.
7. Vitamin C is available as a second-line agent if patients cannot tolerate methylene blue or are not responding to treatment as expected.
8. Vitamin E in doses above 400 international units daily has been shown to increase all-cause mortality in some studies.
9. Patients with paroxysmal nocturnal hemoglobinuria will lyse RBCs preferentially when they are sleeping because the acid–

base state when one sleeps is respiratory acidosis and that state favors complement lysis when a patient has RBC membrane defects in CD55 and CD59 as do the PNH patients.

10. Polycythemia vera can lead to hepatic vein thrombosis (Budd-Chiari syndrome).

16.33 Year 2—Week 11—Day 2

1. Methotrexate has been noted in the literature as a cause of diffuse large B-cell lymphoma.
2. Blastomycosis can cause skin and lung lesions and examination of KOH smear would show broad-based budding.
3. Wellens sign involves deep T-wave inversions in the leads V2–V4 especially and is associated with critical stenosis of the left anterior descending artery.
4. Intracranial hemorrhage can lead to deep, inverted symmetrical T-waves over the anterior leads of the EKG as well.
5. Adult Still's disease (adult-onset juvenile rheumatoid arthritis) can present with ferritin values in the tens of thousands (felt to be due to overproduction of IL-6).
6. The most common cause of supraventricular tachycardia is AV-nodal reentrant tachycardia.
7. Follow free T4 levels in patients with hypothyroidism who have had total pituitary resection in the past. It is also the most useful test to follow to see if you are heading in the right direction in correcting hyperthyroidism (as TSH may take a long time to correctly show a recovering clinical state).
8. Drug-induced BOOP (bronchiolitis obliterans with organizing pneumonia which is also now known as cryptogenic organizing pneumonia) is caused by D-penicillamine, amiodarone, and busulfan.
9. Cimetidine and sulfamethoxazoletrimethoprim can cause false elevations of the serum creatinine.
10. Klinefelter's syndrome is associated with gynecomastia and an increased risk of male breast cancer.

16.34 Year 2—Week 11—Day 3

1. The rash of facial erysipelas can be distinguished from malar rash of lupus as the latter does not involve the nasolabial fold.
2. Cryptococcus and Penicillium infections are fungal infections that can mimic the appearance of molluscum contagiosum (pearly umbilicated centered papules).
3. Condyloma lata are flat, wart-like lesions that can appear in the anal area of patients with secondary syphilis.
4. Hemorrhagic pustules on erythematous bases, usually found on the dorsum of the hand, are the usual skin manifestation of disseminated gonorrhea.
5. Treatment of disseminated gonorrhea is with at least one week of IV ceftriaxone.
6. IV ceftriaxone is also used to treat severe carditis and severe neurological complications of Lyme disease.
7. Ehrlichiosis is marked by splenomegaly, thrombocytopenia, transaminitis, and WBC inclusions. Treatment is doxycycline.
8. Babesiosis is marked by hemolytic anemia and RBC inclusions. Treatment of this condition is usually with atovaquone and azithromycin (although quinine and clindamycin could be used).
9. Anthrax can present with widened mediastinum but usually no pulmonary infiltrates are seen unlike tularemia which has a marked predisposition to involve the lung parenchyma.
10. Listeria meningitis needs to be treated with IV ampicillin as third-generation cephalosporins are ineffective.

16.35 Year 2—Week 12—Day 1

1. Random serum tryptase levels can be used to screen for systemic mastocytosis. These patients can have eosinophilia.
2. Bone marrow biopsy is often required to finalize the diagnosis of systemic mastocytosis.

3. Exercise-induced urticaria can occur. Other urticaria states include cold-induced urticaria and cholinergic urticaria.
4. Epinephrine is preferred to be given by intramuscular route in the treatment of anaphylaxis and the thigh muscle is the preferred site.
5. Scombroid poisoning can occur after eating seafood especially tuna and mackerel and is marked by flushing due to histidine release.
6. Ciguatera is another seafood poisoning state and classic symptom of this poisoning is "hot-cold" reversal where warm liquids feel cold and vice versa.
7. Obstructive sleep apnea can lead to both pulmonary hypertension and systemic hypertension.
8. Always check a TSH level in patients with atrial fibrillation, especially in the elderly, looking for hyperthyroidism.
9. Hypercalcemia, eosinophilia, normochromic/normocytic anemia, mild non-gap metabolic acidosis, and hyperkalemia are among the lab manifestations of adrenal insufficiency.
10. The most common worldwide cause of primary adrenal insufficiency with large adrenal glands noted on CT scan is tuberculosis. Addison's disease (autoimmune adrenalitis) is the most common cause of adrenal insufficiency with small adrenal glands noted on CT scan.

16.36   Year 2—Week 12—Day 2

1. Giant keratoacanthoma syndrome may respond to cis-retinoic acid therapy.
2. There is a retinoic acid syndrome where patients getting trans-retinoic acid develop pulmonary infiltrates and need to be taken off the medication for a short time and steroids can be considered for treatment.
3. Jaw claudication is a classic feature of temporal arteritis. Polymyalgia rheumatica symptoms can be seen in quite a few patients as well.

4. Acute paronychia is usually caused by *Staphylococcus aureus*. Chronic paronychia is caused by *Candida* species.
5. If someone has a paronychia (nailbed infection) due to chronic nail biting, consider *Eikenella corrodens* as a pathogen. This bug is resistant to clindamycin and only partially responsive to Keflex (use Augmentin).
6. Augmentin is the first-line treatment for cat and dog bites.
7. Valproic acid is the most common antiepileptic causing alopecia.
8. Lupus is associated with non-scarring alopecia, unless one has the discoid variant which is associated with scarring.
9. Sarcoid can cause anterior uveitis, hypercalcemia, disfiguring skin lesions (known as lupus pernio), and Lofgren's syndrome.
10. Lofgren's syndrome involves erythema nodosum, ankle arthritis, and bilateral hilar lymphadenopathy.

16.37   Year 2—Week 12—Day 3

1. Factor 12 deficiency patients have a prolonged PTT but do not bleed if challenged with surgical procedure.
2. Patients with antiphospholipid antibody syndrome are also prone to have a prolonged PTT and they do not have history of bleeding but rather thrombosis.
3. The standard of care has shifted to aspirin and heparin for treatment of most patients with antiphospholipid antibody syndrome during pregnancy.
4. Tetracyclines and fluoroquinolones are to be avoided during pregnancy.
5. Alpha-methyldopa is first-line drug therapy for HTN during pregnancy with hydralazine being second-line agent.
6. Anagrelide is a megakaryocyte maturation inhibitor that is used to decrease the platelet count in patients with myeloproliferative disorder who do not respond to hydroxyurea.
7. Among causes of a low MCV and anemia, do not forget about hemoglobin E disease, anemia of chronic disease, and thalassemias.

8. Among causes of high MCV and anemia, do not forget about liver disease, alcohol abuse, hypothyroidism, and myelodysplasia.
9. Vertical nystagmus should always trigger a workup for a central cause such as a head bleed, stroke, or brain tumor.
10. Patients with pontine infarcts will usually have a history of HTN and have small pupils on physical examination.

16.38   Year 2—Week 13—Day 1

1. Application of a magnet to a single chamber pacemaker always results in asynchronous pacing, but this does not always happen with dual chamber pacing.
2. TENS unit may cause spikes in the EKG that resemble pacemaker spikes.
3. Dual chamber pacing has been used in treating patients with IHSS that are not responding to drug therapy.
4. Atropine may not work in the treatment of second-degree heart block if the patient has a transplant, denervated heart.
5. Ventricular escape rhythms will have wide QRS complexes and have a slower rate than the atria.
6. Consider pacemaker placement for episodes of asystole greater than 3 seconds in duration or an escape rate less than 40 in an awake, asymptomatic patient.
7. Patients with myotonic dystrophy and AV block should be considered for pacemaker therapy more liberally as their progression of AV-nodal disease is quite unpredictable.
8. Treatment of epididymitis is with 10–14 days of fluoroquinolone therapy.
9. Prehn's sign is positive if lifting the scrotum relieves scrotal pain in patients where epididymitis is being considered as a diagnosis.
10. Klinefelter's syndrome patients have increased risk of cryptorchidism (undescended testis) and male breast cancer. The chromosome analysis is 47 XXY in this patients and they have a high incidence of anxiety and depression states as well. Life expectancy is close to normal in these patients.

16.39   Year 2—Week 13—Day 2

1. Parasitemia with *Plasmodium falciparum* of greater than 15% should trigger RBC exchange transfusion therapy.
2. Sickle cell disease indications for RBC exchange transfusion include priapism, acute chest syndrome, and stroke syndrome.
3. Steroids should be used in treating patients with neurosarcoidosis and heart disease with conduction blocks.
4. Sjogren's syndrome can present with distal RTA and increased risk of lymphoma and pseudolymphoma.
5. There is an increased risk of lymphoma in patients with rheumatoid arthritis and Sjogren's disease.
6. Serotonin syndrome can present with trismus, teeth chattering, myoclonus, and fever.
7. Low uric acid levels are seen in patients with SIADH and Wilson's disease.
8. Any young patient with liver disease who has a hemolytic anemia should be worked up for Wilson's disease
9. Allopurinol can lead to a granulomatous hepatitis as well as a hypersensitivity syndrome.
10. Amiodarone and methotrexate can cause restrictive lung disease.

16.40   Year 2—Week 13—Day 3

1. *Enterobacter cloacae* infections do not respond to metronidazole but do respond to trimethoprim-sulfamethoxazole.
2. There is an increased incidence of community-acquired MRSA in the USA. Doxycycline and trimethoprim-sulfamethoxazole are amongst the antibiotics that work well in treatment of uncomplicated community acquired MRSA infections.

3. Efavirenz is relatively contraindicated for use during pregnancy and can cause CNS side effects.

4. Use of zidovudine alone starting in the second trimester of pregnancy in HIV positive patients cuts down the rate of transmission to child from 33% to 8%.

5. Atovaquone/proguanil can be used for malaria prophylaxis in chloroquine resistant areas in patients who cannot use mefloquine.

6. Mefloquine is absolutely contraindicated to be used in patients with cardiac conduction blocks.

7. Amoxicillin is the second-line therapy for patients with Lyme disease who cannot use doxycycline.

8. Streptococcus pneumoniae can lead to purpura skin findings in disseminated disease.

9. Deficiencies in properdin and factor D can lead to recurrent *Neisseria meningitidis* infections just like late complement deficiencies.

10. If CH50 level is normal, there is no reason to check individual complement levels in most situations.

16.41   Year 2—Week 14—Day 1

1. Lipodystrophy can occur in patients with HIV disease regardless of whether they are taking protease inhibitors.

2. Thiazolidinediones (such as pioglitazone) are being used in patients with HIV lipodystrophy with some success.

3. The gold standard for diagnosis of usual interstitial pneumonitis is an open lung biopsy.

4. Metoclopramide can lead to Parkinson's disease-like symptoms including rigidity and tremor.

5. COMT inhibitors such as entacapone and tolcapone are used for treatment of Parkinson's disease.

6. Avoid dextromethorphan treatment for cough in patients with SSRI as they have increased risk of serotonin syndrome.

7. Sarcoid patients are at risk of uveitis (usually anterior type if symmetric) as well as optic neuritis. Uveitis symptoms in these patients includes pain, photophobia and erythema of the eye.

8. Myopia is the most common reason in the general population for retinal detachment.

9. Cluster headaches can be treated acutely with oxygen. Lithium has been used for suppression of these headaches, along with beta-blockers and calcium channel blockers.

10. Indomethacin is the drug of choice for treatment of headaches of chronic paroxysmal hemicrania.

16.42   Year 2—Week 14—Day 2

1. The rash of subacute cutaneous lupus erythematosus is very photosensitive. The rash may be seen as an annular, polycyclic, or psoriasiform entity.

2. The anti-Ro or anti-SSA antibody will be positive in many cases of subacute cutaneous lupus erythematosus.

3. Choose amoxicillin for therapy of Lyme disease when a patient will not be able to avoid prolonged periods of sun exposure (for instance, they are a lifeguard or outdoors landscape designer).

4. Azithromycin one time dosing may be used to treat gonorrhea and chlamydia STD infections.

5. *Mycoplasma hominis and Ureaplasma urealyticum* are among two causes of nongonococcal urethritis.

6. Amiodarone and minocycline can cause bluish discoloration of skin, with minocycline favoring previously scarred areas.

7. Schistosomes exist in the USA in freshwater rivers and they can cause a very itchy dermatitis.

8. Hot tub folliculitis is usually due to *Pseudomonas aeruginosa.* Usually no pharmacological treatment is needed as condition

will resolve with discontinuation of use of hot tubs.

9. *Aureobasidium* species can cause a hypersensitivity pneumonitis in patients who enjoy taking saunas frequently.

10. There is a link between celiac sprue and selective IGA deficiency as well as T-cell lymphoma.

16.43   Year 2—Week 14—Day 3

1. Aspirin is not to be used in the treatment of thyroid storm as it may increase free thyroid hormone. Use acetaminophen instead for fever control.

2. PTU or methimazole should be used before iodine in the treatment of thyroid storm.

3. One must have fever before a diagnosis of thyroid storm is made. The usual cause of death in these patients is cardiac in nature whether from heart failure or from a fatal arrhythmia. Abrupt discontinuation of antithyroid medication can lead to this condition.

4. Do not forget to rule out adrenal insufficiency before treating any patient who has myxedema coma as they may go into adrenal crises.

5. 5q- syndrome is a good prognostic cytogenetic result for patients with myelodysplasia (MDS) diagnosis.

6. There is a variant of MDS that is associated with fever, pulmonary infiltrates, and cutaneous vasculitis.

7. A good rule of thumb for what the cellularity should be in the bone marrow for a given patient is 100 minus the age, thus a 65-year-old male should have 35% cellularity in the bone marrow. Any number higher than that should raise suspicion for myelodysplasia (MDS).

8. Ringed sideroblasts are a type of MDS that may arise due to alcohol abuse.

9. Chloroma, or granulocytic sarcoma, and Sweet's syndrome (neutrophilic dermatosis) are among the skin manifestations of MDS.

10. Turcot syndrome patients have lesions in the hemispheres of their brain parenchyma as opposed to Gardner's syndrome patients that have lesions in the jaw and skull but not the brain matter itself.

16.44   Year 2—Week 15—Day 1

1. Sulfamethoxazole-trimethoprim is the second-line agent to be used in patients with Listeria infection who cannot take ampicillin due to penicillin allergy.

2. Trisomy 8 and monosomy 7 are poor cytogenetic prognostic factors in dealing with patients with MDS.

3. Ertapenem does not cover Pseudomonas or Acinetobacter organisms reliably. Use imipenem instead.

4. Adrenal insufficiency may present with subtle signs of pigmentation, such as pigmentation of the oral cavity with no other obvious pigmentation sites.

5. There must be greater than 90% bilateral adrenal destruction by tumor before adrenal insufficiency is likely to arise in a patient.

6. Besides use in CML (chronic myelogenous leukemia), imatinib mesylate can be used in treatment of eosinophilic leukemias.

7. Thalidomide can be used in the treatment of multiple myeloma, severe lupus disease, and myelodysplastic syndromes.

8. Morning headaches can occur in patients with COPD who suffer from overnight hypoxemia while they sleep. These patients do not necessarily have obstructive sleep apnea.

9. Pemberton's sign involves the turning of a patient's facial skin into a reddish hue as he holds his arms above his head due to compression of a substernal goiter on central vasculature.

10. Propranolol, PTU, and dexamethasone are three drugs which block the peripheral conversion of T4 to T3.

16.45 Year 2—Week 15—Day 2

1. Patients with hepatic hydrothorax are at risk of developing spontaneous bacterial empyema from infection translocation from the peritoneal to the pleural space. Treatment of this condition is with IV antibiotics, preferably a third- or fourth-generation cephalosporin.
2. Chest tube placement in patients with hepatic hydrothorax, even with empyema, will usually lead to adverse events given continual volume of fluid that will translocate to the pleural space from the peritoneal space.
3. One thing that can be done to check effectiveness of treatment of spontaneous bacterial empyema is repeat thoracentesis checking results of glucose and pH values.
4. Most common organism as expected for spontaneous bacterial empyema is *Escherichia coli*. Third generation cephalosporin therapy is the treatment of choice similar to spontaneous bacterial peritonitis.
5. Celiac sprue is among the most popular causes of persistent transaminitis not due to an infectious process.
6. Hepatitis C patients may not have much of a transaminitis despite fibrosis or cirrhosis as hepatocyte death occurs from both necrosis and apoptosis in this condition.
7. Patients with acute hepatitis B can present with serum sickness symptoms including a hemorrhagic rash known as the Arthus reaction.
8. Gingival hyperplasia most commonly occurs from dilantin, cyclosporine, and calcium channel blockers.
9. Cutaneous T-cell lymphoma can be misdiagnosed as psoriasis due to similar clinical appearance.
10. The rash of pustular psoriasis is very similar to the rash of keratoderma blennorrhagica that is seen in patients with reactive arthritis.

16.46 Year 2—Week 15—Day 3

1. Patients with Wilson's disease are acutely treated with D-penicillamine and then chronically treated with zinc usually.
2. D-penicillamine is safe to give to patients with penicillin allergy. It can cause a neurological syndrome similar to myasthenia gravis, as well as nephrotic syndrome.
3. The AST and ALT lab values in acute alcoholic hepatitis are rarely above 400 IU/L.
4. Starvation and chronic alcohol abuse patients do worse in acetaminophen toxicity than patients who do not have those conditions. This is due to chronic depletion of glutathione.
5. Patients with refeeding syndrome will have hypophosphatemia, hypomagnesemia, metabolic alkalosis, and even cardiac arrest/pulmonary edema.
6. Distinguish patients with Bartter's syndrome and chronic vomiting state (such as bulimia) by getting a urine chloride level which is low in the former.
7. Bartter's syndrome patients have normal blood pressure with juxtaglomerular apparatus hyperplasia mechanism as physiology cause.
8. Patients with renal tubular acidosis (RTA) type 4 will have a state with low renin and low aldosterone levels.
9. Patients with RTA type 1 get kidney stones due to low urinary citrate levels (hypocitruria) which leave calcium free to supersaturate with oxalate. This does not happen in RTA type 2 disease.
10. Sjogren's syndrome is classically associated with type 1 RTA, while multiple myeloma is generally associated with RTA type 2.

16.47 Year 2—Week 16—Day 1

1. AST level is usually above the ALT level in patients with alcohol use due to (a) pyridoxine is depleted in chronic alcohol use leading to less ALT formation and (b) AST is both a cytosolic and mitochondrial enzyme leading

to increased release when alcohol takes effect.

2. Allopurinol can cause a granulomatous hepatitis and an interstitial nephritis.

3. NSAIDs can cause significant liver toxicity, usually presenting as a hepatitis.

4. Ceftriaxone can cause a significant drug-induced cholestasis.

5. Be aware that many over the counter sleep preparations contain a significant amount of acetaminophen.

6. An interesting phenomenon is that the alkaline phosphatase will rise after a large meal in patients with type O or type B blood type.

7. Do not forget that pregnant patients will have a rise in alkaline phosphatase levels as they approach the third trimester due to contribution from the placenta.

8. Distinguishing where the alkaline phosphatase comes from can be done by ordering separate isoenzymes. If this is not available and the liver origin is to be ruled out, order a 5' nucleotidase level or GGT level. If normal, then the liver is ruled out as source.

9. Do not forget that Q-fever, caused by *Coxiella burnetii*, can present with acute liver failure. Treatment is with doxycycline.

10. CMV and EBV can also cause acute liver failure even outside of a mononucleosis clinical syndrome.

16.48 Year 2—Week 16—Day 2

1. Patients with acute glaucoma can present with a wide range of symptoms including an acute abdomen presentation (yes, usually they have the red eye at the same time).

2. Timolol can cause significant bradycardia and even congestive heart failure has been reported once the medication was started.

3. Latanoprost has been associated with significant myalgias as a side effect. Consider switching to another class of agents for treatment of glaucoma if the symptoms are intractable.

4. The pupil may be constricted in patients presenting with acute anterior uveitis and there may also be a whitish layer of cells present known as hypopyon iritis.

5. Roth's spots occur mostly in association with endocarditis but similar lesions have been noted to occur in patients with fungemia and with acute leukemia.

6. Central retinal artery occlusion is manifested by a cherry red spot in the macula and can be seen with hypercoagulable states or infectious states.

7. Central retinal vein occlusion is noted by a fundoscopic exam noting "blood and thunder" throughout the retina.

8. Rheumatoid arthritis patients can get a variety of eye disorders including corneal melt, corneal ulcers, and scleromalacia perforans, as well as scleritis and episcleritis.

9. Angioid streaks are disruptions of Bruch's membrane that can be visualized on fundoscopic exam and can be seen in diseases such as acromegaly, Paget's disease, pseudoxanthoma elasticum, sickle cell disease, and Ehlers-Danlos syndrome.

10. Sunflower cataracts and Kayser-Fleischer rings (involving Descemet's membrane) are among the manifestations of Wilson's disease.

16.49 Year 2—Week 16—Day 3

1. The most common finding on fundoscopic exam in patients with temporal arteritis is a pale, slightly swollen optic disc, but about 10% of patients can present with central retinal artery occlusion.

2. Hyperthyroidism can lead to thickening of the extraocular muscle belly but usually the tendon of the muscle is spared.

3. There is a tendon sheath inflammation of the superior oblique muscle that occurs in patients with rheumatoid arthritis that may lead to what appears to be a CN 4 palsy on

physical exam. This is termed Brown's syndrome.

4. There can be retinal involvement in Behcet's syndrome along with the more familiar symptoms of genital ulcers, mouth ulcers, arthritis, pathergy, and vascular complications.

5. Sickle cell disease can lead to retinal hemorrhage usually appearing in a sea-fan shape. This is an ocular emergency when it occurs.

6. Transient cortical blindness has been described as one of the possible ocular complications of migraine headaches.

7. The most common eye finding in HIV retinopathy is cotton-wool exudates.

8. Patients presenting with ptosis and blurry vision late in the day with better vision in the early morning should be worked up for myasthenia gravis.

9. Blurry vision with heat (such as with taking a hot shower) in a young patient should trigger workup for multiple sclerosis. This effect of worsened nerve conduction with heat in multiple sclerosis patients is termed Uhthoff's effect.

10. Optic neuritis and trigeminal neuralgia recurrent attacks should raise the suspicion of multiple sclerosis.

16.50   Year 2—Week 17—Day 1

1. Yellow deposits called drusen can be found in patients with dry macular degeneration.

2. The prevalence of macular degeneration increases with age and is the most common cause of visual loss with advancing age.

3. Macular degeneration patients have typically normal peripheral vision while having trouble seeing at a distance, recognizing faces, and distinguishing between colors.

4. Wet macular degeneration is less common than the "dry" form and is marked by subretinal fluid accumulation with neovascularization, retinal pigment epithelial detachment, and subretinal hemorrhage possible. Symptom onset is typically rapid.

5. Among the possible side effects of systemic carbonic anhydrase inhibitors (such as dorzolamide), which are topically used for glaucoma, are bitter taste, headaches, nausea, and even the rare description of kidney stones.

6. Among the sympathomimetic topical agents for glaucoma, brimonidine works similar to clonidine and is contraindicated in patients taking MAO-inhibitors.

7. Loss of color vision is among the earliest signs of ethambutol toxicity when being used for treatment of tuberculosis.

8. Band keratopathy has been described in patients with chronic hypercalcemic states as well as patients with juvenile rheumatoid arthritis.

9. Patients with juvenile rheumatoid arthritis are at risk as well for iridocyclitis.

10. New onset of floaters in a patient with diabetes mellitus should trigger an ophthalmologic evaluation as the patient may be at risk of retinal detachment.

16.51   Year 2—Week 17—Day 2

1. In a patient with oral and genital ulcers who has a CXR showing "prominent pulmonary arteries," think of Behcet's disease as the prominent pulmonary arteries are likely aneurysmal disease.

2. In patients with renal transplant, the ratio of squamous cell cancer of the skin to basal cell cancer of skin is reversed in 2 to 1 fashion unlike the general population.

3. Squamous cell cancers of the skin involving the lower lip and the ear have a very high metastasis rate.

4. Squamous cell cancer of the skin that arises from an actinic keratosis usually has a low transformation rate.

5. Group A streptococcus, but not *Streptococcus pneumoniae,* is known to exacerbate guttate psoriasis.

6. Steroids are known to worsen the skin disease of pustular psoriasis.

7. Whereas polyarteritis nodosum rarely if ever involves the lung, microscopic polyangiitis is an entity that affects both lung and kidney.
8. Phosphodiesterase-4 inhibitors such as apremilast are second-line agents to use in Behcet's disease not responding to colchicine or if colchicine is contraindicated due to medical comorbid diseases.
9. D-penicillamine and amiodarone are culprits in causing drug-induced BOOP.
10. Terbutaline and nitrofurantoin can cause interstitial pulmonary edema and fibrosis, respectively, in women if used during pregnancy.

16.52   Year 2—Week 17—Day 3

1. L-asparaginase can induce protein S deficiency.
2. Although the anticoagulation for antithrombin III is lifelong after a clot, patients with protein S and protein C deficiency may be able to come off anticoagulation after a year if no further clots are noted.
3. Treatment of antiphospholipid antibody patients with previous episode of clotting or miscarriage events should be with heparin (or LMWH) and low-dose aspirin.
4. There is a catastrophic antiphospholipid antibody variant that requires corticosteroids and plasma exchange for treatment.
5. All vertical nystagmus should be worked up for central cause with at least an MRI or MRA.
6. Marchiafava-Bignami disease is a variant of alcoholic neurological disease which causes atrophy of the white matter tracts.
7. Acute disseminated encephalomyelitis may occur after post-vaccination state such as for influenza or MMR.
8. Myoclonus, fever, and rigidity (in about 50% of patients) can be seen in those patients afflicted with serotonin syndrome.
9. Adrenal leukodystrophy can present with encephalopathy and adrenal insufficiency. Genetic aminoacidurias can present with

encephalopathy as well—long chain fatty acids can be tested.
10. Any rapid demyelinating process will lead to elevation of myelin basic protein. This is not specific to multiple sclerosis.

16.53   Year 2—Week 18—Day 1

1. The murmur of mitral regurgitation is increased with isometric hand grip (this will increase afterload mostly through increased peripheral vascular resistance).
2. Do not forget to include aortic dissection in the differential of a patient with severe chest pain and ST-segment elevation in the inferior leads.
3. Marked ST-segment elevation that diminishes shortly after nitroglycerin or calcium channel blocker administration should raise suspicion of coronary vasospasm.
4. Cerebral vasospasm might occur for up to 21 days post-subarachnoid bleed; thus, most authorities recommend calcium channel blocker (usually nimodipine) in this time.
5. Plasmacytomas are usually associated with similar abnormal findings in bone marrow aspirate and biopsy.
6. Lymphoplasmacytoid lymphomas might be noted on bone marrow biopsy of patients with Waldenstrom's macroglobulinemia.
7. Doubt diabetes mellitus as the cause of nephropathy in patients with lack of retinopathy.
8. Fabry's disease, morbid obesity, chronic vesicoureteral reflux, chronic heroin abuse, and hepatitis C are among the causes of focal segmental glomerulosclerosis.
9. Always measure uric acid level in patients with bulky lymphoma tumor burden as they will be at risk of tumor lysis syndrome once chemotherapy begins.
10. Syringomyelia is the most common cause of upper extremity Charcot joint.

16.54 Year 2—Week 18—Day 2

1. Celiac sprue should be ruled out in all patients that are being considered for a diagnosis of irritable bowel syndrome.
2. Isolated hematuria should make one consider GU malignancy and endocarditis.
3. Smoking markedly increases the risk of bladder cancer.
4. Proximal myopathy considerations include polymyositis, dermatomyositis, steroid myopathy, and hypothyroidism.
5. HIV disease needs to be ruled out in all patients with pneumonia and pneumothorax (as pneumocystis is likely infectious culprit).
6. Celiac disease should be ruled out in all patients with diarrhea and an unexplained transaminitis.
7. Suspect heparin contamination as the cause of a prolonged PT and PTT if these labs are drawn in an asymptomatic patient before surgery.
8. Erysipelas is a well demarcated form of cellulitis commonly caused by group A streptococcus.
9. Psoriasis is notorious for causing nail pitting in combination with an arthritis that favors the distal interphalangeal (DIP) joint over the proximal interphalangeal (PIP) and usually does not involve the metacarpophalangeal (MCP) joints.
10. Patients with discoid lupus will have scarring features to their disease as opposed to subacute cutaneous lupus erythematosus (SCLE) patients who generally do not have scarring complications after their rashes.

16.55 Year 2—Week 18—Day 3

1. Hydrocortisone in excess of 100 mg daily will usually have mineralocorticoid effects as well making mineralocorticoid administration unnecessary in patients with primary adrenal insufficiency at that given dose of hydrocortisone.
2. The half-life of levothyroxine is about a week, thus usually it does not need to be given during the post-operative period where a patient may not be able to take oral medications.
3. There must be edema and proteinuria before entertaining the diagnosis of pre-eclampsia in a patient with hypertension.
4. Hydralazine is a nice adjunct agent to use in patients already on alpha-methyldopa for blood pressure control.
5. Vitamin K administration is the first step in evaluation in a patient with an elevated PT value.
6. Factor 12 deficiency patients will have a prolonged PTT value but do not clinically bleed in surgery.
7. The treatment for acute fatty liver of pregnancy is immediate delivery of baby.
8. Scurvy is vitamin C deficiency and can be marked by congestive heart failure and by gastrointestinal bleeding due to collagen synthesis problems.
9. T-wave inversion can be seen in patients as the natural evolution of acute pericarditis.
10. Increased fremitus is a finding in patients with bronchopneumonia.

16.56 Year 2—Week 19—Day 1

1. Morbid obesity is a risk factor for development of pulmonary hypertension, atrial fibrillation, and even kidney stones.
2. A kidney stone that is stuck at the right uteropelvic junction may mimic acute cholecystitis. If it is stuck in the right lower ureter, it may mimic acute appendicitis.
3. Alkalinization of the urine may help acutely in dealing with ureteral uric acid stones but actually may increase stone size if the stone is a calcium phosphate stone.

4. Extracorporeal shock wave lithotripsy is most effective for stones that are less than 2 cm but greater than 6 mm in size, located in the renal pelvis, and composed of one of the following: calcium oxalate, apatite, uric acid, or struvite.

5. Thiazide diuretics are helpful in preventing calcium stone formation as they reduce urine calcium excretion.

6. The goal of what is the correct amount of hydration to prevent urine stones is enough 8 ounce glasses of water to produce 2 L of urine daily.

7. Studies show that parenteral NSAIDs (such as toradol) are as effective as opioid analgesics in dealing with the acute pain of kidney stones.

8. Kidney stones are associated with distal RTA's (type 1) but not classically with the other RTAs. Sjogren's syndrome is the disease to remember in association with type 1 RTA.

9. Most kidney stones less than or equal to 6 mm will pass spontaneously. Alpha blockade therapy may help in the passage of the stone.

10. Gout, primary hyperparathyroidism, and primary hyperoxaluria are among other common conditions associated with kidney stones.

16.57 Year 2—Week 19—Day 2

1. Quinine and doxycycline is the most common drug combination to treat acute *Plasmodium falciparum* malaria, which may mimic acute fulminant hepatic failure.

2. Exchange red blood cell transfusions must be performed on patients with greater than 15% parasitemia in the setting of *Plasmodium falciparum* malaria.

3. Of patients who suffer from both angioedema and urticaria, 75% continue to suffer episodes for the next 5 years, whereas 20% continue to suffer symptoms over the next 20 years.

4. Chronic idiopathic urticaria is defined by episodes of urticaria that recur for a duration of over 6 weeks and generally lack identifiable triggers.

5. Nearly 50% of patients with chronic urticaria have angioedema.

6. In comparison to chronic urticaria, lesions of urticarial vasculitis last longer than 72 h, may have pruritis or burning sensation, and can demonstrate features of purpura or hyperpigmentation as they vanish.

7. The C4 level is low in both hereditary angioedema types 1 and 2. They also both have low C1-INH function, but type 2 has a normal C1-INH antigen level.

8. The inheritance pattern of hereditary angioedema is autosomal dominant.

9. Steroids are rarely needed in the treatment of chronic urticaria and angioedema.

10. Anabolic steroids, such as stanozolol and danazol, are used in treatment of hereditary angioedema.

16.58 Year 2—Week 19—Day 3

1. A common mistake in missing celiac sprue is failing to order the IGG isotypes of the antibodies (such as tissue transglutaminase) as this condition may be accompanied by IGA deficiency.

2. Washed RBCs can be used in transfusion of patients with IGA deficiency to decrease chance of reaction.

3. Consider IGA deficiency testing in patients who have an anaphylactic reaction to fresh frozen plasma.

4. The best blood product to give to a patient who has a very low VWF (von Willebrand factor) level that needs a surgical intervention is cryoprecipitate, not fresh frozen plasma.

5. Celiac disease is believed to affect 1% of the general population in the United States.

6. Among the diseases/states associated with celiac sprue are Addison's disease, alopecia areata, migraine disease, cerebellar ataxia, idiopathic dilated cardiomyopathy, Sjogren's disease, iron deficiency anemia, and osteoporosis.

7. Behavior therapy (such as bladder training techniques) is preferred over oxybutynin or tolterodine as initial treatment of urge incontinence.

8. Oxybutynin is an anticholinergic agent, so be wary of mental status changes in the elderly.

9. West-Nile virus encephalitis can present with poliomyelitis type symptoms due to disease affecting the anterior horn cells of the spinal cord.

10. Community-acquired MRSA severe infections should probably be treated initially with IV daptomycin. More moderate infections usually respond to two drug therapy choosing among doxycycline, rifampin, and trimethoprim-sulfamethoxazole.

16.59 Year 2—Week 20—Day 1

1. Sulfamethoxazole-trimethoprim and doxycycline are among the most common causes of fixed drug eruption.

2. Clinicians should monitor CPK levels weekly while treating patients with daptomycin.

3. There is a link between hyperopia (farsightedness) and glaucoma.

4. Patients with Meniere's disease should first be treated with low salt diet and if that fails, try thiazide diuretics.

5. Hoarseness can be seen with left atrial enlargement as seen in mitral stenosis (due to compression of left recurrent laryngeal nerve).

6. Among signs of multiple sclerosis are trigeminal neuralgia, optic neuritis, shooting pains down the spine (Lhermitte's sign), and blurry vision or weakness after heat is introduced (Uhthoff's effect).

7. The most common cause of nephrotic syndrome in the general population from an idiopathic standpoint is membranous nephropathy amongst Caucasians.

8. Cimetidine and sulfamethoxazole are two medications that can increase the creatinine level without truly affecting the glomerular filtration rate.

9. The FENA in acute glomerulonephritis may be falsely less than 1%. This phenomenon is felt due to abnormal intrarenal handling of sodium in this condition.

10. The differential of a patient with pulmonary infiltrates and acute renal failure includes the following: granulomatosis with polyangiitis, lupus disease, Goodpasture's syndrome, and microscopic polyangiitis. Remember that polyarteritis nodosum does not affect the lung.

16.60 Year 2—Week 20—Day 2

1. Among the causes of PR interval prolongation is endocarditis with perivalvular abscess and Lyme disease carditis.

2. Methadone is the only analgesic shown to significantly prolong the QT interval.

3. Salicylate poisoning can cause both respiratory alkalosis and anion gap metabolic acidosis.

4. NSAIDs are a common cause of lithium levels becoming elevated when patients start taking them for pain relief.

5. Lithium should be discontinued in patients who develop nephrogenic diabetes insipidus (DI) if possible with amiloride as a treatment choice if the drug must be continued to try to overcome the DI state. One can treat through the hypothyroidism caused by this drug (by replacing with Synthroid).

6. If a patient develops hematuria three days after onset of a viral URI, suspect IgA syndrome (Berger's disease) as the cause of the hematuria.

7. Clozaril and the antithyroid meds (PTU and methimazole) can lead to agranulocytosis.

8. One can use doxycycline as second-line agent for treatment of actinomycosis if a significant PCN allergy is present.

9. Solitary bone plasmacytomas most commonly occur in the vertebral bodies. Radiation therapy is the treatment of choice in isolated plasmacytomas.
10. *Nocardia asteroides* can cause disseminated subcutaneous skin lesions in addition to brain and lung involvement.

16.61   Year 2—Week 20—Day 3

1. Evan's syndrome, which is ITP (idiopathic thrombocytopenic purpura) with autoimmune hemolytic anemia, is treated with steroids and marked by spherocytes.
2. Bernard-Soulier syndrome is marked by giant platelets and involves a problem with platelet adhesion.
3. Consider obtaining platelet function testing in patients with normal platelet counts who keep bleeding for unexplained reasons (stuff like ASA and NSAIDs and clopidogrel can cause an abnormal PFA). Treatment of the bleeding if test is abnormal is to transfuse platelets even if normal platelet count is present.
4. Steroids are used in the treatment of catastrophic antiphospholipid antibody syndrome (marked by CNS events).
5. Among the drugs with level 1 evidence for causing thrombocytopenia are acetaminophen, tamoxifen, haldol, digoxin, quinidine, methyldopa, and amiodarone.
6. TTP (thrombotic thrombocytopenic purpura) and ITP are among the hematological states associated with HIV disease.
7. If a patient with HIV disease and active toxoplasmosis is sulfa-allergic, use pyrimethamine and clindamycin in treatment of the condition.
8. Haptoglobin levels may be low in patients with liver disease. Thus, in these patients, use a reticulocyte count as a best marker for hemolytic anemia.

9. Lupus, inflammatory bowel disease, and beta-lactam antibiotics are among the causes for autoimmune hemolytic anemia.
10. The LDH level is followed in making decisions about when to stop plasmapheresis in patients with TTP.

16.62   Year 2—Week 21—Day 1

1. Heparin-induced thrombocytopenia can develop weeks after the heparin is discontinued.
2. Isoproterenol is an anti-arrhythmic agent that can be used in the treatment of torsades des pointes (it sort of induces a chemical overdrive pacing).
3. Amiodarone's side effects include hyperthyroidism, hypothyroidism, liver dysfunction, bluish skin discoloration, corneal toxicity, interstitial lung disease, and, of course, pro-arrhythmic effects.
4. Patients on IV daptomycin need weekly check of CPK levels. Adjust the dose in renal insufficiency.
5. Ebstein's anomaly, which causes an arterialization of the right ventricle, is associated with WPW and use of lithium during pregnancy.
6. Scarring alopecia is a hallmark feature of discoid lupus.
7. Hydroxychloroquine is the first-line drug of choice for treatment of lupus arthritis and skin manifestations.
8. Always check a PPD skin test before starting treatment with TNF-alpha receptor blocker agents.
9. Bacteremia is most associated with platelet transfusion among all blood product transfusions as platelets are stored at room temperature.
10. Patients receiving plasmapheresis are at risk of citrate toxicity which can lead to hypocalcemia.

16.63   Year 2—Week 21—Day 2

1. Consider checking a CPK level if there is an isolated AST elevation without elevated GGT level in a patient's lab as the AST may be elevated from muscle damage.
2. Hyperthyroidism has been noted to increase the AST and ALT without specific liver injury. Also, with very elevated AST and ALT levels, and concomitant high LDH and alkaline phosphatase levels, consider ischemic hepatitis.
3. One condition to consider when the ALT to AST ratio is greater than 4 to 1 is Wilson's disease. The next test would be a ceruloplasmin level. These patients also frequently have low or low normal alkaline phosphatase levels.
4. In central vertigo, there is no latency before the onset of vertigo when performing a Dix-Hall-Pike maneuver (also known as Nylen-Barany test), whereas peripheral vertigo will have a latency anywhere from a few seconds out to about half a minute.
5. The duration of nystagmus during such a test as described in #4 is usually less than 1 min in peripheral vertigo but may be longer than a minute in central vertigo.
6. Modified Epley maneuvers are employed to overcome the vertigo in benign positional vertigo.
7. There is an association between migraine headache and vertigo.
8. In renal tubular acidosis type 1 and 2, there is generally the inability to acidify urine to a pH less than 5.5 value.
9. Levodopa may give a false positive glucose test on a urinalysis in a patient with no hyperglycemia.
10. Phenazopyridine may give a false positive bilirubin test in the urine in patients with normal bilirubin levels.

16.64   Year 2—Week 21—Day 3

1. Glomerular causes of hematuria include Fabry's disease, Alport's syndrome, nail-patella syndrome, and thin basement membrane disease.

2. Medullary sponge kidney, renal vein thrombosis, sickle cell disease, papillary necrosis, and polycystic kidney disease are all also associated with hematuria.
3. Besides tuberculosis, other causes of sterile pyuria include urethritis, bladder tumors, kidney stones, steroid/cyclophosphamide use, and even exercise.
4. Glycosuria generally develops when the serum blood glucose level exceeds 180–200 mg/dl.
5. Brown muddy granular casts are the hallmark finding in the urine for patients with acute tubular necrosis.
6. Hyaline casts in urinalysis may be a normal finding. It is also seen with pyelonephritis and chronic renal disease.
7. Ethambutol is associated with optic neuritis and with drug-induced gout disease states.
8. Premedication with diphenhydramine and steroids can cut down on the chills and rigors associated with amphotericin-B administration.
9. Demerol is never to be given to a patient on a MAO (monoamine oxidase) inhibitor, including selegiline which is used for Parkinson's disease. Seizures or hypertensive crisis may develop if both used together.
10. The crystals in a urinalysis associated with Proteus infections are colorless and have a "coffin-lid" appearance.

16.65   Year 2—Week 22—Day 1

1. There is no cross-reactivity between honeybees and hornets/yellowjackets.
2. Large local insect reactions should be treated with steroids and antihistamines. They are not predictive of future anaphylactic reaction.
3. The most important first step in managing a patient with anaphylaxis even on a beta-blocker is to administer epinephrine. If no response, then administer glucagon.
4. Macrolides and fluoroquinolones are among the medications that can prolong the QT interval.

5. Factor 8 inhibitor can present in the elderly and be marked by retroperitoneal bleeds and impressive bruising.
6. Treatment of factor 8 inhibitor is based on Bethesda titers. If the Bethesda titer is low, can try purified porcine factor 8. If it is high, you likely should treat with recombinant factor 7.
7. Dapsone provides Pneumocystis prophylaxis coverage but needs to be combined with pyrimethamine to provide adequate toxoplasmosis coverage.
8. Myopia provides the greatest risk for retinal detachment in the general population.
9. Goodpasture's disease involves an abnormality in type 4 collagen, while Ehlers-Danlos involves an abnormality in type 3 collagen.
10. Patients with Ehlers-Danlos disease frequently develop secondary osteoarthritis.

16.66 Year 2—Week 22—Day 2

1. Jervell-Lange Nielsen is a prolonged QT syndrome with autosomal recessive inheritance that is associated with deafness.
2. Romano-Ward syndrome is a prolonged QT syndrome with autosomal dominant inheritance that is not associated with deafness.
3. Patients with liver disease can get hyponatremia independent of hepatorenal syndrome as the body perceives the present vasodilation as "dehydration" and causes a non-osmotic secretion of antidiuretic hormone.
4. Goodpasture's syndrome is associated with renal failure and pulmonary disease (including hemoptysis). Treatment is plasmapheresis.
5. Granulomatosis with polyangiitis also is associated with renal failure and pulmonary disease, with treatment being cyclophosphamide and steroids.
6. Behcet's syndrome is marked by vascular complications (pulmonary artery aneurysms and DVT), genital ulcers, oral ulcers, and arthritis.
7. The differential for periorbital edema includes hypothyroidism, trichinosis, and nephrotic syndrome.
8. Rule out mitral stenosis and ostium secundum ASD in all pregnant patients with heart failure who do not have cardiomyopathy.
9. If a patient is on carbamazepine during pregnancy with good seizure prevention outcomes, then it is best simply to continue that medication rather than try to switch the patient to a safer agent as you run the risk of provoking a seizure during the transition.
10. The treatment for acute fatty liver of pregnancy is to induce delivery.

16.67 Year 2—Week 22—Day 3

1. Retinal detachment is most commonly seen in patients who have severe myopia.
2. In a diabetic who complains of marked increase in eye "floaters," the next event may be retinal detachment.
3. Papillitis (painless visual loss) may be a presenting sign of methanol toxicity.
4. Central retinal vein occlusion presents with a "blood and thunder" appearance to the retina.
5. Central retinal artery occlusion presents with a cherry red spot in the macula on fundoscopic exam.
6. Patients with glaucoma present with a dilated pupil with a steamy cornea and circumcorneal injection (thus the red eye title).
7. Uveitis can be seen in patients with ankylosing spondylitis and with sarcoidosis.
8. A Marcus-Gunn Pupil (lack of afferent response in contralateral eye when light is shined in one eye) is seen in patients with multiple sclerosis.
9. Patients with myasthenia gravis might complain of blurry vision and ptosis as the day progresses.

10. Amiodarone (mostly corneal), tamoxifen (both corneal and retinal), and hydroxychloroquine (nearly all retinal) are associated with eye toxicity.

16.68 Year 2—Week 23—Day 1

1. Mitral valve prolapse and cardiomyopathies are among the causes of a prolonged QT interval.
2. Pentamidine can also cause a prolonged QT interval, along with its side effects of hyperglycemia, hypoglycemia, and pancreatitis. Also, consider organophosphate poisoning in farmers presenting acutely ill with prolonged QT interval.
3. Cerebrovascular events, such as stroke or intracerebral hemorrhage, can lead to prolonged QT interval.
4. Consider temporarily discontinuing ace-inhibitor therapy in patients with severe URI, such as the influenzae, as they may become dehydrated and be prone to succumb to the effects of vasodilation inherent to the ace-inhibitor.
5. Sacroiliitis needs to be considered in a young man with back pain and morning stiffness. Start with SI joint films.
6. Barter's syndrome is clinically marked by muscle spasm and cramping, and it also can be associated with significant upper gastrointestinal symptoms to include nausea.
7. Consider gastroparesis in diabetic patients who have nausea and vomiting.
8. Among the diseases that can cause a sporotrichoid pattern of infection, consider sporotrichosis, *Mycobacterium marinum*, tularemia, and *Nocardia braziliensis*.
9. Severe vibrio vulnificus and parahemolyticus infections should be treated with both doxycycline and a third- or fourth-generation cephalosporin.

10. Consider NASH (non-alcoholic steatohepatitis) as the cause of liver dysfunction in patients even with mild long-standing history of diabetes mellitus (liver biopsy will likely be needed to establish diagnosis).

16.69 Year 2—Week 23—Day 2

1. Some classic features of autoimmune hepatitis on liver biopsy include interface hepatitis, rosettes, loss of biliary features, and plasma cell presence.
2. More than 90% of patients with hemochromatosis are homozygous for the C282Y mutation on the HFE gene.
3. It is worth repeating that all patients with neuropsychiatric disease or an unexplained hemolytic anemia with concomitant liver disease need to be ruled out for Wilson's disease.
4. Acute treatment of Wilson's disease is usually with D-penicillamine (which can cause a host of side effects including mimicking myasthenia gravis), with eventual transition into zinc therapy.
5. Hartnup disease and carcinoid syndrome can cause niacin deficiency (pellagra).
6. Clindamycin and trimethoprim-sulfamethoxazole remain as the most popular choices for treatment of community-acquired MRSA.
7. Performing a sensitive PTT assay and a dilute Russell Viper Venom Test can help when trying to distinguish whether a low positive IGM anticardiolipin antibody could have clinical significance.
8. Patients with high risk antiphospholipid antibody syndrome and low platelet counts are still recommended to continue warfarin therapy despite a risk of bleeding (benefit still outweighs risk in this situation).

9. Right-sided EKGs are helpful in evaluation of right ventricular infarct as one will see elevation in lead V4R.
10. Neoadjuvant chemotherapy is indicated in patients with breast cancer who present with the inflammatory disease variant (*peau d' orange* discoloration).

16.70 Year 2—Week 23—Day 3

1. The most common cause of upper extremity Charcot joints is the entity known as syringomyelia.
2. Patients with advanced rheumatoid arthritis who begin complaining of weakened hand grip bilaterally need to be ruled out for C1-C2 subluxation with cervical spine films.
3. Parathyroid hormone effect on the kidney consists of phosphaturia and increasing tubular reabsorption of calcium.
4. Magnesium levels need to be normal to have appropriate parathyroid hormone function.
5. Glutamic acid decarboxylase antibodies can be seen in diabetes mellitus type 1 as well as a neurological disease known as Stiff-person's disease.
6. Patients taking anti-epileptic medications require more vitamin D replacement than usual.
7. The frequency of life-threatening penicillin anaphylaxis in the general population is estimated at 0.01–0.05%.
8. Cephalosporin therapy particularly cefepime is used in severe *Vibrio vulnificus* and *Vibrio parahemolyticus* infections of the skin as adjunct therapy to doxycycline.
9. Approximately 75% of all intracerebral hemorrhages are due to the ravages of chronic hypertension.
10. Consider cerebral amyloid as a cause of lobar hemorrhages in the elderly (involving areas not usually affected by hypertension).

16.71 Year 2—Week 24—Day 1

1. Once ATN (acute tubular necrosis) develops from iodine contrast, there is no specific treatment recommended other than observa-tion to make sure the patient does not develop oliguria.
2. Severe lithium toxicity is treated with hemodialysis.
3. HIV and Parkinson's disease need to be considered in young patients who develop seborrheic keratosis.
4. Poxvirus is the causative agent of molluscum contagiosum.
5. Areflexia is a common finding in patients with Guillain-Barre syndrome. Also do not forget to check the FVC in patients with this syndrome even if they are not complaining of shortness of breath as respiratory failure may develop.
6. *Campylobacter jejuni* is the most common worldwide cause of Guillain-Barre syndrome.
7. Consider tuberculosis as a cause for adrenal insufficiency in patients with large adrenal gland size bilaterally on CT imaging.
8. Condyloma lata lesions are flat and caused by syphilis. Condyloma acuminata lesions are larger and cauliflower-like and caused by human papilloma virus.
9. Aldolase is a muscle enzyme which will usually be elevated in patients with dermatomyositis or polymyositis.
10. Consider inclusion body myositis in patients with distal and proximal muscle weakness who have both neuropathic and myopathic abnormalities on EMG testing.

16.72 Year 2—Week 24—Day 2

1. Bilateral axillary freckling is called Crowe's sign when it is associated with neurofibromatosis.
2. The list of medications to consider in hypersensitivity syndrome situations as culprits include abacavir, phenytoin, and allopurinol.
3. Efavirenz is a highly active antiretroviral agent that can cause mental status changes and delirium in pregnant patients.
4. Most cases of reactive arthritis will resolve within 4–6 months even with no treatment.
5. *Escherichia coli* dysentery episodes are not associated with subsequent reactive arthritis

(unlike the potential for this order after episodes of Campylobacter, Shigella, Salmonella, and Yersinia).

6. Tinea versicolor may be marked by either hyperpigmentation or hypopigmentation. The causative organism is Malassezia furfur.

7. Valproic acid is associated with weight gain, alopecia, pancreatitis, and abnormal liver function testing.

8. Aromatic anticonvulsants are associated with elevation of gamma-glutamyl transferase (GGT) lab test from chronic stimulation of the liver microenzyme network.

9. Cladribine or 2-chlorodeoxyadenosine is the treatment of choice for hairy cell leukemia.

10. CD-38 positivity is a poor prognostic marker in patients with chronic lymphocytic leukemia.

16.73 Year 2—Week 24—Day 3

1. Acquired cystic kidney disease is a risk factor for renal cell carcinoma.

2. Medullary sponge kidney is rarely associated with renal failure but can cause kidney stones.

3. Cadmium toxicity may lead to renal failure and to painful bone deposition and fractures (sometimes referred to as "itai-itai").

4. Stauffer's syndrome is the transaminitis of renal cell cancer with no visible lesions on CT scan.

5. Mirizzi syndrome involves dilation of the common bile duct without stone impaction in the common bile duct, but rather due to stone impaction in the cystic duct. Treatment is usually ERCP with drainage as needed and then eventual cholecystectomy.

6. Lead toxicity can lead to abdominal pain, gout, and microcytic, hypochromic anemia.

7. Miliary tuberculosis may present with a normal CXR and granuloma lesions in the liver.

8. 20% of patients with giant cell arteritis may actually have a normal erythrocyte sedimentation rate (ESR).

9. Pancreas divisum afflicts about 7% of the population but only about 5–10% of those patients develop clinical signs of pancreatitis.

10. Calcitonin level is the test to obtain in screening for medullary cancer of the thyroid.

16.74 Year 2—Week 25—Day 1

1. Thyroglobulin level will be elevated in subacute thyroiditis but low normal to low in patients with thyrotoxicosis factitia states.

2. Choriocarcinoma is associated with a high radioactive iodine uptake (RAIU) but struma ovarii is not associated with a high RAIU.

3. Always rule out pheochromocytoma before proceeding to operate on a patient with medullary cancer of the thyroid.

4. Patients with Cushing's syndrome can be hypertensive with hypokalemia with a metabolic alkalosis.

5. Bicarbonate should only be given in diabetic ketoacidosis (DKA) for life-threatening situations such as pH less than 6.90. Routine use in other instances will lead to an "overshoot" metabolic alkalosis as you correct the DKA.

6. Causes of DKA include pregnancy, Graves' disease, myocardial infarction, cocaine use, and infection.

7. Azithromycin is the first-line treatment of legionella infections. Add rifampin if disease is severe requiring ICU admission.

8. A worrisome side effect associated with linezolid is neutropenia.

9. Topiramate is a useful pharmacological agent in the treatment of menstrual period induced migraines.

10. The first-line agent for essential tremor is a beta-blocker.

16.75 Year 2—Week 25—Day 2

1. Initial treatment of organophosphate poisoning is atropine.

2. Atropine is also indicated in acute anterior MI with significant bradycardia compromising cardiac output.
3. Look for gastroparesis in patients with diabetes mellitus who are complaining of nausea and vomiting.
4. High-dose tetracycline and folic acid for 4–6 months is the usual treatment of tropical sprue.
5. Arsenic has been used to treat refractory AML and is associated with QT interval prolongation.
6. Hyperthyroidism and diabetes mellitus can lead to a secretory diarrhea process.
7. Check for hepatitis D serology in patients with chronic hepatitis B who suddenly develop fulminant liver failure.
8. Penicillin G is first-line treatment of tetanus. Metronidazole is a second-line agent.
9. Cardiac arrythmias are extremely common in patients afflicted with tetanus. Opisthotonos refers to the arched back in these patients.
10. Schatzki's ring is a smooth, symmetrical mucosal ring at the gastroesophageal junction which causes dysphagia, and this condition can be treated with mechanical dilation.

16.76 Year 2—Week 25—Day 3

1. Pancreatitis can lead to splenic vein thrombosis which can lead to variceal bleeding. The first line treatment is splenectomy.
2. Azathioprine and 6-mercaptopurine are used as steroid-sparing agents in Crohn's disease. Both agents can lead to drug-induced pancreatitis.
3. Gynecological cancers are associated with Lynch syndrome (hereditary non-polyposis coli) and with Peutz-Jeghers syndrome.
4. Patients with IGA deficiency are at increased risk of Giardia lamblia infections.
5. *Isospora belli* is an opportunistic agent that can lead to diarrhea in HIV positive patients, but unlike other similar parasites, it can be treated with trimethoprim-sulfamethoxazole.

6. Check for iron deficiency anemia in patients with restless leg syndrome.
7. Patients with vocal cord dysfunction will be misdiagnosed as having asthma. Check a flow-volume loop which will reveal a spastic, chaotic inspiratory flow limb in vocal cord dysfunction.
8. Acute hepatitis B is associated with vasculitis, arthritis, and serum sickness.
9. Acute retroviral syndrome might resemble infectious mononucleosis and should be sought after especially in patients with a morbilliform exanthem that spares the palms and soles.
10. CMV is the most common viral pathogen in adults presenting as a mononucleosis after EBV has been ruled out.

16.77 Year 2—Week 26—Day 1

1. Hairy cell leukemia is associated with splenomegaly, leukopenia, and recurrent Legionella infections.
2. CML is associated with basophilia and multiple WBC forms including metamyelocytes, myelocytes, and bands noted on peripheral smear.
3. In patients with unexplained persistent high eosinophil counts, a bone marrow aspiration must be done.
4. Acute tubular necrosis is associated with isosthenuria (the inability to concentrate or dilate urine) as well as muddy brown granular casts noted on urinalysis.
5. The lowest urine osmolality values will be seen in patients with psychogenic polydipsia.
6. Alcohol abuse can cause damage in several areas. If the cerebellar hemisphere is involved, the biggest deficit will be in finger to nose pointing with an outstretched hand and dysdiadochokinesia will be noted. If the damage is to the cerebellar vermis, truncal ataxia will dominate the picture. If the mamillary bodies are affected, then memory loss will be the main feature.

7. Target cells are seen in patients with thalassemia and with liver disease.

8. Hereditary spherocytosis is associated with a positive osmotic fragility test and with risk of pigmented gallstones.

9. Thiazide diuretics should still be considered as first-line treatment of an otherwise healthy person with isolated systolic hypertension.

10. The most common rash of Lyme disease is erythema chronicum migrans.

16.78   Year 2—Week 26—Day 2

1. A cerebral bleed in elderly patients with a distribution not classic for hypertension-related (the classic hypertension-related areas are the pons, the pulvinar of the thalamus, the putamen, cerebellar poles) is usually due to amyloid angiopathy.

2. Detrusor hyperreflexia (instability) is the most common cause of incontinence in patients with Parkinson's disease and in the general population. Treatment is giving an anticholinergic to block bladder contraction or giving an alpha-adrenergic agonist to increase urethral resistance (preferred option).

3. Pelvic muscle exercises (Kegels) are good only for stress incontinence. Estrogen replacement in the elderly has not been shown to affect stress incontinence, but it does improve dysuria and urgency caused by atrophic vaginitis (estrogen vaginal cream could also be used). Hormone replacement therapy is not to be started on any patient with undiagnosed genital bleeding. It is generally held that transdermal estrogen patches help with hot flashes and osteoporosis yet are not associated with the increased thromboembolic risk of oral therapy.

4. Patients with cystocele through the vaginal introitus and the finding of incontinence should be referred for surgery as drugs are unlikely to work.

5. All patients with incontinence should have a urinalysis and rectal exam to rule out infec-tion and impaction. Calcium and glucose levels should also be done to rule out hypercalcemia and diabetes.

6. Post-void residuals should be done on all patients with incontinence. A volume greater than 60 cc is abnormal and suggests retention.

7. If a patient has urinary or fecal contamination of a sacral decubitus ulcer, the ulcer should be cleaned but antibiotics should not be started.

8. Turning a patient every 3 hours in a nursing home while the patient is in bed prevents decubitus ulcers and the development of ileus. Narcotics in elderly patients commonly cause ileus (pseudo-obstruction or Ogilvie's syndrome). Other causes of pseudo-obstruction in the general population are hypothyroidism, scleroderma, bacterial overgrowth syndrome (e.g., scleroderma patients and tropical sprue), and electrolyte disorders (hypokalemia, hypomagnesemia).

9. Although Paget's disease is common in the elderly, it is only those patients who are immobilized that are at increased risk of hypercalcemia.

10. Recurrent otitis media infections may lead to the formation of cholesteatoma (epithelialized sac of contents that may interfere with hearing).

16.79   Year 2—Week 26—Day 3

1. Hypothermia may lead to deflections on the last part of the QRS complex known as J-waves or Osborne waves.

2. A wide fixed split S2 should raise suspicion of atrial septal defect. Endocarditis prophylaxis is not needed in cases of ostium secundum ASD.

3. Periungual fibromas and adenoma sebaceum are physical exam clues to the diagnosis of tuberous sclerosis.

4. Uric acid stones are always radiolucent. Cystine stones will be either radiolucent or radio-opaque depending on their sulfur content.

5. Ciguatera poisoning from fish is marked by hot-cold reversal and teeth-shattering chills. Scombroid poisoning from fish is marked by a flushing presentation with vasodilation.
6. Atropine is the first-line treatment emergently of organophosphate poisoning, which may be marked by prolonged QT interval.
7. Indomethacin is the drug of choice for chronic paroxysmal hemicrania headaches. Cluster headaches are acutely treated with 100% oxygen.
8. Horner's syndrome may appear with a lateral medullary infarct (Horner's syndrome), cluster headaches, or a bronchogenic carcinoma at the apex (Pancoast tumor).
9. Chronic inflammatory demyelinating polyneuropathy is marked by its assocations with hematological disorders such as multiple myeloma, lymphomas, and leukemias.
10. Vertical nystagmus must always be worked up with imaging of the CNS, usually MRI and MRA to start. Horizontal nystagmus is usually from a peripheral source, as seen with BPV and Meniere's disease.

16.80   Year 2—Week 27—Day 1

1. Persistent split of S2 is seen with right bundle branch block on EKG. One may see a left bundle branch block on EKG with paradoxical split of the S2.
2. Low voltage EKG may be seen in amyloidosis, hypothyroidism, COPD, and pericardial effusion.
3. Pontine infarct is seen in the setting of chronic uncontrolled hypertension and may present with small pupils on physical exam.
4. Disturbance by an infarct of the suprachiasmatic area may result in disruption of sleep-wake cycles.
5. Gerstmann syndrome is a lesion of the left parietal lobe involving signs of right/left confusion, finger anomia, acalculia, and agraphia.
6. Wallenberg's syndrome is an infarct of the left lateral medulla which is marked by Horner's syndrome, ipsilateral facial motor

signs, contralateral body hemiparesis, dysarthria, and dysphagia.
7. Carcinoid syndrome causes flushing only if the lesion is found in the liver or in the bronchial area.
8. Carcinoid syndrome may lead to niacin deficiency as tryptophan is shunted to form serotonin rather than niacin.
9. Erythromycin or cimetidine may inhibit the cytochrome P450 pathways in such a way as to lead to theophylline toxicity in patients taking that medication.
10. Avoid quinidine whenever possible in patients taking digoxin. Other class 1a antiarrhythmic agents can also lead to gastrointestinal disturbance. Disopyramide additionally has a large anticholinergic effect so beware in patients with glaucoma.

16.81   Year 2—Week 27—Day 2

1. Patients with chronic alcohol abuse with diets that sometimes are comprised of beer, cola, and hot dogs are susceptible to getting scurvy (vitamin C deficiency). Severe scurvy may even end up in congestive heart failure.
2. Thiamine deficiency (B1) may present with wet or dry variants. Dry beriberi is dominated by neurological signs, whereas wet beriberi is marked by congestive heart failure.
3. Other causes of high output heart failure besides beriberi include multiple myeloma, Paget's disease, and arteriovenous malformations.
4. *Diphyllobothrium latum* is a tapeworm that can cause B12 deficiency.
5. *Strongyloides* infections may resemble asthma in presentation. It easily can be diagnosed with recent travel to affected area and a sputum for larvae. Also beware of gramnegative septicemia that can occur in patients afflicted with this parasite.
6. Personality and behavioral changes can occur in patients with B12 deficiency.
7. Spinal cord swelling and gadolinium enhancement may be seen in patients with

B12 deficiency, as well as abnormal visual evoked potentials.

8. Enterobius vermicularis is the pinworm, and it can actually lead to acute appendicitis if it migrates to that area. About a third of the patients have perianal itching and treatment is with a thiabendazole one time dose with repeat dose two weeks later.

9. The most common location to find a lesion of carcinoid syndrome is in the small bowel/appendix.

10. Iron stores may be depleted real fast once erythropoietin is started. Be sure to follow ferritin levels in these patients.

16.82 Year 2—Week 27—Day 3

1. West-Nile encephalitis is marked by a high CSF protein and can cause symptoms resembling ALS.

2. ALS is never associated with a sensory level. It is marked by both upper motor neuron signs (spasticity and clonus) as well as lower motor neuron signs (fasciculations and atrophy).

3. Proton pump inhibitor therapy may induce B12 deficiency given time due to the resultant state of achlorhydria that the drug induces.

4. Carbon monoxide poisoning patients can have a cherry red spot in the macula noted similar to patients with central retinal artery occlusion. Blood gas with carbon monoxide level will be helpful in this situation.

5. Scleroderma is associated with bacterial overgrowth syndrome. This can be diagnosed with an extended Schilling's test and usually responds to 3–4 weeks of broad-spectrum oral antibiotic therapy.

6. Guillain-Barre syndrome and CIDP are associated with areflexia on physical exam.

7. HSV encephalitis should be suspected in all renal transplant patients with acute change in mental status. Treatment is with high-dose acyclovir intravenously for 14 days.

8. Amyloid angiopathy is a common cause for recurrent CNS lobar hemorrhages in the elderly.

9. Ferrous sulfate may interfere with the absorption of fluoroquinolones and Synthroid so be sure to space the administration of these medications by several hours.

10. Ciprofloxacin has poor to non-existent coverage for *Streptococcus pneumoniae*.

16.83 Year 2—Week 28—Day 1

1. Coarse atrial fibrillation is classically associated with rheumatic heart disease.

2. If you see a tall R-wave in lead V1 and an old EKG when the patient was in sinus rhythm with left atrial enlargement, and now the patient has coarse atrial fibrillation, you can state even further that mitral stenosis is likely present.

3. Mitral stenosis is associated with hoarseness due to left atrial enlargement impinging on the left recurrent laryngeal nerve and this is known as Ortner's syndrome.

4. Antibodies that can be seen in autoimmune hepatitis include anti-smooth muscle antibody titer and anti-liver-kidney-microsomal antibody.

5. Washed RBC products are used in patients with IGA deficiency.

6. NSAIDs are known to cause aseptic meningitis, particularly in patients with lupus.

7. The most common cause of meningitis in the summer months are enteroviruses.

8. Steroids should be given in patients with tuberculous (TB) pericarditis and meningitis (as well as four drug TB therapy).

9. Normal pressure hydrocephalus may cause lower extremity signs of Parkinsonism. Do not forget to exclude drug-induced causes of Parkinsonism, most commonly seen in the medical realm with metoclopramide.

10. Clubbing is not classically associated with bronchial asthma but is commonly seen in COPD.

16.84 Year 2—Week 28—Day 2

1. Primary sclerosing cholangitis is seen with ulcerative colitis and with HIV disease. ERCP is the test to detect this entity.
2. Radioactive iodine and amiodarone may cause either acute hypothyroidism or hyperthyroidism.
3. Meningiomas may become evident during pregnancy as estrogen stimulates growth of this tumor.
4. Gardner's syndrome is FAP with colorful features of jaw osteomas, skull osteomas, and soft tissue skin tumors.
5. Ursodeoxycholic acid can be used to prevent gallstone formation in patients planning to lose a large amount of weight, and of course, for treatment of primary biliary cirrhosis.
6. Porcelain gallbladder is a risk for development of gallbladder adenocarcinoma.
7. U-waves likely represent late repolarization and can be seen with low magnesium and low potassium states, as well as with digoxin toxicity.
8. A negative U-wave can be seen with coronary artery disease and with left ventricular hypertrophy.
9. Choledochal cysts can lead to biliary dilation and are at risk for malignant transformation and thus should be removed.
10. Vocal cord dysfunction is a common mimicker of asthma seen mostly in young females. Treatment is speech therapy.

16.85 Year 2—Week 28—Day 3

1. High CPK and aldolase levels may be seen with polymyositis and dermatomyositis and the treatment is IV steroids initially.
2. Polymyalgia rheumatica is not associated with weakness but rather with pain and stiffness of the hips and shoulders.
3. Although melanoma, choriocarcinoma, and renal cell cancer are the tumors most classically associated with hemorrhage, adenocar-

cinomas can also bleed when presenting with brain metastasis.
4. Patients with glaucoma can actually present with an acute abdomen—mechanism is not totally clear how this happens.
5. Patients with alligator and piranha bites are at risk of Aeromonas infections. Treatment is with IV penicillin therapy.
6. The two poisonous lizards in the USA are the Mexican beaded lizard and the Gila monster.
7. Grover's disease is transient acantholysis and can present with pruritis papules over the trunk and back of patients who are hospitalized (heat and sweating factors).
8. Toxoplasmosis causes ring-enhanced lesions with a predilection for the basal ganglia.
9. Medications that can increase the MCV lab value include dilantin, hydroxyurea, and methotrexate (if folic acid not given with methotrexate).
10. Mucha-Haberman disease is also known as pityriasis lichenoides et varioliformis acuta (PLEVA). The rash of this disease resembles a pattern of pityriasis rosea but has necrotic based features.

16.86 Year 2—Week 29—Day 1

1. Sulfasalazine, cyclosporine, and infliximab are treatment options for pyoderma gangrenosum.
2. Streptococcus is the most common infectious agent to cause erythema nodosum. Other infectious causes include Yersinia, coccidiomycosis, and tuberculosis.
3. Aphthous ulcers can be seen in patients with inflammatory bowel disease.
4. Acrodermatitis enteropathica is the rash that is seen with zinc deficiency.
5. Scurvy is seen with perifollicular plugging and corkscrew hair formation. Treatment is ascorbic acid and complications include left ventricular dysfunction leading to heart failure.

6. Dermatitis herpetiformis and lichen planus lesions are pruritic.
7. Tissue transglutaminase is felt to be the most sensitive and most specific antibody to detect celiac sprue.
8. Oral beta-carotene is the treatment of variegate porphyria, which demonstrates features of both porphyria cutanea tarda and acute intermittent porphyria.
9. Urticaria and vasculitis can be seen with hepatitis A.
10. There has been an association in the literature between hepatitis C and lichen planus.

16.87   Year 2—Week 29—Day 2

1. Antibiotic of choice for Nocardia and Whipple's disease is sulfa-based antibiotic.
2. Antibiotic of choice for actinomycosis and syphilis is penicillin.
3. Antibiotic of choice for *Stenotrophomonas* is sulfa-based antibiotic or ticarcillin-clavulanate.
4. Antibiotic of choice for leprosy is dapsone.
5. Antibiotic of choice for tropical sprue and Q-fever is tetracycline/doxycycline.
6. Antibiotic of choice for ehrlichiosis and Lyme disease is doxycycline.
7. Antibiotic of choice for SPICE organisms (*Serratia, Citrobacter, Proteus* as examples) if inducible beta-lactamase activity suspected is carbapenem therapy.
8. Antibiotic of choice for skin candida infections is nystatin.
9. Antibiotic of choice for septic arthritis due to methicillin sensitive *Staphylococcus aureus* is nafcillin or oxacillin.
10. Antibiotic of choice for Legionella and bacillary angiomatosis is macrolide therapy.

16.88   Year 2—Week 29—Day 3

1. Drug of choice to treat chronic paroxysmal hemicrania headache is Indomethacin.
2. Drug of choice to treat erythromelalgia in myeloproliferative disease is aspirin.

3. Drug of choice to use to lower platelet count if hydroxyurea fails in myeloproliferative disease is anagrelide.
4. Drug of choice to treat lupus skin and arthritis disease is hydroxychloroquine.
5. Drug of choice to treat fistulas in Crohn's disease is infliximab.
6. Drug of choice to treat kidney stones from inflammatory bowel disease patients with terminal ileal resection is calcium carbonate **taken with meals**.
7. Drug of choice to treat primary hypercalciuria is thiazide diuretics.
8. Drug of choice to treat isolated systolic HTN in otherwise healthy individual is thiazide diuretic or dihydropyridine calcium channel blocker.
9. Drug of choice to give to a patient with prolonged QT syndrome is beta-blocker therapy.
10. Drug of choice to give to a patient with hypertrophic cardiomyopathy is beta-blocker therapy.

16.89   Year 2—Week 30—Day 1

1. Clindamycin and gentamicin are an acceptable antibiotic regimen for pelvic inflammatory disease if a patient has severe PCN allergy and cannot tolerate doxycycline.
2. Bacterial vaginosis and Trichomonas are treated similarly with metronidazole.
3. Trichomonas vaginitis features the highest pH of the vaginitis infections. Candida vaginitis features the lowest pH.
4. Tetracycline and fluoroquinolones are contraindicated during pregnancy.
5. Consider alpha-methyldopa first line for HTN control in pregnancy and use hydralazine as an adjunct agent.
6. TTP has a marked rise in incidence during the second trimester of pregnancy.
7. Consider retained placental/fetal products as a cause of persistent vaginal bleeding and hypotension post-delivery.
8. Pre-eclampsia can occur post-partum.
9. Valproic acid is the most frowned upon antiepileptic for a woman planning pregnancy

(incidence of open neural tube defects can be high).

10. Think of tocolytic-induced pulmonary edema in a woman receiving terbutaline who starts complaining of shortness of breath.

16.90 Year 2—Week 30—Day 2

1. Streptococcus is the most likely offending organism of a cellulitis when streaking lymphangitis is noted.
2. Ecthyma gangrenosum are necrotic lesions seen in patients with neutropenia that are usually caused by Pseudomonas.
3. Outdated tetracycline has been associated with type II renal tubular acidosis with Fanconi's syndrome.
4. Cefepime, ceftazidime, ticarcillin-clavulanate, and piperacillin-tazobactam are the beta-lactam drugs with the best action against Pseudomonas.
5. Steroid therapy is to be used in patients with *Streptococcus pneumoniae* meningitis.
6. There is a risk for SBP (spontaneous bacterial peritonitis) in patients with ascites who are to undergo an esophagogastroduodenoscopy (EGD) procedure. Giving prophylactic dose of levofloxacin before procedure is recommended by many authorities.
7. Clindamycin is the second-line drug of choice for endocarditis prophylaxis in patients who are about to undergo dental procedures and are felt at risk of endocarditis.
8. Rheumatoid arthritis can cause aggressive eye disease, such as scleritis and scleromalacia perforans.
9. Conditions such as cryoglobulinemia and endocarditis can cause a positive rheumatoid factor.
10. Epitrochlear lymphadenopathy can be detected in patients with Hodgkin's and non-Hodgkin's lymphomas.

16.91 Year 2—Week 30—Day 3

1. Anemia of chronic disease is usually normocytic in nature but can be microcytic at times.
2. A Coombs positive hemolytic anemia can occur in systemic lupus erythematosus.
3. Patients with Felty's syndrome demonstrate leukopenia, splenomegaly, and signs of rheumatoid arthritis.
4. Leukopenia and lymphopenia are hallmark features on complete blood count of systemic lupus erythematosus.
5. Drug-related interstitial nephritis will cause urine eosinophils to be observed in only about 20% of total cases.
6. Albumin, serum iron, and transferrin are examples of negative acute phase reactants in acute inflammatory states.
7. Only about 10% or less of patients with discoid lupus will demonstrate a positive ANA (anti-nuclear antigen) test.
8. Procainamide can cause a positive ANA in about 50–75% of patients, but only a small percentage of those patients will ever develop symptoms of drug-induced lupus.
9. Papulosquamous and annular are the two most common descriptors used for describing the rash of subacute cutaneous lupus erythematosus.
10. Tietze syndrome describes costochondritis of the second and third costochondral joint.

16.92 Year 2—Week 31—Day 1

1. Vancomycin can worsen the skin disease of linear bullous IGA disease.
2. All the neutrophilic dermatitis states can be treated with dapsone.
3. Lichen planus can be seen with hepatitis B and C. Porphyria cutanea tarda is highly associated with hepatitis C. Lichen planus is

highly pruritic while porphyria cutanea tarda is highly photosensitive.

4. Pemphigus vulgaris has a paraneoplastic association with ovarian and colon cancer.

5. Bullous pemphigoid has no paraneoplastic associations and usually arises in the elderly population (treatment is oral steroids usually).

6. Erythroderma can be seen with psoriasis and cutaneous T-cell lymphoma.

7. Discoid lupus can be treated with hydroxychloroquine as can the subacute cutaneous lupus erythematosus.

8. Dermatitis herpetiformis is associated with celiac sprue. Dapsone helps the associated pruritis but gluten-free diet is the eventual best treatment.

9. Amiodarone and minocycline can cause bluish discoloration of the skin. Minocycline tends to prefer previously scarred areas for its discoloration pattern as opposed to the diffuse usual nature of amiodarone.

10. Gardner's syndrome is a colon cancer syndrome associated with soft tissue skin tumors (especially epidermal inclusion cysts). Screening should include both upper and lower endoscopy for GI carcinoma in these patients.

16.93   Year 2—Week 31—Day 2

1. The RDW (red cell distribution width) lab value will be clearly increased in iron deficiency anemias as opposed to thalassemia where the RDW will be normal. Also, there will be thrombocytosis with iron deficiency anemia as it is the most common cause of thrombocytosis in the general population. The hemoglobin A2 level will be increased with beta-thalassemia trait on hemoglobin electrophoresis as long as there is not a concomitant iron deficiency anemia.

2. The most impressive microcytosis (MCV value below 68 commonly) for a slightly depressed hemoglobin will be seen in patients with hemoglobin E disease. These patients will be of Southeast Asian descent.

3. The most common cause of microcytic anemia in the general population is anemia of chronic disease—but the MCV will almost always be above the value of 74 in these patients. The ferritin level is *high* in this condition, whereas the total iron binding capacity(TIBC) is *low*.

4. Paroxysmal nocturnal hemoglobinuria is an intrinsic acquired anemia commonly seen in patients who are treated for aplastic anemia . The way to diagnose this disease is by flow cytometry (abnormal CD-55 and CD-59). The Ham test and sugar water test are now considered obsolete in diagnosis.

5. Pernicious anemia is best diagnosed by testing for anti-intrinsic factor antibody and anti-parietal cell antibody. It is associated with increased incidence of gastric carcinoid and gastric adenocarcinoma so surveillance EGDs should be done every 2–3 years.

6. Pseudogout can be highly associated with underlying diseases of hyperparathyroidism and hemochromatosis.

7. A Heinz body is denatured hemoglobin and is seen in G6PD deficiency. Remember that G6PD levels are normal in an acute attack and that the time to measure the level is 2 weeks after the acute attack. The most helpful test in the acute attack is the reticulocyte count (as the peripheral smear is almost always already given in a clinical scenario).

8. Hairy cell leukemia is seen with splenomegaly, a "dry" bone marrow tap, and an increased incidence of Legionella infections.

9. HUS (hemolytic-uremic syndrome) is seen in association with mitomycin C chemotherapy used in the treatment of metastatic anal cancer. It is also seen in *E. coli* 0157.H7 infections treated with antibiotics.

10. Bernard-Soulier disease is associated with a low platelet count, giant platelets, and a defect at the von Willebrand 's receptor causing problems with adhesion. Glanzmann's thrombasthenia has normal platelet count and size with a defect at the fibrinogen recep-

tor (glycoprotein 2b-3a) causing a problem with aggregation.

16.94   Year 2—Week 31—Day 3

1. Lead poisoning can lead to an acute gout attack.
2. Adenovirus is associated with GI disturbances as well as myocarditis cases.
3. Chlorpromazine can cause an elevated prolactin level.
4. Most hyperkalemia states caused by renal tubular acidosis type 4 can be handled by switching patients to low potassium diets.
5. Long-standing hypertension can lead to left ventricular hypertrophy of the heart and an increased risk for aortic dissection.
6. Mild bullous pemphigoid disease can be treated with topical steroid therapy.
7. Mild uveitis syndromes can be treated with ophthalmological steroids, thus being able to avoid systemic steroid side effects.
8. Vasoactive intestinal peptide tumors (VIPomas) have decreased pH values on nasogastric aspirate as opposed to gastrinomas which have increased pH value in aspirate.
9. Iris hamartomas are frequently found in neurofibromatosis type 1 as opposed to bilateral acoustic neuromas which are highly associated with neurofibromatosis type 2.
10. Beta-interferon is used in the treatment of multiple sclerosis syndromes. Alpha-interferon is used in the treatment of Mediterranean-type Kaposi's sarcoma.

16.95   Year 2—Week 32—Day 1

1. The DLCO is the key test in the PFTs that is most helpful in distinguishing whether interstitial lung disease is from extrinsic or intrinsic cause (low value in intrinsic cause).
2. Remember that emphysema is an obstructive lung disease that will have a low DLCO value.

3. Pulmonary hemorrhage (as seen in lupus diffuse alveolar hemorrhage) will cause an increased value to the DLCO.
4. High-dose steroid use for prolonged periods greater than four weeks can lead to a higher risk for Nocardia infections and Pneumocystis infections. Prophylaxis with trimethoprim-sulfamethoxazole should be considered.
5. The number one cause of hemoptysis in the USA is bronchitis. The second most common cause is bronchiectasis.
6. Chest physiotherapy has only proven of benefit in patients with underlying bronchiectasis as part of their pulmonary disease.
7. Colistin is an old aminoglycoside that is still used in treatment of cystic fibrosis patients with multidrug resistant Pseudomonas.
8. Patients with *Burkholderia cepacia* infections with underlying cystic fibrosis are generally not candidates for lung transplant.
9. Airway resistance, whether from mucus plugging or from undetected bronchospasm, will lead to significant difference between peak and plateau pressures on a ventilator.
10. Bilateral lung lavage under general anesthesia is the treatment of choice for patients afflicted with alveolar proteinosis.

16.96   Year 2—Week 32—Day 2

1. Patients with HIV disease are at higher risk of a skin condition known as eosinophilic folliculitis.
2. Use of steroids should be employed when treating tuberculous meningitis and pericarditis
3. Beta-2 microglobulin amyloid is the cause of carpal tunnel syndrome in patients with hemodialysis for greater than 5 years.
4. Amyloid is also the cause of cerebral lobar hemorrhages in the elderly in areas not expected to be affected by chronic hypertension.
5. Azathioprine (as well as 6-mercaptopurine) and L-asparaginase are common causes of drug-induced pancreatitis.

6. High-dose tetracycline and folic acid are used together in the treatment of patients with tropical sprue.

7. The tissue transglutaminase assay used in diagnosing celiac sprue is an offshoot of the anti-endomysial antibody.

8. Carbamazepine is the first-line treatment of trigeminal neuralgia.

9. Acetaminophen should still be answered as the boards answer for first-line treatment of osteoarthritis.

10. The presence of morning stiffness greater than 30 min with joint fluid WBC count above 3000 cells/CC makes an inflammatory arthritis (rather than osteoarthritis) the likely culprit in a patient with arthritis.

16.97   Year 2—Week 32—Day 3

1. Somatomedin C (IGF-1) is the screening test for acromegaly. It is confirmed by growth hormone levels before and after a glucose load is given. If hormonally positive test comes back, next step is MRI of the brain with attention to the pituitary.

2. Acromegaly, like all other functioning adenomas except for prolactinoma, is to be treated with transsphenoidal surgery.

3. Bromocriptine is the first-line treatment of prolactinoma EVEN if a visual field cut is present in a patient.

4. Prolactin levels in patients with prolactinoma are generally above 1000 mg/dL and nearly always above 200 mg/dL.

5. The first test to order in a young woman with elevated prolactin level and secondary amenorrhea is a pregnancy test.

6. The most common adenoma of the pituitary is a non-functioning adenoma. Some of these if large enough will cause elevation of the prolactin level by inhibiting dopamine due to compression effect on the pituitary stalk.

7. Severe hypothyroidism can cause elevation of the prolactin level. In this case, treat only the thyroid disease and the prolactin level should come back to normal. The mechanism for this prolactin level is felt to be an excessive level of TRH.

8. Hypophosphatemia can develop in treating a case of DKA, and theoretically, this could cause respiratory depression by not allowing the diaphragm to function appropriately.

9. Sternoclavicular hyperostosis is often associated with the finding of palmoplantar pustulosis.

10. Thiazolidinediones work by the peroxisomal proliferator activating system. Metformin belongs to the biguanide family of drugs.

16.98   Year 2—Week 33—Day 1

1. Acrodermatitis enteropathica is the acral scaly rash that is associated with zinc deficiency, which can be seen in TPN patients and alcohol abuse.

2. Scurvy can lead to severe systolic congestive heart failure if left untreated. Also, treat all patients with scurvy with thiamine as well as they have a high likelihood of concomitant beriberi disease.

3. Patients with chromium deficiency may have glucose intolerance.

4. Patients with selenium deficiency are predisposed to myalgias and hemolytic anemia.

5. Wilson's disease should be thought of in any young patient with liver disease with either neuropsychiatric features or hemolytic anemia present.

6. *Malassezia furfur* and *Candida albicans* are the two fungal organisms which one should be concerned about in cases of fungemia in patients with TPN.

7. Bronchopulmonary aspergillosis is treated with steroids and itraconazole.

8. Condyloma lata is a flat sessile lesion seen in the rectal area of patients with syphilis.

9. Condyloma acuminatum is a cauliflower-like raised warty lesion which can be seen in the genital area of patients afflicted with human papilloma virus.

10. Legionella pneumonia is first treated with azithromycin (rifampin reserved for synergism in only severe cases requiring ICU care). Fluoroquinolone therapy is also effective in those patients with intolerance to macrolides.

16.99   Year 2—Week 33—Day 2

1. Always be wary of atrial flutter in an arrythmia with a heart rate of 150 beats per minute.
2. Disopyramide is a class Ia anti-arrhythmic with significant anticholinergic effects which is used more often now for adjunct treatment of hypertrophic cardiomyopathy.
3. The first-line treatment of hypertrophic cardiomyopathy and prolonged QT syndrome is beta-blockers.
4. The causes of low voltage EKG include amyloid, COPD, obesity, hypothyroidism, and pericardial effusion.
5. Causes of periorbital edema include trichinosis, hypothyroidism, and nephrotic syndrome.
6. Wellen's sign describes critical stenosis of the proximal left anterior descending artery usually seen as deep T-wave inversions over leads V1–V3.
7. Multifocal atrial tachycardia can be seen in cases of theophylline toxicity.
8. Beta-2-microglobulin amyloid is the cause of carpal tunnel syndrome in patients with a long history of hemodialysis
9. Other causes of carpal tunnel syndrome include pregnancy, rheumatoid arthritis, multiple myeloma, diabetes mellitus, acromegaly, and hypothyroidism.
10. Primidone is the second-line agent for essential tremor if there is failure or contraindication to a beta-blocker.

16.100   Year 2—Week 33—Day 3

1. Patients may experience a flare of guttate psoriasis if they have a recent group A streptococcal infection.

2. Adenosine is the first-line drug to give in a patient with suspected SVT as it may break the arrythmia.
3. Bronchiectasis, the second most common cause of hemoptysis in the general population, may be seen in patients with common variable immunodeficiency.
4. Patients with common variable immunodeficiency have a higher incidence of celiac disease so consider this entity in these patients if they have iron deficiency anemia.
5. Selective IGA deficiency is the most common immunodeficiency found in the adult population.
6. Leflunomide is a pyrimidine nucleotide inhibitor which may be added to the treatment of rheumatoid arthritis patients not completely responding to methotrexate.
7. The side effects of leflunomide include liver toxicity and diarrhea.
8. A PPD skin test needs to be checked on all patients before beginning therapy with a TNF-alpha receptor blocker such as infliximab or etanercept.
9. Post-CABG syndrome involves the formation of a left pleural effusion usually within 2–3 months after a CABG is performed. Most of these effusions go away on their own.
10. Patients with ankylosing spondylitis are at risk of anterior uveitis, apical pulmonary fibrosis, aortic insufficiency, IGA syndrome, and amyloidosis.

16.101   Year 2—Week 34—Day 1

1. Patients with pustular psoriasis may experience flares during or shortly after receiving treatment with oral steroids.
2. In general, topical steroids and oral steroids worsen the condition of acne rosacea.
3. Non-comedonal acne usually responds to topical combination of erythromycin/benzoyl peroxide solution. Comedonal acne usually responds to topical retinoic acid.
4. Cystic acne can be treated with oral retinoic acid (accutane). Side effects include birth

defects, hypertriglyceridemia, hypercalce-mia, and pseudotumor cerebri.

5. Lichen planus lesions and pemphigus vulgaris lesions can occur in the oral cavity in patients afflicted with skin disease with these conditions.

6. Bullous pemphigoid, unlike pemphigus vulgaris, does not have a risk for paraneoplastic disease.

7. Enterococcus faecalis is best treated with linezolid. Side effect of that medication is neutropenia.

8. Daptomycin may lead to renal failure with or without rhabdomyolysis, so always check a CPK level if creatinine begins to elevate.

9. There is a drug–drug interaction between azathioprine and allopurinol, so always try to avoid using the two together if possible.

10. Colchicine is used for gouty arthritis management in many transplant patients as single agent treatment.

16.102   Year 2—Week 34—Day 2

1. If a patient has an isolated lung abscess, physicians should not attempt drainage from the exterior as one would do for empyema and physicians should delay bronchoscopy for a few weeks while the patient is on antibiotics. Eventually, all patients with lung abscess should have airway evaluation with bronchoscopy.

2. Infliximab is used in Crohn's disease patients with fistulas with great effectiveness in controlling disease.

3. Smoking worsens Crohn's disease, whereas it is felt to be protective against ulcerative colitis.

4. The anti-Saccharomyces cerevisiae antibodies (ASCA) can be positive in Crohn's disease patients.

5. Autoimmune hepatitis is marked by positive anti-smooth muscle antibodies or anti-liver-kidney-microsomal antibodies. Treatment is steroids.

6. Primary biliary cirrhosis is best treated in early disease state with ursodeoxycholic acid.

7. Stenotrophomonas infections are universally resistant to imipenem. Use trimethoprim-sulfamethoxazole or fluoroquinolone therapy for treatment.

8. Do not forget that ticarcillin-clavulanate has active coverage against Pseudomonas.

9. Chlorthalidone is a thiazide diuretic similar to hydrochlorothiazide that can be used in treatment of isolated systolic hypertension.

10. Avoid NSAID therapy in patients with active congestive heart failure exacerbation (CHF), and one should use only sparingly (if no other agent can be substituted) in those who carry CHF in their past medical history.

16.103   Year 2—Week 34—Day 3

1. Recurrent pneumonia with no evidence of airway obstruction should lead one to exclude common variable immunodeficiency (CVID).

2. Eplerenone is an aldosterone blocker that does not seem to have the side effects of gynecomastia and tenderness to breast area that are part of spironolactone's profile.

3. SBP facts are the following: most common organism is *E. coli* and first-line drug is cefotaxime.

4. Patients on beta-blockers who become anaphylactic may need glucagon if they do not respond initially to epinephrine.

5. The most common cause for a pause in the general population is a blocked premature atrial contraction.

6. Chancroid causes a painful chancre and can lead to lymphadenopathy. Treatment can be with fluoroquinolone or macrolide.

7. Secondary syphilis can lead to a diffuse rash that mimics lichen planus or pityriasis rosea. When in doubt, check an RPR and anti-treponemal antibody.

8. Posterior herniation of the nucleus pulposus is more common that anterior due to the

weaker nature of the posterior longitudinal ligament.

9. Drooping of the toes in heel-walking maneuvers is suggestive of L5 root impingement.

10. Drooping of the ankle in toe-walking maneuver is suggestive of S1 root impingement.

16.104 Year 2—Week 35—Day 1

1. The differential diagnosis for leptomeningeal enhancement in a patient with HIV disease includes syphilis, toxoplasmosis, tuberculosis, sarcoidosis, and cancer (such as lymphoma).

2. The highly HIV-associated cancers are felt to be invasive cervical cancer, systemic non-Hodgkin's lymphoma, and CNS non-Hodgkin's lymphoma.

3. Rhodococcus equi is an organism that can cause cavitary lung disease in patients with HIV disease, and classic history would state something about the patient being near horses or horse farms.

4. Linezolid is used mostly to treat *Enterococcus faecalis* and *Enterococcus faecium*. It can cause drug-induced neutropenia.

5. Osteoarthritis is the most common arthritis in the general population. First-line treatment is acetaminophen. There is no morning stiffness with this condition.

6. Leflunomide can lead to diarrhea and LFT abnormalities and it is used to treat rheumatoid arthritis patients not responding to methotrexate.

7. Gold and D-penicillamine are old drugs used for R.A. which can lead to nephrotic syndrome. Gold can also cause a horrific exfoliative dermatitis.

8. Lupus arthritis is inflammatory but not erosive. Thus, morning stiffness usually occurs but X-rays of the hands are generally unremarkable except for generalized osteoporosis. Ulnar deviation occurs due to ligament laxity from recurrent bouts of inflammation.

9. Hydroxychloroquine is the first-line agent to treat lupus arthritis and skin manifestations. It can cause retinal toxicity.

10. First-line agent to treat psoriatic arthritis is methotrexate. The dose should be pushed to close to 15 mg per week at minimum before the medication is felt to be ineffective in treatment.

16.105 Year 2—Week 35—Day 2

1. Digoxin toxicity is worsened in the setting of hypokalemia. Do not shock patients with digoxin toxicity. Use FAB-ligand therapy if there is a life-threatening arrythmia.

2. Causes of AV dissociation include third-degree AV block, sinus or pacemaker (junctional or sinus), and accelerated rhythms (such as ventricular tachycardia).

3. Meningiomas are dural based, calcified, and usually located along cerebral convexities.

4. Nystagmus can be an associated finding in patients with multiple sclerosis who have lesions of the medial longitudinal fasciculus.

5. There are no sensory findings in patients with amyotrophic lateral sclerosis.

6. There can be sensory findings in about 1/3 of patients with Guillain-Barre syndrome. Do not forget that areflexia is the key to thinking about this syndrome.

7. Plasmapheresis is the treatment of choice for patients with Guillain-Barre syndrome with IVIG as an alternative. Combination treatment has shown no benefit.

8. Phlebotomy helps heart failure symptoms the most in patients with hemochromatosis.

9. Wilson's disease is treated with D-penicillamine acutely and then chronically with zinc.

10. Ursodeoxycholic acid is the first-line treatment for primary biliary cirrhosis.

16.106 Year 2—Week 35—Day 3

1. Amantadine is used for the chronic fatigue syndrome of multiple sclerosis.

2. Drugs that impact the course of multiple sclerosis include mitoxantrone, beta-interferon, and glatiramer acetate.

3. Use methylprednisolone in acute bouts of multiple sclerosis such as treating neurological deficits.

4. Pontine infarcts are marked by history of hypertension, and feature small pupils and the risk of locked-in syndrome.

5. Wallenberg's syndrome is marked by dysphagia, ataxia, and a unilateral Horner's syndrome and involves an infarct at the lateral medulla.

6. Amyloid can cause pinch purpura around the eyelids after a Valsalva maneuver.

7. Raynaud phenomenon is treated with calcium channel blockers as first-line and alpha-blockers as second-line agent.

8. Dermatofibromas should be monitored as if they increase in size acutely, they may transform into dermatofibrosarcomas.

9. Granuloma annulare, diabetic dermopathy, necrobiosis lipoidica diabeticorum, cheiroarthropathy, and diffuse idiopathic skeletal hyperostosis (DISH) are all conditions associated with diabetes mellitus.

10. Mohs microsurgery is used for basal cell cancers involving nose or nasolabial area, and it is also used for Merkel cell cancer.

16.107   Year 2—Week 36—Day 1

1. Merkel cell cancer is a skin neuroendocrine cancer which requires wide margins on excision.

2. Thyroglobulin is a tumor marker for papillary and follicular thyroid cancer.

3. CEA level may be slightly elevated in smokers.

4. Calcitonin levels are useful when working up patients for medullary cancer of the thyroid. Always exclude pheochromocytoma before proceeding to surgery.

5. There is a correlation between coronary vasospasm and migraine headaches.

6. Cluster headaches run higher in males and are treated with 100% oxygen acutely. Pain usually lasts as short as 15 minutes and rarely longer than 2–3 hours. Nasal congestion may be seen during acute attacks.

7. Hemicranium continuum is more common in females and attacks tend to linger for days (uncommon in cluster headaches). Use indomethacin for acute treatment.

8. Screen for acromegaly with somatomedin C level (IGF-2). Surgery is the treatment for acromegaly. Octreotide and radiation therapy are only used for surgery refractory disease.

9. Prolactinomas are always treated medically first, except for very rare cases. Treat these lesions with cabergoline or bromocriptine.

10. Prolactin levels can be elevated between 40 and 200 mg/dL in situations such as pregnancy, phenothiazine use, severe hypothyroidism, and non-functioning adenomas that cause stalk effect.

16.108   Year 2—Week 36—Day 2

1. Carbamazepine and SSRIs are known to lead to drug-induced hyponatremia through an SIADH-like process. Watch out for hyperreflexia, increased temperature, and agitation in patients on SSRIs as they are at risk for serotonin syndrome. Treatment would be with cyproheptadine (peri-actin) and discontinuation of SSRI.

2. Of the seven porphyrias, know only two enzyme deficiencies for testing purposes. One is uroporphyrinogen decarboxylase which is abnormal in patients with porphyria cutanea tarda. The other is an enzyme known by 2 names, HMB (hydroxymethylbilane) synthase or PBG (porphyrobilinogen) deaminase, which is deficient in acute intermittent porphyria.

3. A simple screen for porphyrias is to do a 24-h urine collection for porphyrins.

4. The meningitis classic for an increased opening pressure is cryptococcus.

5. 10% of pheochromocytomas are bilateral, 10% are malignant, and 10% are extra-adrenal.

6. The three cardinal signs of aortic stenosis are angina, syncope, and heart failure. Surgery is indicated when the patient becomes symptomatic with any one of these. The next step in management before surgery is a cardiac catheterization.

7. The anti-Ro antibody is seen in congenital lupus heart block, subacute cutaneous lupus erythematosus, and Sjogren's syndrome.

8. There is a risk for lymphoma with both Sjogren's and rheumatoid arthritis.

9. The drugs causing gingival hyperplasia are dilantin, calcium channel blockers, and cyclosporine.

10. Niacin deficiency must be ruled out in all patients with carcinoid syndrome.

16.109 Year 2—Week 36—Day 3

1. Platelets are stored at room temperature; thus, there is a higher risk for bacteremia associated with this transfusion compared to other blood product transfusions.

2. Most reactions to vancomycin (reddish discoloration of neck and face) can be overcome by slowing the infusion rate.

3. IGA deficiency patients are at risk of anaphylaxis when receiving blood products.

4. Hypoglycorrhachia (low glucose in CSF) is unique to the salicylate toxicities among all the poisonings.

5. Lithium toxicity may cause a false high chloride level elevation.

6. NSAID over the counter use is still one of the most common reasons that patients develop elevated serum lithium levels

7. Centrilobular necrosis is the classic pathology in acetaminophen poisoning, which is treated with N-acetylcysteine.

8. One of the most common reasons for diplopia is a cranial nerve palsy.

9. Diabetics do not get pupillary abnormalities when they have cranial nerve palsies as the afferent fibers run on the outside of the nerve and are unlikely to get affected by infarction. Contrast this to an aneurysm which would cause cranial nerve abnormalities as it compresses the optic nerve and causes a cranial nerve palsy.

10. The most common reason for fever associated with blood transfusion is the febrile non-hemolytic transfusion reaction.

16.110 Year 2—Week 37—Day 1

1. One of the biggest clues to an ABO incompatibility transfusion reaction is pain at the infusion site and back pain.

2. There is a strong correlation between EBV in the CSF and CNS lymphoma of the brain.

3. The most common cause of erysipelas cellulitis is group A streptococcus.

4. Babesiosis presents with RBC inclusions and a hemolytic anemia. Treat with either quinine and clindamycin *or* azithromycin and atovaquone. The disease may be spread by blood transfusion and from mother to child through the placenta but is not transmitted person to person.

5. Ehrlichiosis is marked by WBC inclusions, and one sees thrombocytopenia, splenomegaly, and transaminitis as part of the disease process. A rash is usually not present. Human granulocytic ehrlichiosis is now referred to by the term "anaplasmosis" and is transmitted by the deer tick.

6. Use ceftriaxone to treat endocarditis caused by the HACEK organisms. Use ceftriaxone as well to treat severe Lyme disease carditis and meningoencephalitis.

7. A very high ferritin can be seen in patients with Still's disease. This is likely due to IL-6 over-stimulation.

8. Erysipeloid is a rash usually found on the hands of fish handlers and meat cutters and resembles erysipelas (swollen cellulitis area with violaceous hue and very well demarcated borders). This disease is caused by *Erysipelothrix rhusiopathiae*.

9. Amoxicillin-clavulanate is the drug of choice for significant traumatic cat and dog bites but other options include clindamycin plus ciprofloxacin twice a day as well as doxycycline twice a day.

10. If a fluoroquinolone or trimethoprim-sulfamethoxazole will be used in the treatment of cat and dog bites, it must be combined with metronidazole or clindamycine.

16.111 Year 2—week 37—Day 2

1. Patients with inferior MI with hypotension should be looked at for evidence of right ventricular infarction. Use normal saline to improve preload and improve blood pressure.
2. Beta-blockers and benzodiazepines are excellent choices for pharmacological therapy in treatment of patients with serotonin syndrome.
3. Ziprasidone can increase the QT interval so baseline EKG on all is essential.
4. Prolongation of the QT interval can occur with citalopram therapy.
5. The first-line treatment of inherited prolonged QT syndromes is beta-blocker therapy.
6. Disopyramide has been used as an adjunct to beta-blockers in treatment of hypertrophic cardiomyopathy.
7. Disopyramide and oxybutynin can have significant anticholinergic side effects. This may lead to delirium syndrome in the elderly.
8. Although secondary amine TCAs like nortriptyline and desipramine are better than tertiary amine TCAs, anticholinergic effects and orthostatic hypotension are still possible.
9. Midodrine can cause supine driven hypertension.
10. Avoid using "triptan" medications more than twice a week in a regimen for migraine prophylaxis.

16.112 Year 2—Week 37—Day 3

1. Patients with large cell cancer of the lung might have the finding of gynecomastia and elevated HCG levels.

2. Bronchoalveolar carcinoma of the lung can be quite aggressive and is usually found with bilateral interstitial spread. It can present in non-smokers. It can present with mucoid-like production.
3. Patients with a nodular lesion in the umbilicus might have an internal malignancy, such as gastric cancer. This nodule has been referred as the Sister Mary Joseph nodule.
4. Valproic acid is the anti-epileptic medication most linked to alopecia.
5. Hypothyroidism should be ruled out in all patients presenting with alopecia.
6. Thyroglobulin can be used as a tumor marker for patients with follicular or papillary thyroid cancer.
7. Calcitonin is the tumor marker for patients with medullary cancer of the thyroid.
8. Diffuse alveolar hemorrhage may occur in patients with systemic lupus erythematosus.
9. Pruritis may be noted as one of the earliest signs of patients afflicted with acute myelogenous leukemia.
10. Generalized psoriasis might require the use of methotrexate or TNF alpha inhibitor therapy if there is no improvement with topical therapy.

16.113 Year 2—Week 38—Day 1

1. If inpatient surgery is planned on a patient with medullary carcinoma of the thyroid, then one must have been sure that the diagnosis of pheochromocytoma was ruled out as it could lead to hypertensive crisis during surgery if the diagnosis was not pursued.
2. MEN II is marked by hyperparathyroidism, medullary cancer of the thyroid, and pheochromocytoma. MEN syndromes have autosomal dominant inheritance.
3. Primary hyperparathyroidism can lead to hypercalcemia which may cause pancreatitis. The difficulty in diagnosing this entity is that the serum calcium level will drop in an acute attack of pancreatitis due to saponification process induced by pancreatic enzyme necrosis.

4. The serum phosphorus level is usually low in primary hyperparathyroidism.

5. The serum phosphorus level may theoretically drop in the process of treating the acidosis of diabetic ketoacidosis. The risk of severe hypophosphatemia is of respiratory failure due to inability of diaphragm to properly work.

6. In an inpatient recently started on anticoagulation (within a few days) who suddenly develops hypotension and hyperkalemia, you must think about acute adrenal insufficiency due to adrenal hemorrhage from anticoagulation.

7. In an adult patient admitted to the hospital with diabetic ketoacidosis, one should rule out the following as possible cause for the process of DKA: (1) infection, (2) myocardial infarction or ischemia, (3) early Graves' disease, (4) pregnancy, and (5) drug abuse, particularly cocaine.

8. There is a thyroid bruit associated with most cases of Graves' disease.

9. Propranolol is the beta-blocker of choice when treating the palpitations associated with Graves' disease as it will also block peripheral conversion of T4 to T3.

10. Mineralocorticoid therapy can be used to lower serum potassium level in patients with type 4 RTA.

16.114 Year 2—Week 38—Day 2

1. Patients can be above age 50 and be diagnosed with type 1 diabetes mellitus. Type 1 DKA patients may have positive antibody assays for anti-insulin, anti-islet cell, and anti-glutamic decarboxylase antibodies.

2. The most important management aspect of patients with type 2 diabetes mellitus admitted to the hospital with nonketotic hyperosmolar coma is the fact that they are likely quite dehydrated and will need IV fluid replacement.

3. Ticarcillin-clavulanate can be used for the treatment of diabetic foot ulcers as it does cover Pseudomonas.

4. Isolated cranial nerve palsies with normal pupillary responses can be seen in patients with diabetes mellitus.

5. If a patient is admitted to the hospital with palpitations and a TSH level of less than .001 mg/dL, one should suspect hyperthyroidism. The first step in management is to confirm that the patient is truly in a hyperthyroid state, which is done by obtaining a free T4 level and a total T3 level (at least one should be high).

6. Struma ovarii is associated with low uptake on radioactive uptake study, while choriocarcinoma is associated with high uptake on the study.

7. Metronidazole is the treatment of choice for Giardia, bacterial vaginosis, and Trichomonas.

8. Thyroid storm is actually rarely ever encountered. A fever must be present to make the diagnosis of this state. Other key features include extreme tachycardia (more than would be expected as compensation for fever which is usually 10 beats/minute for every degree above 100 degrees Fahrenheit), central nervous system signs, and marked GI system disturbances.

9. The key to managing thyroid storm is to first administer antithyroid agents at high doses (e.g., PTU at dose of 100mg every 2 h) and soon after that to start stable iodine compounds such as Lugol's solution or SSKI (saturated solution of potassium iodide) which will further inhibit the release of thyroid hormone. An acceptable substitute to the stable iodine is a compound known as sodium ipodate, which can also block conversion to T3 from T4. Propranolol is the beta-blocker of choice, except in really severe cases where IV esmolol needs to be given. As the adrenal gland may be susceptible to the effects of thyroid storm, IV dexamethasone is also given as well.

10. Beta-blockers, lithium, and anti-malarial agents can lead to the worsening state of underlying psoriasis.

16.115 Year 2—Week 38—Day 3

1. Lithium can interact with all NSAIDs, but particularly avoid indomethacin if an NSAID must be used.
2. One can treat through the hypothyroidism induced by lithium.
3. One can use amiloride to try to treat through nephrogenic diabetes insipidus if lithium therapy cannot be discontinued. Lithium use can lead to that renal state.
4. NSAIDs, thiazide diuretics, and cyclosporine can mimic porphyria cutanea tarda and cause a condition known as pseudoporphyria.
5. Patients with pseudoporphyria can present with bullous lesions like porphyria cutanea tarda (PCT), but they do not get hyperpigmentation, hypertrichosis, or the slight tightening of the skin that can be seen with PCT.
6. Chronic kidney disease and hemodialysis itself are rarer associations with porphyria cutanea tarda.
7. Both hepatitis B and hepatitis C can cause cryoglobulinemia. Plasmapheresis may be needed for treatment in severe cases.
8. Serum sickness is only seen in the viral hepatitis in the realm of acute hepatitis B. It may cause a hemorrhagic skin condition known as the Arthus reaction.
9. Always vaccinate patients with chronic liver disease with hepatitis A vaccine if they have no prior history of the disease.
10. Patients with ischemic liver disease can present with AST and ALT levels into the tens of thousands. The clue to this condition is that the ALT will stay persistently elevated a lot longer than the AST and will generally be higher than the AST nearly always in initial presentation.

16.116 Year 2—Week 39—Day 1

1. Osteomalacia may be seen in patients who are frequently admitted to the hospital from nursing homes. Patients with this state have vitamin D deficiency, and the test to check is a 25 hydroxyvitamin D level (not the 1,25 dihydroxyvitamin D level which should be checked in states of toxicity or suspected hypercalcemia). Osteomalacia may lead to bone pain and can even appear as pseudo-fractures on X-rays.
2. Many of you may notice an increased alkaline phosphatase in many of your admissions to the hospital. When these patients have normal liver enzymes, you should suspect that the elevation is likely due to Paget's disease (of bone). These patients generally do not get hypercalcemic unless they are immobilized for a very long period of time (much longer than even a long hospitalization).
3. Paget's disease carries with it a small risk of osteosarcoma so monitor the alkaline phosphatase level.
4. Inpatients with osteomalacia may also have elevated alkaline phosphatase levels and the way to distinguish from Paget's disease is that the patients with osteomalacia will also have low calcium and low phosphorus levels usually.
5. Klebsiella is a common pathogen among nursing home patients with pneumonia. It is associated with currant jelly sputum and can lead to a bulging fissure sign on CXR.
6. Linezolid can be used for the treatment of MRSA pneumonia.
7. Clindamycin is the drug of choice for patients with Lemierre's syndrome who are allergic to penicillin.
8. Desensitization to aspirin can be performed and the patient can be maintained on a certain dose of aspirin or NSAID such that he never needs to be desensitized again
9. Patients desensitized to treat syphilis, for instance, with penicillin must be desensi-

tized again the next time they get an infection and penicillin is thought to be used as they would have needed continual exposure to PCN to avoid a repeat desensitization procedure.

10. Among the paraneoplastic processes in small cell lung cancer are ectopic ACTH syndrome, Eaton-Lambert syndrome, and subacute cerebellar syndrome.

16.117 Year 2—Week 39—Day 2

1. CH50 is a good screening tool to find any complement deficiency that may be present.
2. Factor D and properdin levels may be low in patients with recurrent meningococcal infections (besides the classic C5-C9 you have memorized).
3. Patients with hereditary angioedema will have low C4 levels "**FOUR-ever" (forever).** C2 levels will be low during attacks.
4. Treat hereditary angioedema patients with anabolic steroids.
5. Patients are more likely to get mechanical complications (such as free wall rupture) after their first MI rather than after subsequent MI's.
6. Papillary muscle rupture usually occurs in the setting of an inferior wall MI.
7. Second-degree heart block Mobitz type 1 usually occurs with inferior MIs.
8. Second-degree heart block Mobitz type 2 usually occurs with anterior MIs.
9. Procainamide and hydralazine are associated with drug-induced lupus (anti-histone antibodies).
10. Rheumatoid factor can be positive in conditions such as mixed cryoglobulinemia and endocarditis.

16.118 Year 2—Week 39—Day 3

1. Hypoparathyroidism can be seen in patients admitted with episodes of mucocutaneous candidiasis as these states keep company in the setting of autoimmune polyglandular syndromes (inheritance by autosomal recessive mechanism).
2. Patients with hypoparathyroidism who are admitted to the hospital with papilledema and severe headaches may have pseudotumor cerebri. Pseudotumor cerebri can also be seen in patients with vitamin A toxicity and patients using steroids.
3. Patients admitted in the hospital on "stress dose" steroid regimen, involving doses of hydrocortisone usually above 50 mg every 8 h, do not need additional fludrocortisone therapy, as the high-dose hydrocortisone therapy will provide cross-over mineralocorticoid activity along with the expected glucocorticoid activity.
4. The most common reason for inpatients to have secondary adrenal insufficiency in the hospital is unawareness that the patient was on a maintenance dose of prednisone. After a few days without receiving prednisone (usually above or equal to 7.5 mg a day) in the setting of an acute illness as an inpatient, hypotension will ensue. Hyperkalemia will not ensue as this is not a primary adrenal insufficiency problem.
5. If an inpatient admitted with lower GI bleeding due to colonic polyps is also noted to have prominent jaw features, to have daily unexplained headaches, to have recurrent carpal tunnel syndrome, and to have diabetes mellitus, one should suspect acromegaly. Acromegaly is associated with an increased incidence of colonic polyps.
6. Screening for acromegaly would involve drawing a somatomedin C level (insulin growth factor I level). If this test is positive, then one should proceed to give the patient a glucose load which should suppress the growth hormone level usually below 2 picograms/nL. If growth hormone level is not suppressed, the next step in management is to go ahead and get an MRI with attention to the pituitary gland looking for an adenoma.
7. The treatment of growth hormone adenoma would be surgical therapy via transsphenoidal approach. All functioning adenomas are treated with surgery except for prolactino-

mas, which are managed medically with bromocriptine as usual first-line agent.

8. Patients with severe hypothyroidism (but not yet myxedema coma) may require admission into the hospital if faced with severe bradycardia or shortness of breath which could be due to either a pericardial effusion or a pleural effusion. Pleural effusions with this state tend to be transudative, although they could also be exudative.

9. Patients with severe hypothyroidism can also be noted to have slightly elevated prolactin levels, which come back down to normal without using bromocriptine (simply treat the primary hypothyroidism).

10. Autonomic dysreflexia is a common finding in patients with Guillain-Barre syndrome (acute inflammatory demyelinating neuropathy).

16.119 Year 2—Week 40—Day 1

1. Patients admitted to the hospital with myxedema coma must first receive IV hydrocortisone before starting IV thyroid hormone. The reason for this fact is that there is a high correlation of adrenal insufficiency (usually primary) with severe hypothyroidism in this situation. The term Schmidt's syndrome has been used to further add substance to the common finding of primary adrenal insufficiency with hypothyroidism. It would be disastrous to give IV hydrocortisone without ruling out adrenal insufficiency in a patient with myxedema coma (it would send the patient into a life-threatening adrenal crisis).

2. Death in adrenal crisis is usually due to either a hypoglycemic cerebral crisis or a ventricular arrhythmia in the setting of hyperkalemia.

3. Patients with symptomatic hyponatremia may be admitted to the hospital for an inpatient workup. SIADH (syndrome of inappropriate diuretic hormone) is a common cause of hyponatremia. In SIADH, there is usually a low BUN (classically less than 10 mg/dl), normal creatinine, and a low uric acid with the most classic finding being an inappropri-

ately elevated urine osmolality for a given plasma osmolality.

4. Patients should be ruled out for adrenal insufficiency and hypothyroidism before a diagnosis of SIADH is given. Usually, lung and CNS processes (such as aggressive pneumonia, lung cancer, and head trauma) are responsible for causing SIADH and treating the underlying cause is the key to resolution of the process.

5. The five diseases **most closely** associated with low complement levels (C3 or C4) in the setting of acute renal failure are postinfectious glomerulonephritis, lupus, membranoproliferative glomerulonephritis, cholesterol emboli syndrome, and cryoglobulinemia.

6. In patients with acute hepatitis B, admission to the hospital may be required for monitoring if they present with arthralgias, urticaria, a necrotic skin rash (Arthus reaction), and acute renal failure. These patients have acute renal failure due to antigen–antibody complex deposition in the kidney. This constellation of findings is known as serum sickness and it is a type III allergic reaction.

7. Whipple's disease and Nocardia are treated first-line with sulfa-based antibiotic therapy.

8. Watch out for hyperkalemia when treating patients with *Pneumocystis jirovecii* with IV sulfamethoxazole-trimethoprim.

9. Atovaquone and pentamidine can be used for acutely treating *Pneumocystis jirovecii* infection.

10. Cocaine and cigarette smoke users are at higher risk of pneumothorax than the general population.

16.120 Year 2—Week 40—Day 2

1. NSAID sensitivity is not IGE mediated, so skin testing is not an effective means of ruling out the diagnosis.

2. Of the common NSAIDs used in clinical practice, salsalate is the safest to use in a patient who might have the aspirin triad due to lesser degree of cyclooxygenase inhibition.

3. Patients with a history of penicillin allergy are at risk for anaphylaxis with carbapenems.
4. Monobactams (aztreonam) do not contain the bicyclic ring of the beta-lactams and thus do not cross-react with penicillin. The side chain of aztreonam does cross-react with ceftazidime and this may account for allergic reactions common to both medications.
5. Allergy to radiocontrast media is not IGE mediated (thus it is anaphylactoid) and a history of previous seafood allergy is not predictive of risk.
6. Patients with cholesterol emboli syndrome can be admitted with acute renal failure.
7. Watch out for CLL causing new onset angioedema in the elderly population.
8. Patients with Waldenstrom's macroglobulinemia do not get bone pain. They usually get headaches and visual loss as presenting symptoms.
9. IVIG is the treatment of patients with chronic idiopathic demyelinating polyneuropathy.
10. One can continue treatment with lithium even if a patient becomes hypothyroid on the medication as one can provide supplemental thyroid hormone.

16.121 Year 2—Week 40—Day 3

1. NSAID use will promote sodium reabsorption and in turn lithium reabsorption by the kidney leading to the potential for toxicity states.
2. One of the subtle signs of adrenal insufficiency is hyperpigmentation of the oral mucosa.
3. Renal failure can lead to hypocalcemia and hyperphosphatemia with secondary increase in PTH level and drop of dihydroxyvitamin D levels (1, 25-dihydroxyvitamin D).
4. Think of free wall rupture in a patient with hypotension and syncope who is in the hospital after his first myocardial infarction a few days ago. Immediate CT surgery consultation is required and outcome even with surgery is generally poor.

5. A mechanical complication of inferior wall MI is papillary muscle rupture which can present with acute mitral regurgitation (holosystolic murmur best heard at apex).
6. Peutz-Jeghers syndrome involves freckling of lips with risk for small bowel hamartomas and large bowel adenocarcinoma.
7. Li-Fraumeni syndrome is a familial cancer syndrome associated with adrenal cortical (not medullary) cancer, soft tissue sarcoma, osteosarcoma, and leukemias.
8. Trochanteric bursitis involves pain at the hip when you lie on that affected side and pain at the hip when you abduct the hip.
9. Iliotibial band syndrome is the most common cause of lateral leg pain in the general population. Pain is worsened when one adducts the leg.
10. Marginal joint erosions are classic on X-rays of patients with rheumatoid arthritis.

16.122 Year 2—Week 41—Day 1

1. The most common cause of hemoptysis in the general population is acute bronchitis. Bronchiectasis is the second most common cause.
2. The joint fluid WBC count in osteoarthritis will be under 3000/mL in most circumstances.
3. Bronchoscopy is usually delayed for a few weeks if not longer in patients being treated for lung abscess. No drainage necessary as far as lung a bscess in comparison to empyema.
4. Coccidiomycosis causes thin-walled cavitary disease in lung (less than 4 mm).
5. Anagrelide inhibits megakaryocyte maturation and thus is useful in myeloproliferative disorders with extreme thrombocytosis when hydroxyurea fails.
6. Aminocaproic acid inhibits plasminogen activator substances and thus can help in conditions such as primary systemic fibrinolysis.

7. High output heart failure can be seen in diseases such as Paget's disease, beriberi, and massive hepatic hemangiomas.

8. Etoposide has been associated with increased leukemogenic risk, meaning it can itself lead to AML (acute myelogenous leukemia).

9. Among the entities that should be ruled out in cases of iron deficiency anemia is celiac sprue disease.

10. Activated resistance to protein C is reflected by the genetic test of factor V Leiden.

16.123 Year 2—Week 41—Day 2

1. Wilson's disease can present with a hemolytic anemia along with neuropsychiatric features.

2. Acute treatment for Wilson's disease involves use of D-penicillamine. Zinc is used for chronic treatment of copper binding.

3. There tends to be a decreased tendency to progress to hepatocellular carcinoma with Wilson's disease when compared to other diseases that lead to liver fibrosis and cirrhosis.

4. Patients with polycystic kidney disease can have berry aneurysms of the circle of Willis, hepatic cysts, and diverticular disease.

5. Workup of small cell lung cancer includes a total body bone scan and MRI of the brain.

6. Carcinoid syndrome can involve all right-sided valves, not only the tricuspid valve.

7. The first-line treatment for histiocytosis X (eosinophilic granuloma) is smoking cessation.

8. ALS and myasthenia gravis can lead to restrictive lung disease with normal DLCO measurements.

9. Rifampin can lower dilantin levels so be sure to monitor level during treatment with rifampin.

10. Digital infarcts (on tips of fingers) can be seen with rheumatoid arthritis, scleroderma, and antiphospholipid antibody syndrome.

16.124 Year 2—Week 41—Day 3

1. Patients may suffer severe hypocalcemia post-operatively after parathyroid surgery. The first thing to ensure is that the patient has a normal magnesium level as it is a required factor for normal PTH function.

2. *Mycobacterium marinum* can lead to a sporotrichoid pattern of infection with a distal ulcer that spreads up the arm along the lymphatics.

3. Achalasia, tylosis, and Plummer-Vinson syndrome are risk factors for squamous cell cancer of the esophagus.

4. Gingival hyperplasia can be seen with AML type M4 or M5 and use of dilantin, cyclosporine, or dihydropyridine calcium channel blockers (like nifedipine).

5. Dermatomyositis can be associated with ovarian or lung cancer.

6. Polymyositis can be seen with keratosis of dorsal surface of hands (mechanic's hands) and interstitial fibrosis.

7. Methotrexate is the drug of choice for aggressive psoriatic arthritis.

8. Leflunomide can be added to methotrexate if a patient with rheumatoid arthritis needs a boost in therapy.

9. Morning stiffness duration is probably the best indicator of response to anti-inflammatory therapy in rheumatoid arthritis.

10. The first-line treatment of trochanteric bursitis is a corticosteroid injection into the bursae, rather than systemic NSAID therapy.

16.125 Year 2—Week 42—Day 1

1. Lupus is associated with interphalangeal erythema, whereas dermatomyositis features discoloration directly above the joint areas.

2. Ace-inhibitors are the drug of choice for patients with scleroderma renal crises.

3. The EPHESUS study showed there was benefit to post-MI patients with low ejection fraction in adding aldosterone blockade to ace-inhibitor and beta-blocker therapy.

4. Patients with subacute cutaneous lupus erythematosus can demonstrate a psoriasiform rash. This rash will worsen with sunlight as do nearly all skin manifestations of lupus.
5. The first-line treatment of discoid lupus is hydroxychloroquine.
6. Thalidomide has been used in treatment of refractory cases of discoid lupus and multiple myeloma.
7. Leflunomide is associated with hepatotoxicity besides its better known side effect of diarrhea.
8. Patients with Legionella pulmonary infections can present with abdominal pain, hyponatremia, and elevated CPK values (the constellation of all three being known as Pontiac fever).
9. The most common finding in a patient with primary hyperparathyroidism is to find a single autonomous adenoma.
10. The second most common finding in a patient with primary hyperparathyroidism is to find general parathyroid hyperplasia.

16.126 Year 2—Week 42—Day 2

1. It is safe to perform paracentesis in patients with INRs that are elevated mildly (up to 3.0–4.0) as there is rare bleeding with this procedure.
2. Appendix may lie on left side or retrocecal/pelvis position so don't always look for the classic right sided pain with this condition.
3. Appendicitis in pregnancy may actually present with right upper quadrant pain. Appendectomy is the most common surgery performed during pregnancy.
4. Patients with acute fatty liver of pregnancy generally present with encephalopathy. Patients with intrahepatic cholestasis of pregnancy generally present with itching.
5. Danazol is used in the treatment of hereditary angioedema but also can be used in the treatment of autoimmune hemolytic anemia.
6. The first step in management of relapsed autoimmune hemolytic anemia states is to make sure the steroid dose is up to at least 1mg/kg

daily before considering steroid-sparing agent additions.
7. Temporal arteritis patients may present with aortic dissection years after initial diagnosis.
8. Patients with hepatitis A will generally have a positive hepatitis A IgM titer at the time of presentation.
9. Hepatitis B "e" antigen reflects active replication of virus and confers a very contagious state.
10. Serum sickness is a common cause of acute renal failure in patients with acute hepatitis B infection (not chronic hepatitis B infection).

16.127 Year 2—Week 42—Day 3

1. Abciximab may lead to a pseudo-thrombocytopenia state within several hours of administration. Abciximab is a glycoprotein 2b-3a inhibitor that is used in treatment of acute myocardial infarction and ischemia.
2. Think about TTP in patients with low platelet counts and mental status changes. Treatment of TTP is plasmapheresis.
3. Make sure your patient is at least 24 hours removed from their last dose of ace-inhibitor medication if possible if they are about to receive plasmapheresis as the procedure can prolong the bradykinin half-life and lead to dramatic hypotension.
4. LDL apheresis is used for patients with refractory cases of hyperlipidemia that have not responded to medical therapy.
5. Patients with familial hypercholesteremia have a defect at the LDL receptor and this is associated with LDL usually above 250.
6. Young patients with alopecia should be worked up for primary hypothyroidism as well as syphilis.
7. Patients with secondary syphilis may present with oral lesions (mucous patches) in addition to generalized lymphadenopathy.
8. Tendon xanthomas are a physical finding associated with familial hypercholesteremia.
9. Eruptive xanthomas are a physical finding associated with familial hypertriglyceridemia.

10. After 48 hours of a ruptured Baker's cyst of the knee, there is an increased incidence of secondary deep venous thrombosis that can occur.

16.128 Year 2—Week 43—Day 1

1. Buerger's disease patients should have definitive angiograms performed to look for abrupt vascular cutoff usually at the wrists and ankles, unlike antiphospholipid antibody syndrome which can mimic this entity.
2. Erysipelas is a form of group A streptococcal cellulitis that may be associated with bullous formation upon resolution.
3. Erysipelas may involve the facial area and be markedly tender.
4. True posterior MI (ST depression of 1–2 mm usually in V1 or V2 with possible tall R-wave in lead V1) is an indication for acute coronary catheterization procedure.
5. New onset LBB is equivalent to ST-segment elevation for MI purposes.
6. Ashman's phenomenon, which is associated with aberrant conduction, may mimic ventricular arrythmias.
7. Always check thyroid tests in patients with atrial fibrillation.
8. WPW and hypertrophic cardiomyopathy are causes for inferior Q waves without active ischemia.
9. Constrictive pericarditis may be seen in patients with rheumatoid arthritis.
10. Patients with drug-induced lupus should overall lack any renal manifestations unlike systemic lupus erythematosus.

16.129 Year 2—Week 43—Day 2

1. The most common antibody ordered in celiac sprue workups is the anti-tissue transglutaminase antibody, which is derived from the anti-endomysial antibody.
2. Antireticulin and antigliadin antibodies are also seen in celiac sprue.

3. Celiac sprue has an epidemiological link to a higher risk of small bowel lymphoma.
4. Imatinib mesylate (Gleevec) was first described in use against the gastrointestinal stromal tumors (GIST tumors).
5. Heparin can cause adrenal insufficiency by interference with aldosterone receptors.
6. An early sign of drug-induced adrenal insufficiency is unexplained, persistent hyperkalemia.
7. Continued excessive testosterone replacement can lead to excessive hemoglobin increases with a risk for thrombotic events.
8. Control hypertension first before starting patients on erythropoietin.
9. Control hypertriglyceridemia first before starting a female on hormone replacement therapy.
10. Valproic acid is the anti-epileptic most linked to hair loss and weight gain.

16.130 Year 2—Week 43—Day 3

1. Untreated hidradenitis suppurativa is a risk factor for development of squamous cell cancer of the skin.
2. Erythema ab igne is a rash that resembles livedo reticularis which can be induced with chronic heating of an area (as with a warming blanket) and can lead to squamous cell cancer of the skin.
3. Schistosoma haematobium bladder infection can lead to squamous cell cancer of the bladder.
4. Achalasia, tylosis, and Plummer-Vinson syndrome are among the esophageal disorders that can lead to squamous cell cancer of the esophagus.
5. GERD does NOT lead to squamous cell cancer of the esophagus.
6. A methylmalonic acid should be elevated in cases of vitamin B12 deficiency.
7. Folic acid supplementation needs to be given to all patients with a history of hemolytic anemia.

8. Gingival hyperplasia can be caused by dilantin, cyclosporine, and dihydropyridine calcium channel blockers.

9. Hutchinson's sign is seen in herpes zoster with a vesicle at the tip of the nose when the nasociliary branch of the trigeminal nerve is involved. Next step in management when this is found is to have an ophthalmologist rule out the presence of zoster involvement of the eye.

10. G6PD deficiency is protective against acquiring malaria.

16.131 Year 2—Week 44—Day 1

1. Candidiasis, hypoparathyroidism, and Addison's disease are the most common manifestations of autoimmune polyendocrine syndrome type 1.

2. Addison's disease, type 1A diabetes, and chronic thyroiditis are the most common manifestations of autoimmune polyendocrine syndrome type 2.

3. Patients with Addison's disease and hypothyroidism together are commonly referred to as belonging to the Schmidt's syndrome.

4. Always rule out adrenal insufficiency first before treating a patient for myxedema coma.

5. Hyperkalemia leading to cardiac arrythmia and hypoglycemia leading to cerebral crisis are two common causes of death from an Addisonian crisis.

6. Methimazole and propylthiouracil have been both associated with drug-induced lupus and with severe aplastic anemia.

7. Fever usually accompanies the presentation of a patient with thyroid storm. Mortality can approach 25 percent if not treated immediately.

8. Always give propylthiouracil or methimazole *first* before giving an anti-iodine drug such as Lugol's iodine or sodium ipodate in patients with thyroid storm.

9. Methyldopa, verapamil, reserpine, metoclopramide, phenothiazines, TCAs, and SSRIs are among the causes of drug-induced prolactin elevations.

10. Cocaine and opiates can also lead to an elevated prolactin level.

16.132 Year 2—Week 44—Day 2

1. The most common inherited bleeding disorder is von Willebrand's disease as it is autosomal dominant. It can be treated with DDAVP (as can uremic bleeding) as long as type 2b (low platelet count) is not present by multimeric analysis.

2. Factor 12 deficiency will prolong the PTT as will deficiency of factors 8,9,and 11 but is not associated with bleeding, thus there is no need for treatment.

3. The most common cause of macrocytosis in the general population is alcohol use. Vitamin deficiencies generally cause a macro-ovalocytosis on a peripheral smear.

4. A patient that is post-partum that presents with large bruises could have a factor 8 inhibitor. The most common cause of a Factor 8 inhibitor is a hemophilia patient who has been receiving long-standing bovine recombinant factor 8 concentrates. The treatment of choice in this condition is purified porcine factor 8 concentrates.

5. The two causes of a PTT that does not correct in a 1.1 mixing study is the presence of a factor inhibitor and the antiphospholipid syndrome.

6. Most individuals with Factor V leiden mutation that is heterozygous never develop thromboembolic disease.

7. The first step in management of a lab test with thrombocytopenia is to examine the peripheral smear for clumped aggregates— this pseudo-thrombocytopenia is an EDTA-reagent mediated phenomenon.

8. A McMurray test for a torn meniscus consists of extending the flexed knee while internally or rotating the tibia to produce a click sound.

9. There can be marked elevations of methylmalonic acid in patients with vitamin B12 deficiency.

10. Antibodies in the antiphospholipid syndrome are directed against beta-2-glycoprotein-1. Livedo reticularis is a skin rash that can be seen in this disorder (rash also seen with cholesterol emboli syndrome).

16.133 Year 2—Week 44—Day 3

1. Patients with mixed connective tissue disease have a good outcome and have high titers of U1 ribonucleoprotein antibodies.
2. Inclusion body myositis patients have only mild elevation of their CPK levels and have EMG studies with both neuropathic and myopathic features. They do not respond well to immunosuppressive therapy.
3. Patients with polymyositis with high titers of anti-histidyl TrNA synthetase antibodies are at high risk for interstitial lung disease.
4. Steroids and colchicine can lead to a myositis/myopathy state with long-term use.
5. Etanercept and other TNF-alpha receptor blockers cannot be initiated for treatment until a PPD is checked to make sure the patient is not at high risk of reactivating tuberculosis.
6. The "saddle nose deformity", where there is a flattened nasal bridge, can be seen in patients with nasal septal inflammation continuously and is found in diseases like granulomatosis with polyangiitis, relapsing polychondritis, lethal midline granuloma, and congenital syphilis.
7. Lethal (idiopathic) granuloma of the midline is a disease that is felt to be moderated by natural killer cells.
8. Ethylene glycol poisoning patients may be noted to have oxalate crystals in the urine.
9. Methanol poisoning patients are at risk of developing blindness due to optic neuritis (papillitis).
10. Urticaria is the rash most closely linked to acute hepatitis C (not porphyria cutanea tarda).

16.134 Year 2—Week 45—Day 1

1. Limbic encephalitis is a paraneoplastic process that has been described with testicular cancer, breast cancer, and Hodgkin's lymphomas and involves an attack on the limbic system (amygdala, hippocampus, etc.) by an unknown effect created by the underlying tumor. Helpful antibody to order would be the anti-Hu or anti-neuronal antibodies.
2. Myasthenic syndrome (Eaton-Lambert syndrome) is a paraneoplastic process of small cell lung cancer. Repetitive action makes a patient stronger rather than weaker as in myasthenia gravis.
3. Respiratory failure and cranial nerve palsies are *unusual* in Lambert-Eaton syndrome (unlike myasthenia gravis).
4. Patients with pontine infarcts can present with small pupillary size.
5. Patients with acute alcoholic hepatitis should have transaminases no higher than 400 mg/dL in most cases.
6. Mollaret's meningitis is caused by HSV and can cause recurrent episodes of meningitis.
7. Recurrent Neisseria meningitis infections calls for one to work up a patient for late complement deficiency.
8. The CH50 level is the first step in management in looking for complement deficiency.
9. Monitor the alkaline phosphatase in patients with Paget's disease as they are at risk of osteosarcoma.
10. Perform an ERCP in a patient with ulcerative colitis who develops increased alkaline phosphatase levels in the serum as they are at risk of primary sclerosing cholangitis.

16.135 Year 2—Week 45—Day 2

1. WBC inclusions are usually classically seen in histoplasmosis and Ehrlichiosis infections.
2. RBC inclusions are classically seen in Babesia and malaria infections. A Maltese cross formation is seen in babesiosis while

banana shaped formation is seen in *Plasmodium falciparium.*

3. Whipple's disease patients require at times up to 18 months of trimethoprim-sulfamethoxazole therapy to completely eradicate symptoms.

4. Cardiogenic shock is a complication of acute myocardial infarction that can be seen upon presentation of the patient into the hospital.

5. Acute papillary muscle dysfunction and rupture is seen in cases of inferior myocardial infarction.

6. A loud systolic murmur that radiates from the left sternal border to the right sternal border a few days after a patient has his first myocardial infarction should draw suspicion of ventricular septal rupture.

7. Sarcoid can present with two acute fever syndromes with one being marked by ankle arthritis and erythema nodosum (Lofgren's) and the other is marked by parotid gland enlargement and uveitis (Heerfordt's).

8. HACEK (Cardiobacterium, Kingella, Eikenella as examples of organisms in the class) endocarditis infections need ceftriaxone for treatment.

9. Horner's syndrome is seen with the following: Pancoast tumor destroying the sympathetic plexus near the apex of the lung, cluster headaches, and Wallenberg's syndrome.

10. Wallenberg's syndrome is a lateral medullary infarct that is marked by dysarthria, ataxia, loss of facial sensation ipsilateral to the lesion, Horner's syndrome, and loss of body sensation contralateral to the lesion.

16.136 Year 2—Week 45—Day 3

1. Dejerine-Roussy syndrome is the name of the post-thalamic stroke syndrome marked by the worst pain syndrome of all the post-stroke entities. Patients have hemisensory sensation of "acid bathing their skin" or "skin being torn from flesh."

2. Classic areas for hemorrhage from a pontine infarct are the pons, putamen, pulvinar nucleus of the thalamus, and occipital poles.

3. Atrial fibrillation and hypertension are the two largest risk factors for stroke in this country. Strokes with atrial fibrillation patients tend to have bad outcomes.

4. Do not stop anticoagulation in a patient with atrial fibrillation just because they suffer one or two falls. Many times, these patients can get a walker or other assist support or even physical therapy to markedly decrease their risk for falls and thus continue anticoagulation.

5. There are several syndromes (Benedict, Weber) that involve a stroke of the midbrain that presents with cranial nerve three palsy and either ataxia or hemiparesis.

6. Patients with cerebellar stroke fall to the same side of their lesion.

7. Patients with stroke are most likely to have dysphagia due to abnormal oropharyngeal transfer. A dynamic video esophagogram is the test of choice to diagnose this state.

8. Carbamazepine if the drug of choice to treat trigeminal neuralgia. Repeated episodes of trigeminal neuralgia should raise suspicion of multiple sclerosis.

9. Patients with paroxysmal hemicrania headache syndromes need to be treated with indomethacin.

10. Hypertrophic pulmonary osteoarthropathy is associated with non-small cell lung cancer. It is marked by new onset clubbing within a few months.

16.137 Year 2—Week 46—Day 1

1. D-penicillamine therapeutic use can mimic the disease of myasthenia gravis.

2. A useful test for myasthenia gravis is to have the patient sustain upward gaze and ptosis should ensue shortly thereafter.

3. Patients with myasthenic syndrome (Eaton-Lambert) do not demonstrate respiratory muscle weakness.

4. Patients with myasthenia gravis crisis and Guillain-Barre syndrome maintain normal PAO2 until the very end at which time they crash quickly. Thus, routine measurements of FVC (forced vital capacity) and negative inspiratory force are needed to know when to protectively intubate.

5. Aminoglycosides are the most notorious antibiotics to cause a myasthenia gravis crisis.

6. Plasmapheresis plus steroids is commonly used in the treatment of myasthenia gravis crisis.

7. Patients with myasthenia gravis may have positive acetylcholine receptor antibodies.

8. Reflexes are normal in myasthenia gravis, whereas patients with Guillain-Barre syndrome have areflexia.

9. Patients with myasthenia gravis not responding to medical therapy may need thymectomy even in absence of a thymoma.

10. Patients with myasthenia gravis have fatigable weakness that improves with rest as seen with diplopia and difficulty in speech that develops during the late stages of the day in patients.

16.138   Year 2—Week 46—Day 2

1. Atrial flutter with symptomatic patients (hypotension, mental status changes) requires synchronized cardioversion therapy.

2. Overdrive pacing is a strategy that can be used for torsades des pointes. Isoproterenol is used for chemical overdrive pacing usually first before temporary transvenous pacer is placed.

3. Magnesium levels should be checked in all patients with parathyroid surgery who are not raising their calcium levels with calcium supplementation.

4. Distal RTA (type 1) have an association with kidney stones due to hypocitraturia.

5. Sjogren's syndrome and rheumatoid arthritis both carry a risk for lymphoma.

6. Pravastatin is the statin of choice in patients with multiple drugs that work through the cytochrome P-450 3a4 system.

7. Cameron lesions are ulcer lesions found in hiatal hernias. Surgical correction of hiatal hernia is the next step in management in these patients.

8. Dieulafoy lesions are aberrant submucosal, usually gastric, vessels that can bleed quite briskly.

9. Flow cytometry of red cells is the gold standard test to rule out paroxysmal nocturnal hemoglobinuria.

10. The osmotic fragility test is the gold standard to rule out hereditary spherocytosis.

16.139   Year 2—Week 46—Day 3

1. Dilantin can cause a marked drop in vitamin D levels with chronic use.

2. Vitamin B12 levels need to be checked in all patients with states of achlorhydria such as VIPOMA.

3. Patients can have elevated calcitonin levels for reasons other than medullary cancer of the thyroid (such as in VIPOMA).

4. Patients with Whipple's disease will often present with hyperpigmentation of the skin and they are at risk of systemic endocarditis as a complication.

5. Look out for laxative abuse as a cause of chronic diarrhea.

6. Patients with carcinoid syndrome can have a wide variety of manifestations including tricuspid valve disease, flushing, and significant liver disease.

7. Mastocytosis can cause bone pain and abdominal pain after meal ingestion, features that distinguish it from carcinoid syndrome.

8. The skin-limited mastocytosis variant is urticaria pigmentosa which features brown macules urticate when the lesions are manipulated.

9. The sweat test is the gold standard to rule out cystic fibrosis.

10. Hypersplenism is a common reason for low hemoglobin and low platelet levels in patients with liver disease.

16.140 Year 2—Week 47—Day 1

1. Intravenous metronidazole should be added as an adjunct therapy to oral vancomycin in patients with severe *Clostridium difficile* infections.
2. Patients with severe penicillin allergies can safely receive aztreonam.
3. Patients with severe streptococcal skin infections with streaking should be given clindamycin to acutely bind streptococcal toxin.
4. Scombroid is a cause of flushing through histidine toxic compounds found in the affected fish.
5. Ciguatera is the most common cause of fish food poisoning syndrome in the USA. Hot-cold reversal and teeth chattering chills are among the features of this state. Flushing is not characteristic of this condition.
6. Cluster headaches tend to affect males much more than females. Paroxysmal hemicranium headaches tend to favor females more than males.
7. Indomethacin is the treatment for paroxysmal hemicranium headaches.
8. 100% oxygen is the treatment for cluster headaches acutely.
9. Lithium can be used in the prophylaxis of cluster headaches.
10. Patients with history of CAD cannot use ergotamine or serotonin agonist/antagonist therapy in the treatment of migraine headaches.

16.141 Year 2—Week 47—Day 2

1. Beta-blockers can lead to hyperkalemia and to nightmares as side effects.

2. Patients with "scars" noted on nuclear medicine heart stress tests are at risk for ventricular tachycardia even if they have normal ejection fraction and this entity should be considered in patients with recurrent syncope.
3. Meckel's diverticulum can still be in the differential of an older adult with bright red blood per rectum.
4. Paget's disease can lead to osteosarcoma thus need monitoring of alkaline phosphatase levels.
5. A patient with ulcerative colitis who starts having a rising alkaline phosphatase level needs ERCP for ruling out primary sclerosing cholangitis.
6. Patients with osteomalacia will have low 25-dihydroxyvitamin D levels with low calcium and low phosphorus levels.
7. Patients taking phenobarbital are also at risk of vitamin D deficiency.
8. Patients with multiple myeloma usually have SPEPs showing monoclonal spike with decrease in the levels of the other components. MGUS (monoclonal gammopathy of unknown significance) patients usually do not have the latter finding on serum protein electrophoresis.
9. Hemoglobin electrophoresis is the test to order if suspecting a thalassemia.
10. An increased hemoglobin A2 level is seen in patients with beta-thalassemia trait. Target cells are frequently seen on the blood smear with thalassemia.

16.142 Year 2—Week 47—Day 3

1. Dysfunctional uterine bleeding in young females should raise the suspicion of von Willebrand's factor deficiency.
2. Type 2b von Willebrand's disease patients may present with thrombocytopenia.
3. First-line treatment of prolonged QT syndrome is beta-blocker therapy.

4. Prolonged ST-segment can be seen in patients with hypocalcemia, whereas a shortened segment is seen in hypercalcemia.

5. Hypocalcemia in the setting of previous thyroid surgery should raise the suspicion of damage or injury to the parathyroid glands.

6. Thiazide diuretics are used to treat calcium-based kidney stones as they lead to decreased calcium excretion.

7. Dilantin levels need to be corrected in the setting of a low albumin state.

8. Calcium replacement in the setting of hypokalemia and digoxin toxicity could worsen the digoxin toxicity; thus, all patients should be on monitored floor if calcium is planned to be given in this setting.

9. Gitelman's and Bartter's syndrome patients have normal blood pressure levels and both involve pathophysiology with juxtaglomerular apparatus hyperplasia.

10. Amiloride is the first-line treatment of Lidle's syndrome, which mimics hyperaldosteronism except there are no detectable aldosterone levels in these patients.

16.143 Year 2—Week 48—Day 1

1. Fusarium is a fungus with acute angle branching hyphae (similar to Aspergillus) which tends to have a very aggressive course.

2. Aspergillus likes to cause aggressive pulmonary disease particularly in those patients who have been neutropenic for over 10 days.

3. Gram-negative organism that can cause aggressive cellulitis in liver disease patients. It is marked by bullous lesions. Treatment is doxycycline and a third-generation cephalosporin if inpatient.

4. The shawl sign of dermatomyositis is an erythema that involves the anterior neck and shoulders. It is associated with a better outcome than those without this sign. Antibody MI-2 is usually present.

5. Patients with dermatomyositis or polymyositis who have interstitial lung disease will usually have positive anti-Jo 1 titers (histidyl TRNA synthetase).

6. Ursodeoxycholic acid can be used for patients with primary biliary cirrhosis. It has also been used in patients planning rapid weight loss in hopes to avoiding gallstone formation.

7. Cutaneous larval migrans is most commonly caused by *Ancylostoma braziliense* in the western world.

8. The complement levels in patients with renal failure due to Goodpasture's syndrome are usually normal. Another consideration in patients who are neutropenic for over a week and develop lower right quadrant pain is typhlitis. Treatment is with metronidazole.

9. Aeromonas is a freshwater bacteria that can cause an aggressive cellulitis in patients with liver disease.

10. Consider Strongyloides infection in patients presenting with acute onset new asthma symptoms particularly if they have had recurrent episodes of gram-negative bacteremia that have gone unexplained.

16.144 Year 2—Week 48—Day 2

1. Think of Q-fever if a patient presents with liver failure and endocarditis. *Coxiella burnetii* is the offending organism.

2. Milk-alkali syndrome involves intentional or unintentional excess use of calcium carbonate which results in alkalosis and hypercalcemia.

3. Lithium can lead to many metabolic abnormalities such as hypercalcemia, nephrogenic diabetes insipidus, and hypothyroidism.

4. The most common inherited bleeding disorder is von Willebrand's disease.

5. Excessive bruising in an elderly patient should raise concern about a factor 8 inhibitor presence.

6. Disseminated CNS histoplasmosis should be treated initially with amphotericin B.

7. Itraconazole suspension is an option for long-term treatment of patients with disseminated histoplasmosis. PPI therapy will interfere with itraconazole absorption and thus cannot be used.

8. Patients with end-stage liver disease (ESLD) with pre-existing cirrhosis are at risk of infection of pleural space if they have hepatic hydrothorax. The pleural fluid infection when it occurs is called spontaneous bacterial empyema and treatment is medical with antibiotics geared toward the most common organism, which is still *Escherichia coli.*

9. Patients with Hashimoto's thyroiditis will usually have high anti-TPO (thyroid peroxisomal) titers.

10. Remember to exclude secondary syphilis in all patients who present with a rash similar to pityriasis rosea and have risk factors for syphilis.

7. With a cellulitis with severe pain and fever, suspect group A streptococcal necrotizing fasciitis.

8. Venous stasis is the most common factor leading to recurrent episodes of cellulitis.

9. Necrotizing fasciitis caused by group A streptococci can begin in deep muscles and not show any cutaneous manifestations until much later in the disease course.

10. Hydroxychloroquine is the treatment of choice for subacute cutaneous lupus erythematosus, similar to the other cutaneous manifestations of the diseases in the lupus spectrum. Patients on this medication need eye exams one to two times a year by an ophthalmologist.

16.145 Year 2—Week 48—Day 3

1. Primaquine is used to treat the hepatic phase of *Plasmodium vivax* and ovale.

2. The most common cause of macrocytosis in the general population is chronic use of alcohol.

3. Poxvirus is the cause of molluscum contagiosum, which can also be seen in immunocompetent patients. The classic description of the lesion is a central umbilicated papule.

4. Erysipelas is a cellulitis with sharply demarcated borders with a violaceous hue discoloration and group A streptococci is the most common cause. Treat with IV penicillin initially (only need 7–10 days of treatment).

5. Erysipeloid is a mimicker of erysipelas, except it is caused by *Erysipelothrix rhusiopathiae*, and this organism affects meat handlers and fish handlers. Treatment is IV penicillin (sometimes it is better to be lucky than good, as you would treat this infection with penicillin without recognizing its true nature and the patient still would get better).

6. Clindamycin should be part of the treatment plan in treating patients with gas gangrene by *Clostridium perfringens* and necrotizing fasciitis by group A streptococci.

16.146 Year 2—Week 49—Day 1

1. Epiphrenic esophageal diverticulum can be quite large so as to mimic a lung abscess or a mass. Use a barium swallow to exclude this as a possibility.

2. CMV disease can cause an inflammatory demyelinating polyneuropathy in patients with advanced HIV disease (such that it can mimic Guillain-Barre syndrome).

3. Acute treatment of toxoplasmosis is with sulfa medication and pyrimethamine (use clindamycin instead of sulfa if there is an allergy to sulfa). Toxoplasmosis can involve the basal ganglia.

4. If a patient had a CD4 count above 200 for at least six months, then prophylaxis against PCP and toxoplasmosis can be discontinued.

5. Cryptococcal meningitis might lead to increased intracranial pressure more so than any other meningitis. Initial treatment is with amphotericin B (not the liposomal complex) and 5-flucytosine.

6. Hemiparesis, ataxia, seizures, cranial nerve palsies, and mental status changes can occur in patients with progressive multifocal leukoencephalopathy.

7. Atrial myxomas can cause distal emboli to brain and to the lower extremities.

8. The treatment for the vascular complications of Behcet's syndrome is chlorambucil.
9. Eruptive xanthomas can be seen with familial hypertriglyceridemia. Most patients with pancreatitis with this disorder have triglyceride levels above 1000mg/dl.
10. Herpes gestationis is a blistering disorder of pregnancy marked by large bullae usually located around the umbilicus.

16.147 Year 2—Week 49—Day 2

1. Acute hepatitis B can present with urticaria, arthritis, fever, serum sickness, and even cryoglobulinemia.
2. Serum sickness is *not* seen in patients with acute hepatitis C infection. Low serum ceruloplasmin levels may be seen at times and may lead to an unnecessary workup for Wilson's disease.
3. Parvovirus B19 can lead to aplastic anemia and a rash known as livedo reticularis.
4. Granuloma annulare, necrobiosis lipoidica diabeticorum, and Candida infections are among the cutaneous problems seen in patients with diabetes mellitus.
5. TPN patients are at risk of fungemia from Candida species infections and from Malassezia furfur when lipid emulsions and fatty acid emulsions are being used as part of the nutrition.
6. Colchicine can cause renal dysfunction and bone marrow suppression.
7. Trichomonas is not felt to be a cause of upper genital tract disease in women; thus, PID should never be labeled as secondary to trichomonas.
8. Clindamycin and gentamicin are an acceptable treatment regimen for patients with pelvic inflammatory disease infections.
9. Actinomycosis can cause fistula formation in whichever anatomical area it attacks. The pelvic, thoracic and mandibular areas are common locations for fistulas. Treat with PCN.

10. The risk of hemorrhagic dengue fever is highest in patients with previous dengue fever attack.

16.148 Year 2—Week 49—Day 3

1. Periosteal elevation on plain films can be seen late in the course of osteomyelitis in adults as opposed to children where it is seen early in the course of disease.
2. Mycoplasma can cause transverse myelitis, bullous myringitis, and cold agglutinin hemolytic anemia.
3. Chlamydia pneumonia infections are classically associated with hoarseness.
4. Patients with *Chlamydia psittaci* infections usually are quite ill on presentation.
5. Diffuse large B-cell lymphoma is the most common NHL to afflict adults.
6. Guttate psoriasis is worsened by acute streptococcal infections but this exacerbation is much more commonly seen in patients under the age of 30 while older patients usually have this variant due to medication effects or excessive alcohol use.
7. Pustular psoriasis usually worsens as a patient is being weaned from systemic steroids.
8. Erythroderma is seen in patients with psoriasis, cutaneous T-cell lymphoma when associated with Sezary syndrome, and pityriasis rubra pilaris.
9. Hypertriglyceridemia is the most common lipid disorder of chronic renal failure.
10. Intussusception in adults is usually due to a solid lesion (such as a polyp or tumor) and thus evaluation for malignancy is always indicated.

16.149 Year 2—Week 50—Day 1

1. Diabetes mellitus, liver disease, and renal insufficiency are all risk factors for development of Legionella infections.
2. Listeria infections are found in greater number in patients with leukemias, in pregnancy, and with liver disease. Treat Listeria with

ampicillin as cephalosporins do not work. Use Septra if PCN allergic.

3. Steroid therapy will not work in patients with cold agglutinin disease.
4. Warm agglutinins can be seen in patients with HIV disease, SLE, inflammatory bowel disease, and in patients with Evan's syndrome (hemolytic anemia with spherocytes noted and with ITP).
5. Mycoplasma and certain lymphoproliferative disorders can cause cold agglutinin disease.
6. Trimethylaminuria is an amino acid disorder that can be seen in young adults. Patients with this disorder smell like rotting fish.
7. Patients with isovaleric acidemia as an amino acid disorder will complain of excessive sweaty feet.
8. Danazol is an anabolic steroid that could be used in the treatment of warm autoimmune hemolytic anemias. It is also used in treating hereditary angioedema.
9. Splenectomy does not help in treating patients with cold agglutinin disease.
10. Splenectomy is helpful in managing patients with refractory cases of warm agglutinin disease and has even been tried in patients with recurrent TTP.

16.150 Year 2—Week 50—Day 2

1. A patient with acute right sided upper and lower extremity weakness should have stat MRI looking for epidural abscess or hematoma that may require stat laminectomy and drainage by neurosurgery.
2. Acute rheumatic fever is associated with carditis, arthritis, erythema marginatum, subcutaneous nodules, and fever.
3. *Serratia marcescens* infections may cause reddish pigmentation of sputum that resembles hemoptysis.
4. Potts puffy tumor describes frontal bone osteomyelitis which may arise as a complication of sinusitis.
5. *Klebsiella pneumonia*, which has an increased incidence in nursing home

patients, can cause hepatic abscess disease which will respond effectively to drainage and oral fluoroquinolone therapy (intravenous antibiotic therapy not necessary).

6. Patients with tuberculosis who have aggressive pericarditis need glucocorticoid therapy along with treatment with antibiotics.
7. Patients with cranial nerve palsies due to diabetes mellitus will have sparing of pupillary function.
8. Transverse myelitis is usually associated with multiple sclerosis but can be seen in patients after hepatitis B vaccination, lupus, and other selected post-infectious states.
9. Inclusion body myositis presents with distal muscle weakness as well as proximal muscle weakness and responds poorly to anti-inflammatory treatment.
10. Never forget to consider concomitant thiamine deficiency in a patient with underlying scurvy deficiency diagnosis.

16.151 Year 2—Week 50—Day 3

1. Hypothyroidism is the most common endocrine disorder to present with periorbital edema.
2. A patient who is a smoker and has a positive low anterior cervical lymph node or a supraclavicular node needs a CXR as the next step in management (before lymph node biopsy).
3. Post-tussive rales heard best in the supraclavicular area with the bell is the classic auscultatory sign with active tuberculosis.
4. Most cases of fever of unknown origin declare themselves in the next 2 years from initial start of symptoms. One strong entity to always consider is Hodgkin's disease, and consider CT scan of thorax even when CXR is unremarkable.
5. Consider going to CT scan of chest even with normal CXR if there is recurrence of an elevated thyroglobulin in a patient with history of follicular or papillary thyroid cancer.
6. Systemic fibrinolysis can be seen in patients with acute pancreatitis.

7. Argatroban is a direct thrombin inhibitor that will artificially increase INR to a higher level than expected for a given dose of coumadin. Continue argatroban until INR level is 4.0 value or above when using argatroban.

8. Lepirudin and hirudin are options for anticoagulation in patients with HIT (heparin-induced thrombocytopenia).

9. Antibodies are not necessary to diagnose HIT (heparin-induced thrombocytopenia) as the platelet count drop is so dramatic that the diagnosis becomes evident easily.

10. Patients with HIT can develop arterial clots (white clot syndrome).

16.152 Year 2—Week 51—Day 1

1. Cholesteatoma is a cause of conductive hearing loss.

2. Multiple sclerosis and stroke are among the causes of a internuclear ophthalmoplegia. Multiple sclerosis tends to present with bilateral findings.

3. The structure involved in internuclear ophthalmoplegia is the medial longitudinal fasciculus (MLF).

4. Unilateral persistent nasal bleeding should raise suspicion of a tumor in the nares in the absence of cocaine use or trauma.

5. Unilateral serous discharge from one ear in a smoker should raise suspicion of squamous cell cancer involving the nasopharynx and blocking the opening of the Eustachian tube.

6. Persistent shoulder pain in a smoker should raise the suspicion of a Pancoast tumor.

7. Among the causes of Horner's syndrome are Wallenberg syndrome, cluster headaches, and Pancoast tumor.

8. The most important lab test to perform in a patient with lupus is to ensure there is no proteinuria noted in urinalyis of patients as early treatment with Ace-inhibitor therapy or Angiontensin receptoer blocker therapy would be essential to preservation of kidney function.

9. When suspecting drug-induced lupus, the first step in management is to order an ANA (then, if positive, order anti-histone antibodies).

10. Hydroxychloroquine remains the first-line drug of choice for patients with lupus skin and joint disease.

16.153 Year 2—Week 51—Day 2

1. Hypothyroidism can elevate CPK levels and LDH levels and present with proximal weakness and myalgias.

2. Hypothyroidism can also lead to an increased LDL level.

3. Ortner's syndrome occurs when an enlarged left atrium in the setting of mitral stenosis impinges on the left recurrent laryngeal nerve causing hoarseness.

4. Brown's syndrome is the inability to gaze downward and in which affects patients with rheumatoid arthritis due to tenosynovitis of the superior oblique muscle.

5. A common cause of painless cranial nerve palsy is uncontrolled diabetes mellitus.

6. Patients with diabetes mellitus can also have problems accommodating their pupils leading to night vision problems.

7. Lofgren's syndrome involves sarcoidosis with features of ankle arthritis, bilateral hilar lymphadenopathy, and erythema nodosum.

8. Patients with psoriasis can have onycholysis in addition to nail pitting.

9. Patients with reactive arthritis get manifestations of circinate balanitis, keratoderma blennorrhagica, and conjunctivitis.

10. Patients with ankylosing spondylitis get anterior uveitis which may lead to a layer of white cells in the anterior chamber of the eye (hypopyon iritis).

16.154 Year 2—Week 51—Day 3

1. Fitz-Hugh-Curtis syndrome is an infection characterized by right upper quadrant pain and it is seen in association with pelvic inflammatory disease (PID) whereby the infection ascends and causes inflammation

and "violin string" adhesions around Glisson's capsule surrounding the liver.

2. Fitz-Hugh-Curtis syndrome, though classically due to gonorrhea, may be caused by Chlamydia as well.

3. Waterhouse-Friderichsen syndrome is acute, usually bilateral, hemorrhage of the adrenal glands most often caused in the setting of Meningococcemia.

4. Waterhouse-Friderichsen syndrome may also be caused by *Streptococcus pneumoniae*, *Staphylococcus aureus*, and *Capnocytophaga canimorsus* all of which have been well described in the medical literature.

5. Asplenic patients are at increased risk of both Waterhouse-Friderichsen and Purpura Fulminans because of increased infections with Meningococcus, Streptococcus, and Capnocytophaga.

6. Purpura Fulminans is a term used to describe a hemorrhagic condition associated with bacterial sepsis and DIC characterized by purpura, petechiae, bullae, and necrotic skin lesions.

7. Purpura Fulminans classically associated with meningococcemia but may also be seen with severe *Staphylococcus aureus* and Streptococcal infections among others.

8. One must consider late complement deficiency, C5–C9 deficiency, in persons with recurrent *Neisseria meningitides* infections.

9. Ampicillin is used to treat *Listeria monocytogenes* which is a gram-positive rod that can cause meningitis particularly in newborns and commonly infects foods.

10. Approximately 10–20% of all sporadic viral meningitis in the USA is due to Herpes simplex virus which has a predilection for temporal lobes and is best diagnosed using PCR.

16.155 Year 2—Week 52—Day 1

1. "Trench fever" now sometimes called "urban trench fever" because of its predilection for inner-city dwellers is caused by *Bartonella quintana*.

2. Trench fever is characterized by fever, maculopapular rash, hepatosplenomegaly, arthralgias, bone pain, and may have endocarditis.

3. Trench fever is treated with doxycycline (first line), erythromycin, or azithromycin.

4. Cat scratch disease which is characterized by papules at the site of inoculation, lymphadenopathy, fevers, malaise, and headaches is caused by *Bartonella henselae*.

5. Cat scratch disease is treated with azithromycin (first line) or doxycycline.

6. There is a greater chance of getting cat scratch disease from kittens than adult cats as they carry a greater concentration of the bacteria.

7. Peliosis hepatis, more often seen in HIV patients and patients with advanced cancer, is characterized by cystic, blood-filled spaces in the liver.

8. Bacillary angiomatosis, a disease caused by the organisms of *Bartonella quintana* or *Bartonella henselae*, is characterized by multiple nodules of vascular proliferation that appear as tumor like masses wither subcutaneous or in other organs.

9. Bacillary angiomatosis is treated with doxycycline or macrolide therapy.

10. Oroya fever is caused by *Bartonella bacilliformis*.

16.156 Year 2—Week 52—Day 2

1. Whipple's disease is caused by *Tropheryma whipplei*, a small gram+ bacillus that can be seen on Periodic-Acid Schiff (PAS) staining of small intestine biopsies inside and outside macrophages.

2. Whipple's disease is characterized by malabsorption, steatorrhea, ab pain, migratory large joint arthralgias, transient fevers, and ophthalmologic and neurologic (CNS, dementia) symptoms.

3. Certain neurologic findings, seen in less than 20% of cases of Whipple's, are pathognomonic for the disease—these include vertical supranuclear ophthalmoplegia and oculomasticatory myorhythmia.

4. *M. avium complex* can also be seen with PAS staining of the small intestine and have similar GI symptoms (but the neurologic symptoms would be atypical).

5. *Actinomyces* is an anaerobe where infection if marked by "yellow sulfur granules" which are clumps of organisms. Tx. PCN or Ampicillin.

6. *Actinomyces* is classically caused by a preceding dental infection and has cervicofacial involvement but may also be seen in pelvic inflammatory disease caused by IUD use.

7. *Cryptosporidium* and *Isospora* are acid-fast parasites that can cause chronic, profuse watery diarrhea in AIDS patients.

8. *Cyclospora* are Coccidian parasites that can cause infection in immunocompetent hosts as well and have been reported in outbreaks in both Texas and Florida related to infected berries. It is usually self-limited, though the secretory diarrhea can last as >1month.

9. *Microspora* are intracellular spore forming parasites and thus require small bowel biopsy for diagnosis.

10. Charcot joint of the foot is most evident in the mid-tarsal area and can lead to "rocker bottom" foot with widening of the mid-foot.

16.157 Year 2—Week 52—Day 3

1. Amongst the causes of nodular lymphangitis are sporotrichosis, *Nocardia brasiliensis*, *Mycobacterium marinum*, *Leishmaniasis*, and *Francisella tularensis*.

2. Streptococcal infections can also cause nodular lymphangitis as a manifestation of disease.

3. Ulcerated or supparated lymph nodes can occur with Nocardia.

4. *Francisella tularensis* can also cause oculoglandular syndrome and pneumonia.

5. *Francisella tularensis* and *Yersinia pestis* are treated with streptomycin first line (although gentamicin more widely available).

6. Streptomycin can cause renal failure and ototoxicity.

7. Chlamydia trachomatis is the leading cause of blindness in the world.

8. There are four main serogroups of Shigella starting with the most common (*soneii*) followed by three others which are *dysenteriae*, *bydii, and flexneri.*

9. Shigella can cause severe dysentery and may be treated with fluoroquinolones, sulfa-based antibiotics, and azithromycin.

10. Shigella toxin is associated with HUS (hemolytic-uremic syndrome).

Further Reading

Abboud H, Henrich WL. Clinical practice. Stage IV chronic kidney disease. N Engl J Med. 2010;362(1):56–65. https://doi.org/10.1056/NEJMcp0906797.

Bartalena L, Tanda ML. Clinical practice. Graves' ophthalmopathy. N Engl J Med. 2009;360(10):994–1001. https://doi.org/10.1056/NEJMcp0806317.

Bilezikian JP, Silverberg SJ. Clinical practice. Asymptomatic primary hyperparathyroidism. N Engl J Med. 2004;350(17):1746–51. https://doi.org/10.1056/NEJMcp032200.

Brickner ME, Hillis LD, Lange RA. Congenital heart disease in adults. First of two parts. N Engl J Med. 2000a;342(4):256–63. https://doi.org/10.1056/NEJM200001273420407.

Brickner ME, Hillis LD, Lange RA. Congenital heart disease in adults. Second of two parts. N Engl J Med. 2000b;342(5):334–42. https://doi.org/10.1056/NEJM200002033420507.

Brugge WR, Lauwers GY, Sahani D, Fernandez-del Castillo C, Warshaw AL. Cystic neoplasms of the pancreas. N Engl J Med. 2004;351(12):1218–26. https://doi.org/10.1056/NEJMra031623.

Carragee EJ. Clinical practice. Persistent low back pain. N Engl J Med. 2005;352(18):1891–8. https://doi.org/10.1056/NEJMcp042054.

Dienstag JL. Hepatitis B virus infection. N Engl J Med. 2008;359(14):1486–500. https://doi.org/10.1056/NEJMra0801644.

Edlow JA, Caplan LR. Avoiding pitfalls in the diagnosis of subarachnoid hemorrhage. N Engl J Med. 2000;342(1):29–36. https://doi.org/10.1056/NEJM200001063420106.

Fenollar F, Puechal X, Raoult D. Whipple's disease. N Engl J Med. 2007;356(1):55–66. https://doi.org/10.1056/NEJMra062477.

Freedman DO. Clinical practice. Malaria prevention in short-term travelers. N Engl J Med. 2008;359(6):603–12. https://doi.org/10.1056/NEJMcp0803572.

Garcia-Tsao G, Bosch J. Management of varices and variceal hemorrhage in cirrhosis. N Engl J Med. 2010;362(9):823–32. https://doi.org/10.1056/NEJMra0901512.

Garovic VD. Hypertension in pregnancy: diagnosis and treatment. Mayo Clin Proc. 2000;75(10):1071–6. https://doi.org/10.4065/75.10.1071.

Gilhar A, Etzioni A, Paus R. Alopecia areata. N Engl J Med. 2012;366(16):1515–25. https://doi.org/10.1056/NEJMra1103442.

Hartzell JD, Wood-Morris RN, Martinez LJ, Trotta RF. Q fever: epidemiology, diagnosis, and treatment. Mayo Clin Proc. 2008;83(5):574–9. https://doi.org/10.4065/83.5.574.

Hesketh PJ. Chemotherapy-induced nausea and vomiting. N Engl J Med. 2008;358(23):2482–94. https://doi.org/10.1056/NEJMra0706547.

Hoffman RM. Clinical practice. Screening for prostate cancer. N Engl J Med. 2011a;365(21):2013–9. https://doi.org/10.1056/NEJMcp1103642.

Hoffman RM. Clinical practice. Screening for prostate cancer. N Engl J Med. 2011b;365(21):2013–9. https://doi.org/10.1056/NEJMcp1103642.

James WD. Clinical practice. Acne. N Engl J Med. 2005;352(14):1463–72. https://doi.org/10.1056/NEJMcp033487.

Kales SN, Christiani DC. Acute chemical emergencies. N Engl J Med. 2004;350(8):800–8. https://doi.org/10.1056/NEJMra030370.

Kamal AH, Tefferi A, Pruthi RK. How to interpret and pursue an abnormal prothrombin time, activated partial thromboplastin time, and bleeding time in adults. Mayo Clin Proc. 2007a;82(7):864–73. https://doi.org/10.4065/82.7.864.

Kamal AH, Tefferi A, Pruthi RK. How to interpret and pursue an abnormal prothrombin time, activated partial thromboplastin time, and bleeding time in adults. Mayo Clin Proc. 2007b;82(7):864–73. https://doi.org/10.4065/82.7.864.

Kumar A, Cannon CP. Acute coronary syndromes: diagnosis and management, part II. Mayo Clin Proc. 2009;84(11):1021–36. https://doi.org/10.1016/S0025-6196(11)60674-5.

Kumar S, Sarr MG, Kamath PS. Mesenteric venous thrombosis. N Engl J Med. 2001;345(23):1683–8. https://doi.org/10.1056/NEJMra010076.

Labelle CA, Kitchens CS. Disseminated intravascular coagulation: treat the cause, not the lab values. Cleve Clin J Med. 2005;72(5):377–8, 383-375, 390 passim. https://doi.org/10.3949/ccjm.72.5.377.

LeWinter MM. Clinical practice. Acute pericarditis. N Engl J Med. 2014;371(25):2410–6. https://doi.org/10.1056/NEJMcp1404070.

Maron BJ. Sudden death in young athletes. N Engl J Med. 2003;349(11):1064–75. https://doi.org/10.1056/NEJMra022783.

Paige NM, Nagami GT. The top 10 things nephrologists wish every primary care physician knew. Mayo Clin Proc. 2009;84(2):180–6. https://doi.org/10.1016/S0025-6196(11)60826-4.

Pirzada NA, Ali II. Central pontine myelinolysis. Mayo Clin Proc. 2001;76(5):559–62. https://doi.org/10.4065/76.5.559.

Plaut M, Valentine MD. Clinical practice. Allergic rhinitis. N Engl J Med. 2005;353(18):1934–44. https://doi.org/10.1056/NEJMcp044141.

Pritt BS, Clark CG. Amebiasis. Mayo Clin Proc. 2008;83(10):1154–9; quiz 1159-1160. https://doi.org/10.4065/83.10.1154.

Rahman A, Isenberg DA. Systemic lupus erythematosus. N Engl J Med. 2008;358(9):929–39. https://doi.org/10.1056/NEJMra071297.

Roden DM. Drug-induced prolongation of the QT interval. N Engl J Med. 2004;350(10):1013–22. https://doi.org/10.1056/NEJMra032426.

Rosenblatt JE. Antiparasitic agents. Mayo Clin Proc. 1999;74(11):1161–75. https://doi.org/10.4065/74.11.1161.

Ryan ET, Kain KC. Health advice and immunizations for travelers. N Engl J Med. 2000;342(23):1716–25. https://doi.org/10.1056/NEJM200006083422306.

Ryan ET, Wilson ME, Kain KC. Illness after international travel. N Engl J Med. 2002;347(7):505–16. https://doi.org/10.1056/NEJMra020118.

Stanley JR, Amagai M. Pemphigus, bullous impetigo, and the staphylococcal scalded-skin syndrome. N Engl J Med. 2006;355(17):1800–10. https://doi.org/10.1056/NEJMra061111.

Tapson VF. Acute pulmonary embolism. N Engl J Med. 2008;358(10):1037–52. https://doi.org/10.1056/NEJMra072753.

Trentham DE, Le CH. Relapsing polychondritis. Ann Intern Med. 1998;129(2):114–22. https://doi.org/10.7326/0003-4819-129-2-199807150-00011.

Wallace DV, Dykewicz MS, Oppenheimer J, Portnoy JM, Lang DM. Pharmacologic treatment of seasonal allergic rhinitis: synopsis of guidance from the 2017 Joint Task Force on Practice Parameters. Ann Intern Med. 2017;167(12):876–81. https://doi.org/10.7326/M17-2203.

Walport MJ. Complement. First of two parts. N Engl J Med. 2001;344(14):1058–66. https://doi.org/10.1056/NEJM200104053441406.

Whitley RJ. A 70-year-old woman with shingles: review of herpes zoster. JAMA. 2009;302(1):73–80. https://doi.org/10.1001/jama.2009.822.

Wigley FM. Clinical practice. Raynaud's Phenomenon. N Engl J Med. 2002;347(13):1001–8. https://doi.org/10.1056/NEJMcp013013.

Wilder-Smith A, Schwartz E. Dengue in travelers. N Engl J Med. 2005;353(9):924–32. https://doi.org/10.1056/NEJMra041927.

Young NS, Brown KE. Parvovirus B19. N Engl J Med. 2004;350(6):586–97. https://doi.org/10.1056/NEJMra030840.

Year 3: Internal Medicine Learning using "1,2,3 Methodology"

17

17.1 Introduction

As the internal medicine learner begins the third year of residency, the focus shifts much greater to the outpatient arena with less time spent in the ICU and general wards of most residencies in the country. The book is designed in this section to focus more on the outpatient facets of care of all the specialties to include the gastroenterology, cardiology, and infectious diseases topics which were much more focused in year 1 of this section on inpatient pearls of wisdom. There are still key inpatient pearls that are introduced and others that are repeated from year 1 and year 2 of this section. This year 3 of this section also emphasizes pearls in the areas of dermatology, ophthalmology, and otolaryngology that were not as frequently discussed in the first 2 years of this section.

17.2 Year 3—Week 1—Day 1

1. Patients with HIV disease presenting with odynophagia should be empirically treated for Candida albicans with fluconazole for 1 week before EGD is even considered. If not better in a week, then proceed with EGD. Do not have to have thrush to have Candida esophagitis.
2. Syphilis in pregnancy and in setting of neurosyphilis must be treated with IV penicillin.

If penicillin allergy exists, the patient must go through desensitization.
3. Secondary syphilis can present with a rash in the palms and soles, **generalized** lymphadenopathy, and with oral mucosal lesions. Primary syphilis presents with a painless genital chancre. Painful genital chancres are associated with *Hemophilus ducreyi* (chancroid).
4. Empiric treatment of early prosthetic valve endocarditis (less than 2 months) is with vancomycin, rifampin, and gentamicin.
5. Treatment of severe cardiac Lyme disease (manifested by substantial AV block) is with IV ceftriaxone. Treatment of the skin lesion (erythema chronicum migrans) is with oral doxycycline.
6. The tick *Ixodes scapularis* (also known as *Ixodes damini*) can carry Lyme disease (Borrelia burgdorferi), Babesiosis (higher risk in asplenic patients), and Ehrlichiosis (splenomegaly and thrombocytopenia are associated).
7. Human bites causing a cellulitis of the hands need to be admitted with urgent referral to hand surgeon for debridement and initiation of IV ampicillin-sulbactam. Dog bite patients with significant injury should at least receive oral amoxicillin-clavulanate.
8. HACEK organisms are slow growing taking up to 1 week to grow positive cultures and

should be treated with IV ceftriaxone and aminoglycoside when causing endocarditis.

9. IV drug abusers can develop tricuspid valve endocarditis with the most common organism for this valve being *Staphylococcus aureus*.

10. Patients without a spleen are at risk of infections with Babesiosis, encapsulated organisms (Streptococcus, Neisseria), and DF-2 (also known as *Capnocytophaga canimorsus* from dog bites presenting with widespread purpura and DIC), and Salmonella.

17.3   Year 3—Week 1—Day 2

1. Patients with hairy cell leukemia have abnormal lymphocytes with projections (hair-appearing) from their membranes. The only other situation where cells may mimic those of hairy cell leukemia are the cells of splenic marginal zone lymphoma.

2. Suspect constrictive pericarditis in patients with significant dyspnea on exertion yet normal ejection fraction and no valvular heart disease.

3. Patients with WPW (Wolff Parkinson White) having symptomatic episodes need radiofrequency ablation.

4. Consider WPW heavily in the differential of a young patient with atrial fibrillation with a very rapid ventricular rate.

5. The most common supraventricular tachycardia seen in the general population is an AV-nodal reentrant tachycardia.

6. Nitrofurantoin can cause a pulmonary toxicity marked by interstitial pneumonitis.

7. Amoxicillin-clavulanate can potentiate the INR in patients taking warfarin. Patients with amoxicillin alone do not seem to have this effect.

8. The preferred dose of clindamycin as an adjunct in therapy when treating a toxin-state such as aggressive streptococcal and clostridial infections is 600 to 900 mg every 8 hours.

9. A Horner's syndrome may be noted in patients with lateral medullary infarction (as part of the Wallenberg's syndrome).

10. Gerstmann syndrome is marked by acalculia, finger anomia, left-right confusion, and dysgraphia.

17.4   Year 3—Week 1—Day 3

1. Lymphoproliferative disorders and autoimmune disorders are among the most common causes for acquired angioedema disease states.

2. The test to order to detect any deficiency in the complement system is CH50. Late complement deficiencies are highly associated with recurrent *Neisseria* infections.

3. The precise test to order to distinguish hereditary from acquired angioedema is the C1q level, which is low in acquired angioedema.

4. The treatment of hereditary angioedema is danazol or stanozolol.

5. Fresh frozen plasma (FFP) therapy could be used in an emergent state in patients with angioedema attacks.

6. Patients with angioedema can have urticaria associated with their condition, although urticaria is noticeably absent in nearly all cases of ACE-inhibitor angioedema.

7. Progesterone can lead to angioedema and urticaria.

8. NSAIDs are frequently overlooked as a cause of angioedema.

9. Patients with angioedema can have the clinical picture of acute abdomen as they can get angioedema of the small bowel.

10. A symptom commonly seen in temporal arteritis patients is jaw claudication, in which a person is unable to eat much as they quickly tire from using their muscles of mastication. In the setting of new onset severe headaches, this should strongly lead to suspicion of temporal arteritis.

17.5   Year 3—Week 2—Day 1

1. The most common ocular complication of rheumatoid arthritis is secondary Sjogren's syndrome (dry eyes).

2. Other ocular complications that are not as common as dry eyes in RA include episcleritis, scleritis, and scleromalacia perforans.

3. Scleritis is an ocular emergency and should be referred immediately to the ophthalmologist. Episcleritis can be observed for a brief period of time.

4. Patients with CNS lymphoma will have positive EBV titers in the CSF. CNS lymphoma is a difficult disease state to obtain tissue positive for the disease.

5. The most common infection worldwide causing Guillain-Barre syndrome is *Campylobacter jejuni*. It can also be seen with Mycoplasma infections.

6. Pustular psoriasis can resemble the keratoderma blenorrhagicum rash of reactive arthritis, but the latter condition is not worsened by use of corticosteroids.

7. Guttate psoriasis can appear as a psoriasis variant in older individuals due to excessive stress, severe sunburn or heavy alcohol use.

8. The most common cause of erythema nodosum is streptococcal infection.

9. Other causes of erythema nodosum include leprosy, tuberculosis, oral contraceptive medications, pregnancy, and inflammatory bowel disease.

10. Pregnancy can lead to worsening of perioral dermatitis and underlying melasma states in women. It also tends to worsen underlying systemic lupus erythematosus.

17.6   Year 3—Week 2—Day 2

1. Hypothyroidism can lead to transudative or exudative pleural effusions and can cause pericardial effusions.

2. Amyloidosis and hypothyroidism are two diseases to cause low voltage on an EKG.

3. Patients with mitral valve prolapse and redundant, myxomatoid valves on 2D echo or with mitral regurgitation need endocarditis prophylaxis before high-risk procedures such as dental cleaning or colonoscopy.

4. Mitral valve prolapse is the leading cause of isolated mitral regurgitation in the USA.

5. Chronic aortic insufficiency will cause wonderful physical exam signs such as water-hammer distal pulses, bobbing of the head (De Musset's sign), pulsation of the iris, and bobbing of the uvula (Muller's sign). Acute aortic insufficiency will not cause these signs.

6. Nitroprusside is an effective agent for very temporary afterload reduction in acute aortic insufficiency while a patient is awaiting imminent aortic valve repair/replacement.

7. Young patients with pneumonia and associated pneumothorax need to be worked up for PCP pneumonia and HIV disease.

8. HIV disease and Parkinson's disease patients can be afflicted with seborrheic dermatitis at a very young age.

9. The most common cause of erysipelas (a form of cellulitis) is group A beta-hemolytic streptococcus.

10. Fabry's disease is marked by a deficiency of alpha-galactosidase and is associated with angiokeratoma corporis diffusum, heart disease, eye disease, and focal segmental glomerulosclerosis.

17.7   Year 3—Week 2—Day 3

1. Multicentric reticulohistiocytosis is a rheumatological disease marked by DIP arthritis (usually asymmetrical and destructive) with associated reddish-brown periungual papulonodules.

2. Psoriasis can also cause a destructive DIP arthritis in young patients and can present initially without skin rash (and even 10% of patients never ever get a skin rash).

3. Occult areas to look for the rash of psoriasis include the scalp, the umbilical area, and the gluteal cleft.

4. Among all the neoplasms, the most common histology to spread to the skin is adenocarcinoma.

5. Merkel's cell cancer is a neuroendocrine skin cancer that is very aggressive and has a poor prognosis. Treatment is wide local excision and chemotherapy.

6. The most common skin finding in patients with endocarditis is petechiae.
7. Patients with dermatitis herpetiformis frequently have IGA identified when immunofluorescence is done on skin biopsy.
8. Darier's sign occurs when one rubs the macule of a patients with urticaria pigmentosa and a wheal and flare reaction occurs around the macule.
9. Urticaria pigmentosa is skin-limited mastocytosis.
10. Mastocytosis can present with widespread systemic signs such as flushing, bone pain, early satiety, nausea, and even leukemic involvement.

17.8 Year 3—Week 3—Day 1

1. *Vibrio vulnificus* and *Vibrio parahemolyticus* infections can present with hemorrhagic bullous lesions over the lower extremities.
2. Besides Vibrio species, *Listeria, Aeromonas, and Yersinia* can infect patients with end-stage liver disease at a higher rate than the general population.
3. Patients with Listeria meningitis need treatment with IV ampicillin as cephalosporins will not work.
4. If a patient has decerebrate posturing, then the midbrain has likely suffered injury. If the patient has decorticate posturing, then the patient likely has suffered thalamic injury.
5. Patients with elevated prolactin level must have pregnancy ruled out. Other causes for elevated prolactin level due to medications include amitriptyline, phenothiazines, and metoclopramide.
6. Severe hypothyroidism can also cause an elevated prolactin level. Treatment is to take care of the underlying hypothyroidism without any specific dopamine receptor agonist therapy.
7. Non-functioning pituitary adenomas can elevate the prolactin level due to "stalk" effect by inhibiting dopamine and thus raising prolactin.
8. Women who are having irregular periods or are truly amenorrheic and are noted to have clitoromegaly on physical exam need to be ruled out for androgen secreting tumor of the adrenal gland or ovary.

9. Patients with polycystic ovarian disease will have acne, hirsutism, and obesity.
10. Sural nerve biopsy can be used as part of making a diagnosis of polyarteritis nodosum. Churg-Strauss vasculitis needs to be considered in all patients with adult-onset asthma and allergic rhinitis, especially if they are having neurological symptoms such as foot drop.

17.9 Year 3—Week 3—Day 2

1. One might see *Streptococcus pneumonia* occasionally engulfed by a white blood cell on peripheral smear when there is a high bacterial component.
2. Klebsiella lung infections can be associated by a bulging minor fissure sign best seen on a lateral X-ray.
3. Pituitary adenomas generally cause bitemporal hemianopsia if they are encroaching on the optic chiasm.
4. TSH secreting pituitary tumors will cause symptoms of hyperthyroidism with elevated free T4 and total T3 levels, but the patient will have normal to elevated TSH levels (instead of the usual TSH less than 0.001 mg/dL which is what one would expect).
5. If one does not treat hyperthyroidism, atrial fibrillation and osteoporosis might ensue.
6. Patients with pheochromocytoma generally need a few liters of normal saline when first diagnosed as they are generally clinically dehydrated.
7. Patients with adrenal insufficiency might demonstrate hyponatremia, hypoglycemia, eosinophilia, and hypercalcemia and may be even hyperkalemia if it is primary adrenal insufficiency.
8. Patients started on anticoagulation can be afflicted with adrenal insufficiency if they suffer adrenal hemorrhage.
9. Coumadin administration can cause cholesterol emboli syndrome in the first week or two of treatment severe enough to cause acute renal failure necessitating hemodialysis.
10. Primary hypogonadism is marked by low testosterone and elevated LH level.

17.10   Year 3—Week 3—Day 3

1. Asthma symptoms usually precede the GI symptoms of eosinophilic gastritis by at least 8–10 years.
2. Oral fluticasone slurry preparation is the treatment of eosinophilic esophagitis as opposed to eosinophilic gastroenteritis where the treatment is oral steroids.
3. Microcytic to normocytic anemia can be commonly found with eosinophilic gastroenteritis, whereas macrocytic anemia should not be found (but can be found in tropical sprue patients).
4. Doxepin is a tricyclic antidepressant that has proven useful for eosinophilic esophagitis and it also has proven useful for patients with insomnia who cannot sleep due to itching.
5. There is an increased incidence of peptic ulcer disease in patients with myeloproliferative disorders.
6. Howell-Jolly bodies are seen in patients with functional asplenia as well as those with history of splenectomy.
7. Target cells are seen in a variety of conditions including thalassemia trait and hemoglobinopathies, as well as patients with liver disease.
8. Basophilic stippling is a feature of lead poisoning, which may also present with acute abdominal pain and acute gout.
9. Adie's (tonic) pupil is a constricted pupil usually due to a ciliary ganglion problem and one can see decreased peripheral reflexes with this condition.
10. Patients with alpha thalassemia trait who develop iron deficiency anemia will have their elevated hemoglobin A2 levels brought back down to normal.

17.11   Year 3—Week 4—Day 1

1. Dermatitis herpetiformis resembles herpes infection and is extremely pruritis and can be seen in patients with celiac sprue.

2. Tinea versicolor infections are caused by *Malassezia furfur* and can be treated with local ketoconazole.
3. Crusted Scabies (Norwegian variant) infection should trigger an HIV test in the afflicted patient.
4. Molluscum contagiosum is marked by umbilicated pearly papules and is caused by poxvirus.
5. Bullous pemphigoid can occur in the elderly and should not trigger an age-appropriate neoplastic workup.
6. Pemphigus vulgaris can be associated with malignancy, especially colonic and ovarian cancer.
7. Superficial spreading melanoma is the most common melanoma of all types.
8. Nodular melanoma tends to have the worst prognosis of all the melanomas, while lentigo maligna melanoma can be present for decades and still be caught before significant invasion.
9. Rheumatoid arthritis patients afflicted with vasculitis usually have a high titer rheumatoid factor, rheumatoid nodules, and rheumatoid lung disease.
10. Secondary syphilis can mimic pityriasis rosea and can cause flat sessile anal lesions known as condyloma lata.

17.12   Year 3—Week 4—Day 2

1. Squamous cell cancer is the lung cancer most associated with hypercalcemia.
2. Hypercalcemia in patients with squamous cell cancer is mediated usually by release of PTH-related peptide.
3. Patients with small cell lung cancer need an MRI of the brain and bone scan to complete staging. Patients with non-small cell lung cancer need an MRI of the brain if they have a high thoracic burden of disease (either a large mass or bulky mediastinal nodal disease).
4. Endocarditis and atrial myxoma are two disease states that can embolize to the brain and mimic metastatic cancer to the brain.

5. Sarcoidosis is another disease state that can have pulmonary and CNS involvement. Treatment of neurosarcoidosis involves corticosteroid therapy.
6. The most common lung cancer to have cavitary lung features is squamous cell cancer of the lung.
7. Adenocarcinoma of the lung can present with new onset clubbing (sometimes as quickly as 3–4 months in origin) and can cause knee pain by the process of tibial periostitis. This is a paraneoplastic process known as hypertrophic pulmonary osteoarthropathy.
8. Bronchoscopy is the next test of choice in trying to get a diagnosis in a patient with a centrally located lung mass.
9. Initial treatment of symptomatic hypercalcemia is aggressive hydration with normal saline (rates at 250 mL/h are not that unusual).
10. Short-term treatment of hypercalcemia includes calcitonin which does not work for long after 24 h and bisphosphonate therapy (pamidronate).

17.13 Year 3—Week 4—Day 3

1. EKG findings of hypercalcemia include shortened QT interval.
2. Small cell lung cancer can be associated with subacute cerebellar degeneration, which is a paraneoplastic syndrome whereby there is truncal ataxia and there is dysdiadochokinesia and abnormal finger to nose testing.
3. Unlike patients with ovarian cancer, patients with small cell lung cancer with subacute cerebellar degeneration usually do not have anti-Yo antibodies (anti-Purkinje cell antibodies).
4. The hallmark of treatment of extensive small cell lung cancer is chemotherapy and prophylactic whole brain irradiation.
5. Patients with proven malignancy present in pleural effusions who have non-small cell lung cancer are generally not surgical candidates.

6. Meningiomas can be found in young patients, and they generally are found in the cerebral convexities and are dural based. They can initially present with seizure.
7. Glioblastoma multiforme is the most aggressive of all the primary CNS tumors.
8. Anticoagulation is absolutely contraindicated in patients with CNS disease that is metastatic from renal cell carcinoma, melanoma, and choriocarcinoma lesions.
9. The cerebral edema from a malignancy will generally respond to steroid therapy and is termed vasogenic. The cerebral edema from stroke does not respond to steroid therapy and is termed cytotoxic.
10. *Nocardia asteroides* is a gram-positive organism that can cause cavitary lung lesions and involve the CNS as well.

17.14 Year 3—Week 5—Day 1

1. Beta-blockers should be avoided in patients with underlying Wolff–Parkinson–White (WPW) disease given the fact that AV-nodal blockade will lead conduction down the aberrant pathway.
2. Amoxicillin is an acceptable second-line oral treatment agent for mild Lyme disease in patients who cannot take doxycycline therapy.
3. Patients with lupus anticoagulant will have an elevated PTT lab value and will also demonstrate a positive Russell Viper venom test.
4. Xanthelasma and xanthomas are skin findings that can be elicited in patients with underlying primary biliary cirrhosis even with normal lipid panels.
5. The first-line treatment of plantar fasciitis is the use of stretching exercises of the Achilles tendon and orthotic devices to offload pressure on the plantar fascia.
6. Patients diagnosed with Morton's neuroma should be referred to podiatry for a neurectomy procedure.
7. Glucagon is the antidote for both beta-blocker and calcium channel blocker overdose situations.

8. Stauffer's syndrome involves the paraneoplastic driven elevation of the AST and AST levels of the liver from underlying renal cell carcinoma. Treatment of the renal cell carcinoma will resolve the situation.

9. Patients with underlying dermatomyositis have unchanged deep tendon reflexes.

10. Patients with hypothyroidism can present with periorbital edema similar to patients with nephrotic syndrome and trichinosis infections.

17.15 Year 3—Week 5—Day 2

1. Rapid quantitative ELISA D-dimer assays have a high negative predictive value for deep venous thrombosis and pulmonary embolism.

2. ST-segment elevation in lead AVR is highly suggestive of left main coronary artery disease.

3. Clopidogrel should never be started in patients with ST-segment elevation in lead AVR as emergent/urgent CABG may be needed in these patients, and platelet dysfunction may last for 5–7 days due to clopidogrel.

4. A qR complex morphology for right bundle branch block is suggestive of underlying pulmonary hypertension.

5. Treatment of Alzheimer's disease with acetylcholinesterase inhibitors can temporarily alleviate symptoms but does not modify disease progression.

6. In Alzheimer's disease, there is an increased number of neuritic (amyloid) plaques and neurofibrillary tangles in the hippocampus, amygdala, and association neocortex.

7. Hypothyroidism is in the differential diagnosis of patients with low voltage on EKG. These patients can have elevated LDH, CPK, CPK-MB levels but should not have elevated troponin I levels due to the thyroid state.

8. When encountering patients intolerant of ACE-I and ARB therapy, clinicians can use nitrates and hydralazine with proper titration of hydralazine dosing occurring as long as tolerated by the patient.

9. Patients with Nocardia asteroids infections who are sulfa-allergic can be treated with minocycline and amikacin.

10. Wide mouthed pseudo-diverticulae and "water-melon stomach" are target organ manifestations of scleroderma.

17.16 Year 3—Week 5—Day 3

1. Patients with HIV disease can have any presentation of tuberculosis, including diffuse interstitial infiltrates and the miliary version of the disease (millet-seed lesions throughout the lung).

2. The fast-growing atypical mycobacteria are the following. Chelonae, fortuitum, and abscessus.

3. *Mycobacterium marinum* is a common organism found in in freshwater and it can lead to a nodular lymphangitis (sporotrichoid) presentation.

4. Nocardia can cause brain abscess disease as well as lung disease. IV amikacin is used by many physicians along with Septra if a brain abscess is present.

5. Whipple's disease patients may need up to 12-18 months of therapy with doxycycline before they are clinically cured of their disease.

6. Anterior mediastinal widening can be caused by "terrible" lymphoma, thymoma, teratoma, or substernal thyroid gland. Anthrax is also associated with anterior mediastinal widening.

7. Posterior mediastinal widening is usually due to neurogenic or esophageal cysts processes but can be caused by histoplasmosis.

8. Q-Fever is caused by *Coxiella burnetii* and can cause endocarditis and liver failure.

9. Rifampin is used in treatment of severe Legionella lung infections as an adjunct to primary therapy with azithromycin.

10. The treatment of Lemierre's syndrome is with penicillin. If penicillin allergic, then use clindamycin.

17.17 Year 3—Week 6—Day 1

1. Omeprazole is the only proton pump inhibitor to significantly affect the INR in patients taking coumadin (tends to potentiate the INR).
2. Patients with restless leg syndrome may have iron deficiency anemia that is correlated with their condition.
3. Dopamine receptor agonist has replaced benzodiazepine therapy as first line for restless leg syndrome.
4. Reserpine is the anti-hypertensive agent most linked to depression.
5. Patients with erythromelalgia (burning and redness of extremity relieved with aspirin, usually involving the digits) need a workup for myeloproliferative diseases.
6. An elevated adenosine deaminase level can be found in the pleural fluid of patients with tuberculosis.
7. Patients with tuberculosis do not have greater than 5% mesothelial cells in the pleural fluid.
8. About 20% of patients with pulmonary embolism will present with pleural effusion. These effusions can be rather large in nature in these patients.
9. Patients with post-CABG exudative effusions generally resolve within weeks after surgery. The effusions are exudative and can be bloody, usually involving the left side.
10. Patients with rheumatoid arthritis can have low glucose in the pleural fluid due to disruption of the capillary glucose transporter in the pleural membrane (this is generally not seen in lupus).

17.18 Year 3—Week 6—Day 2

1. Mefloquine is the recommended drug to take for prophylaxis of malaria to most parts of the world.
2. Both Aspergillus and Nocardia should be considered in patients with lung and brain infection who are taking high doses of steroids.

3. Patients with recurrent episodes of *Neisseria meningitidis* should be worked up for late complement deficiency.
4. Patients with recurrent episodes of sinusitis and pneumonia should be worked up for common variable immunodeficiency.
5. IGA deficiency is the most common immunodeficiency worldwide.
6. Patients with IgA deficiency are at risk for anaphylaxis when receiving FFP or blood products. Washed blood products are useful in markedly decreasing this risk.
7. H2 receptor antagonists can cause mental status changes and hallucinations in the elderly.
8. Oxybutynin is an agent for urge incontinence that has anticholinergic effects. Tolterodine is another option that does not have that side effect.
9. Disopyramide is a class IA arrhythmic that can be used for the treatment of hypertrophic cardiomyopathy as an adjunct to beta-blockers and it can lead to anticholinergic side effects.
10. Disopyramide is the most negative inotrope of the class IA anti-arrhythmics.

17.19 Year 3—Week 6—Day 3

1. Patients with isolated cranial nerve 3 palsy should be ruled out for diabetes mellitus.
2. An oral glucose tolerance test is sometimes needed to be done to definitively rule out diabetes mellitus as the cause of erectile dysfunction, peripheral neuropathy, and other diabetes-associated conditions.
3. Gastroparesis should be sought after in all patients with diabetes mellitus who start to show new pattern of instability in blood sugar measurements.
4. Scleredema is a condition mimicking scleroderma which can be seen in patients with diabetes mellitus.
5. Avoid using metformin in patients with ischemic cardiomyopathy.
6. There is a small cell cancer variant that can involve the prostate gland.

7. Legionella pneumophilia can cause Pontiac fever, which is a febrile state associated with myositis with lack of pneumonia.
8. Sjogren's syndrome is the autoimmune disease most linked to renal tubular acidosis type 1.
9. Acetazolamide is a carbonic anhydrase inhibitor that can cause a non-gap metabolic acidosis.
10. The urine chloride level is the most helpful test in seeing if a patient with metabolic alkalosis will respond to a fluid challenge.

17.20   Year 3—Week 7—Day 1

1. Focal segmental glomerulosclerosis is the most common histology affecting patients with HIV nephropathy.
2. The best treatment for HIV nephropathy is the use of HAART therapy (highly active antiretroviral treatment).
3. Abacavir is associated with a hypersensitivity syndrome and testing for HLA B 57 allele variant should be done before initiating therapy.
4. If HIV disease is diagnosed early in pregnancy, most authorities would choose to start or continue three drug therapy.
5. Patients with cervical cancer at a young age should be worked up for HIV disease.
6. Patients with *Candida krusei* infections will not respond to fluconazole therapy. Other antifungal agents such as amphotericin-B may need to be used in these situations.
7. Hypothyroidism and hypercalcemia are two simple things that should be ruled out in patients with severe constipation.
8. One of the best prophylaxis regimens for cluster headaches involves the combination of lithium and calcium channel blocker (verapamil).
9. Beta-blocker is the first-line therapy for essential tremor. Primidone is second-line agent.
10. Lamotrigine is the drug of choice for patients with atonic seizures (drop attacks) by stabilization of membranes in neural network

through action at voltage sensitive sodium channels.

17.21   Year 3—Week 7—Day 2

1. Nodular lymphangitis is also known as sporotrichoid pattern dermatitis. A distal ulcerative lesion is mimicked up the lymphatic chain of the arm or leg by similar lesions. Causes include sporotrichosis, *Mycobacterium marinum*, tularemia, other atypical mycobacteria, and *Nocardia braziliensis* infections.
2. Sporotrichosis is treated first-line with itraconazole. Use SSKI (potassium iodide) if LFT's or QT interval prolongation do not allow for use of itraconazole.
3. Do not use isoniazid to treat *Mycobacterium marinum* as it is very ineffective. Medications such as rifabutin, clarithromycin, and ethambutol will work.
4. A side effect of ethambutol is optic neuritis. Color vision loss is the first warning sign of this phenomenon. It can cause gout as well, but to a lesser degree than pyrazinamide.
5. Although the anti-histone antibody is classically linked to drug-induced lupus, patients with real SLE can also have a positive antibody.
6. Autoimmune hemolytic anemia is marked by the presence of spherocytes and a positive direct Coombs test. No schistocytes are seen with this disease.
7. Wilson's disease, chronic lymphocytic leukemia, systemic lupus erythematosus, and inflammatory bowel disease are among the most common causes of an autoimmune hemolytic anemia.
8. Hepatitis B testing must be done on all patients with rheumatological or hematological diseases before they are treated with rituximab therapy. Failure to do so can cause reactivation of Hepatitis B.
9. A reactive arthritis can occur with tuberculosis known as Poncet's arthritis. This has also been noted with local BCG therapy for bladder cancer.

10. Pyrazinamide and ethambutol are both known to cause drug-induced gout in the treatment of tuberculosis but only ethambutol is associated classically with optic neuritis.

17.22 Year 3—Week 7—Day 3

1. Itraconazole is the first-line treatment of patients with Sporotrichosis. Beware of QT interval prolongation.
2. Atypical Mycobacterium infections will need at least 12 months to 18 months of prolonged therapy for eradiction with 2-3 drug therapy (usually need clarithromycin plus rifabutin and may be even ethambutol).
3. Bullous pemphigoid is a condition marked by tense bullae, usually arising in the elderly, with no paraneoplastic association.
4. Pemphigus vulgaris does have paraneoplastic association in most literature, particularly to ovarian cancer in females.
5. Among the causes of bilateral carpal tunnel syndrome are amyloidosis, hypothyroidism, multiple myeloma, acromegaly, pregnancy, and rheumatoid arthritis.
6. Consider first carpometacarpal osteoarthritis and De Quervain's tenosynovitis in patients presenting with pain at the anatomical snuffbox.
7. Fever associated with thyroid storm is best treated with acetaminophen rather than salicylate therapy.
8. Hydatidiform mole must be considered in pregnant women presenting with clinical signs of pre-eclampsia in the first trimester of pregnancy.
9. Gilbert syndrome is the most common cause of an unconjugated bilirubin increase in the general population.
10. Second and third metacarpal disease can be seen in patients with hemochromatosis.

17.23 Year 3—Week 8—Day 1

1. Patients with significant liver failure are at risk for infections with Listeria, Yersinia (pseudoappendicitis), *Vibrio vulnificus* and *Vibrio parahemolyticus* (hemorrhagic bullous lesions), and Aeromonas (also Plesiomonas).
2. Ceftriaxone is associated with a drug-induced liver cholestasis.
3. Cephalosporins with a methylthiotetrazolium ring (MTT) are associated with hypoprothrombinemia and a disulfiram reaction with alcohol.
4. *Stenotrophomonas maltophilia* lung infections are universally resistant to imipenem. Treatment includes levofloxacin and ticarcillin-clavulanate therapy.
5. There is a risk of seizures with high-dose penicillin and imipenem particularly in patients with renal insufficiency.
6. Patients with bite of the brown recluse spider can benefit if given dapsone within the first 48 h to stop the necrosis caused by the sphingomyelinase poison. Dapsone is also used to treat leprosy and to ameliorate the skin lesions of dermatitis herpetiformis.
7. Among the bacterial causes of erythema nodosum are streptococcal infections, Yersinia infection, and tuberculosis. It is also caused by fungal diseases particularly Coccidiomycosis.
8. Chlamydia pneumonia has been associated with hoarseness. Mycoplasma has been associated with bullous myringitis, cold agglutinin disease, and transverse myelitis.
9. Lemierre's syndrome is caused by *Fusobacterium species frequently* and is associated with septic jugular vein thrombophlebitis and septic pulmonary emboli.
10. *Actinomycosis israelii* is associated with finding of "sulfur granules" on histology. It is a fistula forming organism. IUD use for contraception is a risk factor. Treatment of choice is IV penicillin.

17.24 Year 3—Week 8—Day 2

1. Acute appendicitis can come about from traditional infection with fecolith blockage but also can arise from worms (*Enterobius vermicularis*), carcinoid tumor infiltration, and adenocarcinoma infiltration.
2. The most common location for carcinoid tumor is the small bowel. Symptoms of carcinoid do not arise unless there is bronchial carcinoid tumor or there is carcinoid involvement of the liver.
3. One of the most distinguishing features between carcinoid tumor and systemic mastocytosis is the presence of bone pain. This feature is found with mastocytosis but is lacking in carcinoid syndrome. Both entities can cause flushing and both can cause epigastric pain after meals.
4. Mitral valve prolapse is the most common cause of mitral regurgitation in North America, well surpassing rheumatic disease.
5. Granuloma annulare is an entity that commonly afflicts the skin of patients with diabetes mellitus, often occurring in weight bearing areas such as joints. Necrobiosis lipoidica diabeticorum appears differently as it usually is found over the anterior shins as an isolated lesion usually with a yellow, waxy complexion with overlying telangiectasias not unusual to be seen.
6. Leishmaniasis can cause a sporotrichoid pattern (nodular lymphangitis). Treatment is with sodium stibogluconate although ketoconazole has been effective in some cases.
7. Consider neurocysticercosis highly in a young patient from Latin America with new onset seizures and an abnormal finding on CT scan. Treatment is with praziquantel.
8. Retinal detachment generally causes acute painless loss of vision. Most common risk factor is severe myopia.
9. Other causes of acute painless loss of vision include vitreous bleeding, exudative macular degeneration, ischemic neuropathy, and cerebral infarction.
10. Acute painful loss of vision includes endophthalmitis, acute angle glaucoma, corneal ulceration, uveitis, and optic neuritis.

17.25 Year 3—Week 8–Day 3

1. Patients with beta-thalassemia trait will have microcytosis and generally normal RDW values and increased red cell number on the CBC measurements.
2. There is an entity known as benign orthostatic proteinuria in which proteinuria will revert to near-normal value once the patient becomes supine.
3. Tricyclic antidepressants can block the anti-hypertensive effects of clonidine, guanethidine, and reserpine. Guanethidine should be discontinued at least 2 weeks prior to major surgery. Among other anti-hypertensive side effects are the nightmares associated with beta-blockers and peripheral edema/gingival hyperplasia common with calcium channel blockers (especially of the dihydropyridine class). Verapamil is associated with constipation and dizziness.
4. If a patient with proteinuria is found to have an idiopathic cause, the most common histology on kidney biopsy will be membranous glomerulopathy. A solid tumor can arise years after diagnosis. If minimal change disease is found in an adult, consideration to Hodgkin's disease should be given.
5. Patients with beta-thalassemia trait can certainly also develop iron deficiency anemia so whenever in doubt, check a ferritin level. If the ferritin level is non-diagnostic, then check a soluble transferrin receptor, which will be elevated if iron deficiency anemia is present.
6. Thiazides in low doses combined with a strong loop diuretic can have a synergistic effect on increased excretion of calcium, whereas thiazide diuretics alone decreases calcium excretion.
7. Tumor lysis syndrome is associated with increased uric acid, phosphorus, and potassium with decreased calcium level.
8. Acute tubular necrosis is commonly associated with renal failure after use of aminoglycosides or vancomycin and can be associated with increased phosphorus level.
9. Struvite stones (magnesium–ammonium–phosphorus stones) can be seen with staghorn calculi and are caused by recurrent Proteus infections with urinary pH generally above

8.0. Cystine stones have strong family history component and appear as a hexagonal crystal. Hyperoxaluria as a mechanism for calcium oxalate stones is seen in patients with Crohn's disease who have had terminal ileum resections. The radiolucent stones are the cystine and uric acid stones. Probenecid is contraindicated in patients with history of uric acid kidney stones.

10. Other common causes of acute tubular necrosis include heavy metals, hypercalcemia, myoglobinuria, hemoglobinuria, contrast dye, and use of cyclosporine, amphotericin B (which can also cause a type 1 RTA) and cisplatin (which can also cause hypomagnesemia and magnesuria most commonly). The hallmark of ATN is large, muddy brown granular casts and the condition resolves in 1–4 weeks. In ATN, the fractional excretion of sodium is generally well above 1 and the urine osmolality is 300–350 mg/dL with a urine sodium above 20 mg/dL.

17.26 Year 3—Week 9—Day 1

1. Contrast dye is also associated with multiple cholesterol emboli syndrome (can be marked by renal insufficiency, eosinophilia, and rash of livedo reticularis). Kidney biopsy in these patients reveals "ghost clefts."

2. Hemoglobin electrophoresis is performed when suspecting a hemoglobinopathy. Protein electrophoresis is done when suspecting a plasma cell dyscrasia, such as multiple myeloma or Waldenstrom's macroglobulinemia.

3. The fractional excretion of sodium is always less than 1% in glomerulopathies. Acute glomerulopathies are associated with sodium retention due to intrarenal hemodynamic factors.

4. A clue to chronic nephropathies is that they usually have heavy proteinuria and can have "oval fat bodies" noted in urinary sediment.

5. Nephrotic syndrome patients tend to get edema, hypoalbuminemia, hypogammaglob-

ulinemia (increased infections with Streptococcus and Haemophilus species), loss of thyroid and iron binding globulins (low total thyroxine and iron levels), and loss of antithrombin III (leading to pulmonary emboli and renal vein thrombosis).

6. Post-infectious glomerulonephritis is associated with diffuse cellular proliferation and subepithelial humps on kidney biopsy. This is a type 3 reaction causing granular deposits of IGG and C3. The skin infection and pharyngitis both lead to this condition but the skin infection is usually present well before the renal disease occurs. Group A beta-hemolytic strep infections are usually considered the common cause, and malaria and toxoplasmosis are two parasitic causes. Complement levels will return to normal after a short period of time.

7. The most common of the acute glomerulonephritis syndromes is Berger's disease which involves mesangial deposition of IGA. Hematuria can occur after viral illness or after exercise. There is no effective treatment.

8. Causes of rapidly progressive glomerulonephritis include SLE, Wegener's granulomatosis, Goodpasture's syndrome, and polyarteritis nodosa. This is marked by severe renal failure of recent onset. Cryoglobulins is also a cause, and treatment of the cryoglobulinemic glomerulonephritis will be with plasmapheresis and then an alkylating agent. It is marked by crescenteric deposits in the kidney biopsy.

9. Causes of focal segmental glomerulosclerosis include HIV disease, chronic heroin use, chronic vesicoureteral reflux, obesity, Charcot–Marie–Tooth disease (associated with sensorimotor neuropathies and "stork" calves), and Fabry's disease (a lipid storage disorder that is X-linked recessive and associated with).

10. Patients with idiopathic hypercalciuria have calcium oxalate renal stones and should be treated with thiazide diuretics and a low-sodium diet to decrease urine calcium. Low

calcium diets do not work and are not practical with risk of osteoporosis.

17.27 Year 3—Week 9—Day 2

1. The CEA level may be falsely elevated in smokers, sometimes as high as twice the upper limit of normal.
2. Finasteride may falsely lower the PSA level in patients with both BPH and prostate cancer, so caution should be taken with patients whose elevated levels start dropping when placed on this medication.
3. CA-125 can be elevated with other non-malignant conditions such as pelvic inflammatory disease and endometriosis.
4. CA 19–9 has its most use as a tumor marker in pancreatic adenocarcinomas among other adenocarcinomas but it has not been found useful in GI lymphomas.
5. CA 15–3 is a tumor marker that may be helpful in the management of patients with breast adenocarcinomas.
6. CA-15-3 can be elevated in non-malignant conditions such as sarcoidosis, tuberculosis, SLE, and chronic hepatitis.
7. Normal pressure hydrocephalus (NPH) can cause symptoms of Parkinsonism in the lower extremities but avoids giving those findings in the upper extremities, meaning patients will lack cogwheel rigidity and tremor of the upper extremity.
8. Progressive supranuclear palsy is a "Parkinson plus" disease which has minimal tremor and cogwheel rigidity but is marked by excessive falls especially when making turns and when reaching for objects above the head.
9. Treatment of normal pressure hydrocephalus (NPH) is usually to first prove that the patient improves with removal of about 30–40 cc of CSF, and then ventriculoperitoneal shunting can be considered.
10. Patients with UTI with organisms showing "extended spectrum beta-lactamase activity" should be considered for imipenem therapy.

17.28 Year 3—Week 9—Day 3

1. Beta-2 microglobulin levels are useful in following patients being treated for multiple myeloma.
2. Nephrectomy may need to be performed in patients with emphysematous pyelonephritis—there is a marked rise of this condition in diabetic patients.
3. Hematuria can be seen in cases of renal cell carcinoma.
4. An elevated serotonin level can be seen in patients with carcinoid syndrome.
5. Patients with carcinoid syndrome can develop symptoms of pellagra due to niacin deficiency.
6. Urothelial bladder cancer has no good tumor markers that can be followed.
7. Intravesicular BCG has been used in the treatment of localized transitional cell bladder cancers. A reactive arthritis can ensue from treatment with this medication.
8. The reactive arthritis associated with tuberculosis is known as Poncet's disease. The bone disease associated with tuberculosis is known as Pott's disease.
9. Calcitonin is elevated as a tumor marker in patients with medullary carcinoma of the thyroid.
10. Thyroglobulin level can serve as a tumor marker in patients with follicular or papillary carcinoma of the thyroid.

17.29 Year 3—Week 10—Day 1

1. The most aggressive thyroid carcinoma with a poor prognosis is anaplastic carcinoma of the thyroid.
2. In the elderly, there is a marked rise of lymphoma of the thyroid and lymphoma of the testicular glands.
3. Patients with gastrointestinal stromal tumors will generally have positive CD-117 markers and thus can be treated with imatinib mesylate.

4. The more common use of imatinib mesylate is to treat patients with chronic myelogenous leukemia.
5. The CD-38 marker if positive usually portends a poor prognosis for patients with CLL.
6. The CD-25 marker is found positive in many cases of cutaneous T-cell lymphoma (mycosis fungoides).
7. Sezary syndrome refers to the erythroderma and the abnormal cerebriform folded nuclei that can circulate in patients with cutaneous T-cell lymphoma.
8. Patients with chronic alcohol abuse can suffer truncal ataxia due to damage to the midline cerebellar structures (the vermis).
9. There is an interesting dementia syndrome whereby patients have the peculiarity of thinking that their hand does not belong to them, known as the "alien hand" syndrome. This is seen in corticobasal ganglion degeneration.
10. Patients with myasthenia gravis may need thymectomies even if no thymic mass is obviously present on imaging, if there is no response to usual treatment given.

17.30 Year 3—Week 10—Day 2

1. Patients with nephrotic syndrome are at risk of DVT/PE due to loss of antithrombin III.
2. Patients with Behcet syndrome can have bilateral pulmonary artery aneurysms and are at risk of both arterial and venous clots.
3. Patients with heparin-induced thrombocytopenia syndrome (HIT) are at risk of arterial and venous clots similar to patients with underlying Behcet's disease and antiphospholipid antibody syndrome.
4. A tall R-wave can be seen in lead V1 with Duchenne muscular dystrophy, right ventricular hypertrophy, true posterior MI, and WPW.
5. A young person with a fast ventricular rate atrial fibrillation should be thought of having WPW until proven otherwise and these patients can have very fast wide complex

tachycardias if aberrancy is present which can appear as if ventricular tachycardia (but the irregular nature of the atrial fibrillation distinguishes it from ventricular tachycardia).
6. Vertebrobasilar insufficiency very commonly presents with dizziness and ataxia.
7. Vertical nystagmus should concern the clinician about a possible stroke or space-occupying lesion in the brain as the cause of the nystagmus.
8. Young patients with recurrent optic neuritis and trigeminal neuralgia need to be worked up for multiple sclerosis.
9. The treatment of benign positional vertigo is head-maneuvering/head turning exercises to "reposition" the otoliths in the semicircular canal.
10. A true positive Romberg test occurs with the patient's eyes closed and implies posterior column problem.

17.31 Year 3—Week 10—Day 3

1. High-dose fluconazole can be attempted to try to eradicate Candida glabrata.
2. *Candida krusei* will not respond to any dosing of fluconazole and options such as voriconazole should be used in infections of this type.
3. Ticarcillin-clavulanate can be used to treat diabetic foot infections similar to piperacillin-tazobactam.
4. Patients with diabetes who have autonomic dysfunction also tend to be at higher risk of having gastroparesis, erectile dysfunction, and peripheral neuropathy.
5. Cyclophosphamide is the treatment of lupus cerebritis and aggressive glomerulonephritis.
6. Among the most common lung/kidney syndromes that should be in your differential in a patient with involvement of those two organ systems are the following lupus, Wegener's granulomatosis, Goodpasture's syndrome, and microscopic polyangiitis.

7. There are patients with dementia that will present with significant levels of depression and this disease should be screened in all patients with this underlyind disease.

8. Depression is usually marked by early morning awakening in sleep patterns.

9. Evan's syndrome refers to ITP in association with autoimmune hemolytic anemia.

10. Still's disease is the adult version of juvenile rheumatoid arthritis and is associated with very high ferritin levels, sometimes above 10,000 mg/dL with evanescent salmon pink rash present usually during febrile state across the torso of patients.

17.32 Year 3—Week 11—Day 1

1. Patients with chronic hepatitis B and hepatitis C are at risk of hepatocellular carcinoma.

2. All patients with chronic hepatitis B and/or hepatitis C should be vaccinated for hepatitis A as they will have a higher risk of fulminant expression of hepatitis A.

3. Check baseline CPK levels in patients being treated with daptomycin as the medication can cause myositis.

4. Patients with Stenotrophomonas infections can be treated with a variety of medications, most commonly sulfa-based antibiotic, ticarcillin-clavulanate, or the fluoroquinolones.

5. Patients with advanced age and rapid rate atrial fibrillation episodes should be considered for amiodarone therapy.

6. Younger patients with symptomatic rapid rate atrial fibrillation should be considered for propafenone or sotalol, rather than amiodarone due to the long-term side effects of that drug.

7. Small cell (neuroendocrine cancer) of the prostate can occur, and it is usually associated with trivial if any elevation of the PSA level.

8. Staging for small cell lung cancer includes MRI of the brain and total body bone scan.

9. Three phase bone scans are useful in making the diagnosis of reflex sympathetic dystrophy, also known as causalgia syndrome.

10. Among the most common causes of recurrent cellulitis are tinea pedis and venous stasis.

17.33 Year 3—Week 11—Day 2

1. Fasciculations of the tongue in the setting of motor weakness is concerning for ALS.

2. There can be a sensory level present in patients with Guillain-Barre syndrome in up to a third of patients.

3. Very small prolactinomas of the pituitary may be associated with prolactin levels under 200 mg/dL.

4. Bromocriptine should be started at very low doses (1.25–2.5 mg a day) when first starting to treat prolactinomas.

5. Prolactinomas with visual field impairments (due to involvement of the optic chiasm) can still be treated medically.

6. Adenomas that are functioning and are not prolactinomas need surgical treatment.

7. Oral contraceptive therapy is the first-line treatment of polycystic ovarian syndrome.

8. Hyperparathyroidism leads to cortical bone loss greater than trabecular bone loss, so forearm fractures with this condition are usually more likely than in patients with usual, run of the mill osteoporosis.

9. Untreated hyperthyroidism can place a patient at risk of atrial fibrillation and osteoporosis.

10. GnRH analogue therapy can lead to a risk of hot flashes in men as well as osteoporosis.

17.34 Year 3—Week 11—Day 3

1. Fava beans should be avoided for ingestion by patients with the Mediterranean-type of G6PD deficiency.

2. A low leukocyte alkaline phosphatase (LAP) score can help distinguish CML from leukemoid reaction.
3. Patients with methanol abuse can complain of visual loss due to a papillitis. These patients will have osmolar gaps and anion gaps.
4. The pulvinar nucleus is the most common thalamic nucleus to be involved in patients with hypertensive disease infarcts.
5. Colchicine can lead to liver toxicity and muscle toxicity if used in high doses over many months to years.
6. Coxiella burnetii is the cause of Q-fever which can lead to liver failure and endocarditis, and it is treated with doxycycline.
7. About 90% of BOTH adrenal glands need to be involved by hemorrhage or tumor involvement before adrenal insufficiency will ensue.
8. Sepsis is the most common cause of glucose intolerance in patients receiving TPN therapy. Chromium deficiency is only entertained after sepsis is ruled out.
9. Mitral stenosis is the valvular disease most associated with hemoptysis in the initial presentation.
10. LVH can commonly be missed by EKG criteria if one does not look at lead AVL. In that lead, R-wave is greater than or equal to 11 units and the ST segment shows signs of strain, one can make the diagnosis.

17.35   Year 3—Week 12—Day 1

1. Hepatitis A should never be overlooked as a possible cause of fulminant hepatitis in a traveler including pregnant women despite the fact that Hepatitis E is the entity most discussed with acute liver failure of viral cause in pregnancy.
2. Ciprofloxacin at onset of diarrhea and bismuth subsalicylate are among the treatment options for traveler's diarrhea. Antibiotic therapy is favored for patients on travel with underlying inflammatory bowel disease.
3. ETEC (enterotoxigenic *E. coli*) is the most common cause of traveler's diarrhea.

4. Vibrio cholera is associated with non-bloody diarrhea and can affect all patients regardless of immune status.
5. *Isospora belli* and *Dientamoeba fragilis* are the two parasites associated with diarrhea and eosinophilia.
6. Trimethoprim-sulfomethoxazole is the first-line treatment of Nocardia infections.
7. Ascaris lumbricoides has been associated with intestinal obstruction.
8. AML M4 with bone marrow eosinophilia is associated with a good overall prognosis.
9. HIV disease is associated with eosinophilia in the absence of any parasitic or neoplastic concomitant disorder.
10. Eosinophilic folliculitis should be considered as underlying skin disease in HIV patients who are not responding to usual folliculitis treatment.

17.36   Year 3—Week 12—Day 2

1. Patients with polymyalgia rheumatica can have pain and stiffness but weakness is an unusual finding in these patients.
2. Polymyalgia rheumatica can be associated with a symmetrical inflammatory arthritis.
3. Patients with SLE can develop hemolytic anemia which usually responds to steroids. The key test to order is the Coombs test (direct antiglobulin test) to make this diagnosis.
4. Patients with polymyositis can have significant dysphagia and have episodes of aspiration pneumonia.
5. Patients with relapsing polychondritis can die of respiratory failure from tracheal collapse.
6. Polyarteritis nodosa usually spares the lung from involvement. Abdominal pain with this disorder can be from abdominal microaneurysm formation and is best detected with an angiogram.
7. Patients with granulomatosis with polyangiitis may present with a variety of findings, including foot drop, hearing loss, and wrist drop.

8. Hepatitis B serological status needs to be checked in all patients with suspected diagnosis of polyarteritis nodosa.
9. *Staphylococcus aureus* is the most common cause of septic joint in the general population.
10. Sickle cell anemia patients are at higher risk of Salmonella joint infections than the general population, and this is felt to be due to gut microinfarctions leading to bacteremia.

17.37   Year 3—Week 12—Day 3

1. Bernard-Soulier syndrome involves the finding of large platelet size along with bleeding disorder with thrombocytopenia common.
2. Type 2b von Willebrand's disease may not respond well to DDAVP and is associated with thrombocytopenia with only mild to moderate bleeding usually noted despite marked abnormal platelet function testing.
3. Glanzmann's thrombasthenia is a bleeding disorder due to abnormal platelet aggregation. Platelet size is normal in this disease with platelet count also usually normal.
4. The coagulation assays will be normal in TTP, whereas they are abnormal in DIC.
5. The direct Coombs test or direct antiglobulin test is the best assay in looking for autoimmune hemolytic anemia.
6. DDAVP can stimulate von Willebrand factor release from the endothelial cell in most types of von Willebrand disease.
7. Young women with dysfunctional uterine bleeding should be worked up for von Willebrand's disease.
8. The PFA (platelet function assay) will be abnormal whenever severe thrombocytopenia is present.
9. PTU is safe to use in pregnancy, whereas methimazole can cause craniofacial fetal deformities and thus is avoided in pregnancy. Methimazole is reported to have less side effects than PTU if a patient could receive either drug.
10. Check a TSH level in all patients with atrial fibrillation rapid ventricular rate that is not responding to AV-nodal blocking agents.

17.38   Year 3—Week 13—Day 1

1. Guillain-Barre syndrome patients will present with areflexia and they will have wide swings in blood pressure as a manifestation of autonomic dysfunction.
2. DDAVP can be given to patients with Von Willebrand's disease who require an agent to raise factor levels slightly to stop bleeding.
3. DDAVP can also be used in patients with uremic bleeding. If this does not work, give platelets if a platelet function assay comes back abnormal.
4. Always rule out surreptitious heparin administration as the cause of a falsely elevated PTT level.
5. Avoid hydralazine in patients with aortic dissection as it can increase shear stress in these patients.
6. Nitroprusside and low-dose esmolol is an acceptable strategy to control blood pressure in patients with aortic dissection.
7. Patients with Factor 12 deficiency will have prolonged PTT testing but they do not bleed similar to Factor 11 deficiency patients.
8. Patients with back pain and markedly elevated blood pressures should be looked at for acute aortic dissection.
9. Treatment of factor 8 inhibitor is usually based on Bethesda titer measurements. If the titer is low, then one would do porcine factor 8 replacement. If the titer is high, then the best starting place is likely recombinant factor 7.
10. Acute myocardial infarction can occur in patients with aortic dissection, most commonly involving the right coronary artery.

17.39   Year 3—Week 13—Day 2

1. Severe hypothyroidism will lead to elevation of both TSH and prolactin. The prolactin level can be high enough to cause problems such as headaches and galactorrhea. The treatment of this condition is levothyroxine only.

2. The half-life of levothyroxine is 7 days so one can usually omit several doses postoperatively without a problem.

3. If one is suspicious of Cushing's syndrome due to a pituitary source from biochemical lab results, the next step is MRI of the brain. Petrosal venous sampling is helpful in preparing for surgery but should be done after MRI of brain.

4. The ACTH level will be low in patients with an adrenal cause to their Cushing's syndrome.

5. The treatment of prolactinomas is medical with bromocriptine, even if visual field deficits are already present at the time of diagnosis.

6. Phenothiazines, atypical antipsychotics, opioid drug therapy, cocaine abuse, pregnancy, metoclopramide, verapamil, and antidepressant (TCA and SSRI) therapy are amongst the causes of elevation of prolactin level usually under 200 mg/dL.

7. IGF-2 is a paraneoplastic hormone released by various soft tissue sarcomas leading to hypoglycemia.

8. Patients with Waldenstrom's macroglobulinemia rarely have bone pain or bone fractures, and more commonly present with hyperviscosity symptoms, such as headaches or stroke like symptoms.

9. Among the most telling signs that you are dealing with Guillain-Barre syndrome is flaccid weakness in the setting of areflexia. Other clues include the classic albuminocytologic dissociation on lumbar puncture where there is a very high CSF protein but few WBC's if any are seen.

10. Conditions for which plasmapheresis is used include TTP, Goodpasture syndrome, and Guillain-Barre syndrome.

17.40   Year 3—Week 13—Day 3

1. The most common cause of an elevated gastrin level in the general population is the widespread use of proton pump inhibitors.

2. Patients with factitious ingestion of insulin will not have elevated C-peptide levels as compared to those who ingest sulfonylureas.

3. Metformin monotherapy is an acceptable treatment of type 2 diabetes mellitus with hemoglobin A1c levels just above target if lifestyle modifications fail to improve the value.

4. Insulin therapy is recommended for short-term inpatient therapy in patients presenting with symptomatic hyperglycemia.

5. Hydroxychloroquine is the first-line agent of treatment of patients with SLE with skin and joint manifestations.

6. Agents such as dapsone and thalidomide have been used in patients with refractory SLE skin disease.

7. Hemorrhagic bullous skin disease can occur in patients with SLE, as can manifestations of panniculitis.

8. Methotrexate is the first-line therapy for patients with aggressive, erosive joint disease in patients with psoriasis or with rheumatoid arthritis.

9. Bisphosphonate therapy is used after failure of NSAIDS to control pain in patients with Paget's disease of the bone.

10. Histoplasmosis is notorious for posterior mediastinitis of the thorax, splenic calcifications, and calcified nodular lesions of the lung.

17.41   Year 3—Week 14—Day 1

1. Osteomalacia can lead to an elevated alkaline phosphatase level in the setting of low calcium and low phosphorus level. Patients with osteomalacia can complain of bone pain.

2. Patients with Paget's disease typically never have hypercalcemia from that state alone unless they have been immobilized for a period of many months.

3. Spinal cord injury patients are not routinely placed on DVT prophylaxis long-term but do get put on DVT prophylaxis if they become

infected or have a recent surgery (states associated with higher risk of DVT).

4. Patients with pancreatitis and inflammatory bowel disease are more predisposed to DVT than most disease states.

5. Smoking appears to protect patients from development of ulcerative colitis disease, whereas it exacerbates Crohn's disease patients (in addition to increase severity of those relapsed episodes).

6. P-ANCA might be positive in patients with ulcerative colitis much more often that patients with Crohn's disease.

7. The spondylitis and pyoderma gangrenosum that might be seen in inflammatory bowel disease do not wax or wane with active colitis, whereas the arthritis and erythema nodosum attacks do wax and wane with active colitis episodes.

8. The treatment of disseminated gonorrhea (symptoms of RUQ pain, hemorrhagic pustules, arthritis, and tenosynovitis) is with IV ceftriaxone for at least seven days.

9. Patients who have heart failure due to hypertension will commonly have diastolic dysfunction noted on echocardiogram.

10. The most common medications to cause a lupus-like syndrome which could cause pericarditis are hydralazine and procainamide. Please note that these meds may cause a positive ANA without lupus-like disease, and that they do not need to be stopped if the ANA is positive unless the patient has developed bothersome symptoms.

17.42   Year 3—Week 14—Day 2

1. Among the rheumatological drugs that can lead to proteinuria are gold and penicillamine. NSAIDs can also cause proteinuria with a nephritic sediment. NSAIDs decrease the release of renin which can lead to hyperkalemia in patients with hyporeninemic hypoaldosteronism.

2. Chronic interstitial nephritis is associated with papillary necrosis and chronic analgesic abuse (especially mixed analgesics and those

that have NSAIDs) with an incredible cumulative ingestion of the analgesic of greater than 6 pounds. It can also be caused by sickle cell disease, multiple myeloma, Sjogren's disease, and lead/cadmium poisoning.

3. Polycystic kidney disease (usually a mutation in short arm of chromosome 16) can present with progressive renal failure, hematuria, and hypertension. Proteinuria may be absent and if present is usually minimal. In adults, it is inherited in an autosomal dominant fashion.

4. There are two types of medullary kidney disease: medullary sponge kidney (usually diagnosed by IVP and not clinically significant unless kidney stones form) and medullary cystic kidney disease (in which there is usually a normal urinalysis with mild to no proteinuria, hyperkalemia, and hyperchloremic metabolic acidosis.

5. Bartter's syndrome refers to the state of increased renin and aldosterone associated with hypokalemia and metabolic alkalosis in patients with normal blood pressure. This disease is due to hyperplasia of juxtaglomerular apparatus with prominence of medullary interstitial cells. Treatment is with potassium and magnesium supplements (magnesuria is common) and patients are encouraged to have a liberal sodium intake as they can get hypotensive. Spironolactone is the drug of choice to stop potassium wasting.

6. Patients with renal failure are not at increased risk of abortion of a fetus or malformation in the fetus nor is there a risk of progression of kidney disease during the pregnancy. There is an increased risk of pre-eclampsia. As renal failure worsens in a woman, her chance of becoming pregnant significantly decreases and most patients on dialysis cannot become pregnant.

7. RTA type 1 (distal) is the RTA associated with kidney stones, and the RTA type 1 is marked by a urine pH usually greater than 5.5 (unlike the other RTAs), has less than 10% bicarbonate filtered, is not associated with the Fanconi syndrome (distinguishes it from type 2 RTA), and is marked by a positive urine anion gap (like all the RTAs and unlike

the process of GI bicarbonate loss) with low serum potassium (like RTA type 2 but unlike RTA type 4).

8. Urinary alkalinization is used in all stones except struvite and calcium phosphate stones. Citrate therapy is useful in all calcium stones as it chelates calcium.

9. Vitamin C and ethylene glycol can cause calcium oxalate stones if taken in large amounts. Methanol (like ethylene glycol) can cause an osmolar gap and an anion gap metabolic acidosis but it does not cause oxalate crystals but it does cause a papillitis with acute visual loss. Isopropyl alcohol (rubbing alcohol) is not associated with a marked anion gap metabolic acidosis and can have hypoglycemia and a falsely elevated creatinine level. Treatment of all the alcohol related ingestions when severe is with emergent hemodialysis.

10. Lithium can cause a nephrogenic diabetes insipidus as well as a state of hypothyroidism which can be treated with amiloride and levothyroxine respectively without necessarily having to stop the medication. Treatment in severe lithium intoxications is with emergent hemodialysis.

17.43   Year 3—Week 14—Day 3

1. Megakaryocytic proliferation is felt to the cause of the fibrosis in chronic idiopathic myelofibrosis.

2. Nailfold capillaroscopy should be done in all patients with Raynaud's phenomenon as abnormal findings will point to underlying rheumatological disease.

3. Calcium channel blockers are first-line therapy for Raynaud's phenomenon. Alpha-blockers are second-line therapy.

4. Among the causes of male gynecomastia are spironolactone therapy, Klinefelter's syndrome, and use of cimetidine.

5. Giardia lamblia infections are markedly increased in patients with IgA deficiency and common variable immunodeficiency.

6. Excessive chewing gum users can develop a chronic diarrhea from excess sorbitol due to the gum while use of sorbitol can lead to the finding of pneumatosis intestinalis on radiographic imaging.

7. Presence of nasal polyposis in a patient with malabsorption from pancreatic insufficiency should lead one to suspect the diagnosis of cystic fibrosis.

8. Consider protein-losing enteropathy in patients with very low albumin levels who have no demonstratable proteinuria.

9. Patients with pure seminomatous testicular cancers should have AFP negative. 20% of them may have an elevated HCG level.

10. Monostotic Paget's disease most commonly involves the pelvis, but it can involve the skull as well.

17.44   Year 3—Week 15—Day 1

1. Prerenal acute renal failure will generally have a FENA less than 1, a urine osmolality greater than 400, and a urine sodium less than 20 with either normal urine sediment or just hyaline or bland granular casts.

2. Nephrotic syndromes always have a normal C3 level. The C3 level is always low in postinfectious glomerulonephritis and is low about half the time in membranoproliferative glomerulonephritis.

3. Membranous nephropathy is associated with renal vein thrombosis and is marked by subepithelial deposits. It is the most common type of nephropathy after diabetes mellitus.

4. A patient who has hyponatremia and is actively seizing should receive 3% hypertonic saline with monitoring in ICU setting.

5. The urine chloride is a helpful test in metabolic alkalosis. If the level is less than 20 mg/dL, then the process can be treated with normal saline infusion.

6. Conn's syndrome is primary hyperaldosteronism and is associated with urine potassium and chloride levels above 30, hypokalemia, hypertension, and a metabolic alkalosis. Treatment is with spironolactone, or amiloride

if patients cannot tolerate spironolactone. Potassium supplements are generally needed.

7. Acute interstitial nephritis (particularly if drug-induced) can have urine eosinophils noted with a combination of RBCs and WBCs seen. Erythrocyte casts generally are not seen in this process but rather in acute glomerulonephritis, while leukocyte casts are seen in acute pyelonephritis.

8. Young women suspected to have fibromuscular dysplasia should have a renal arteriogram to confirm the diagnosis (beading of the renal artery) and respond to interventional radiologic therapy.

9. In SIADH, there is usually a low BUN (classically less than 10 mg/dL), normal creatinine, and a low uric acid with the most classic finding being an inappropriately elevated urine osmolality for a given plasma osmolality.

10. Patients with Giardia infections will often have marked flatulence as part of their gastrointestinal symptoms.

17.45   Year 3—Week 15—Day 2

1. The most common risk factor for aortic dissection is hypertension. Beware of patients with new onset severe back pain with history of uncontrolled hypertension as they may have aortic dissection distal to the subclavian artery presenting as back pain.

2. Among the genetic diseases causing aortic dissection are the following. Marfan's syndrome, Ehlers-Danlos syndrome, bicuspid aortic valve, and familial aortic dissection.

3. Two-thirds of patients with aortic dissection are male. The mean age is at around 63 years of age.

4. Among the causes of vascular inflammation causing aortic dissection are the following. Temporal arteritis, Behcet's disease, syphilis, and Takayasu's arteritis.

5. The mortality rate with acute ascending aortic dissection goes up 1–2% per hour once the onset of chest pain or back pain starts up.

6. Chronic cocaine use leads to aortic dissection, interestingly with a strong tendency to affect the descending aorta rather than the ascending aorta.

7. The sudden onset of severe, "knife-like" chest pain remains the most common presenting symptom of aortic dissection.

8. When syncope occurs with aortic dissection, it usually reflects a state that could include cardiac tamponade, cerebral vessel obstruction, or cerebral baroreceptor activation.

9. The patients who do worse with aortic dissection as far as presenting symptoms are those who present with initial symptom of back pain likely because it does not make the differential diagnosis.

10. Ten to 20% of patients with aortic dissection will have a completely normal chest X-ray. Mediastinal widening is the most common abnormal X-ray finding when there is an abnormal finding present.

17.46   Year 3—Week 15—Day 3

1. Protease inhibitors tend to cause a marked rise in triglycerides, sometimes above 1000 mg/dL. Interestingly, indinavir is better known for LDL elevation than triglyceride elevation, as opposed to the other protease inhibitors.

2. Lipodystrophy can occur due to advanced HIV disease itself even if no protease inhibitor therapy has been used in the past treatment of the patient.

3. Never give simvastatin with protease inhibitors given marked rise in myositis rate. Atorvastatin may be used but the lowest dose possible needs to be started and there is still a significant risk of myositis. Pravastatin is the recommended HMG-CoA reductase inhibitor when co-administering with protease inhibitor.

4. No dose reduction in niacin or fibrates needs to be done in patients taking protease inhibitors. One should not give bile acid sequestrants to patients with HIV disease.

5. Epistaxis is the first symptom of 90% or more patients with Osler-Weber-Rendu disease (hereditary hemorrhagic telangiectasia syndrome). Major gastrointestinal bleeding likely occurs in about 20% of patients eventually.

6. The diagnosis of Osler-Weber-Rendu disease requires two of the following features: (a) telangiectasias at the face, lips, oral cavity, or fingers, (b) family history of the disease, (c) visceral AVM formation, or (d) epistaxis.

7. Psoriasis has been reported as triggered by many states. Among the most interesting ones are staphylococcal infection (generalized psoriasis), group A beta-hemolytic streptococcus presenting with pharyngitis or perianal dermatitis (guttate psoriasis), oral steroid use (pustular psoriasis), and HIV infection (generalized psoriasis).

8. Medications known to worsen generalized psoriasis include beta-blockers, lithium, certain NSAIDS, and anti-malarial agents.

9. The first-line medication for aggressive psoriatic arthritis is methotrexate, but other medications such as cyclosporine have also been found to be effective.

10. The Auspitz sign of psoriasis refers to punctate bleeding that occurs at the site of removal of the scale of a psoriatic lesion.

17.47 Year 3—Week 16—Day 1

1. An anion gap needs to be calculated in all acid-base problems as a hidden anion gap metabolic acidosis could be missed if there are multiple acid-base disorders. An anion gap greater than 20 almost assuredly indicates that there is a metabolic acidosis with anion gap.

2. The urine chloride level is the most helpful test in seeing if a patient with metabolic alkalosis will respond to a saline challenge.

3. Although BPH can present with microscopic hematuria, this is a diagnosis of exclusion and a urinary tract malignancy must be first looked for.

4. Patients with liver cirrhosis rarely have BPH due to a high level of circulating estrogens in these patients relative to the amount of androgens present in these patients.

5. Patients on finasteride who are having their PSA levels followed must take into consideration that this medication can theoretically cut the pre-existing value by half. Thus, a patient on finasteride who has a PSA level of 3.5 mg/dl should be considered to have a level of 7.0 mg/dL.

6. It is now recommended to start alpha-blockers and finasteride together in treating patients with BPH. From studies, it appears to reduce the rate of acute urinary retention and the need for prostate surgery.

7. The following are the recommendations for what to do with phosphodiesterase drugs and alpha-blockers. Sildenafil (Viagra) doses of greater than 25 mg should not be taken within 4 h of an alpha-blocker. Also, patients taking alpha-blocker should never take vardenafil. Tadalafil can only be taken with one alpha blocker, tamsulosin, and never at a dose greater than 0.4 mg of tamsulosin.

8. Alpha-blockers should never be used for monotherapy in treating hypertension. They are useful as second line agent for Raynaud phenomenon if calcium channel blockers prove ineffective.

9. The first-line drug for control of hypertension in pregnancy is alpha-methyldopa. Hydralazine is the second-line agent.

10. Among the side effects of alpha-methyldopa is that it can cause a hemolytic anemia with a positive direct Coombs test. Among the most annoying effects of alpha-methyldopa is that it can cause a false positive direct Coombs test.

17.48 Year 3—Week 16—Day 2

1. The most common lung cancer to cavitate is squamous cell lung cancer.

2. The most common lung cancer to have associated hypercalcemia is squamous cell lung cancer by release of PTH-related peptide.

3. Bronchioalveolar carcinoma is associated with rapid onset of lymphangitic spread and patients describe copious "sputum" with this carcinoma. It has a poor prognosis.
4. Large cell carcinoma of the lung is associated with gynecomastia through release of HCG in a paraneoplastic fashion.
5. Horner's syndrome is seen with cluster headaches, lateral medullary infarction (Wallenberg's syndrome), and bronchogenic carcinoma of apex of lung (Pancoast tumor).
6. Venous stasis ulcers will heal more effectively if the legs are lifted above the level of the heart for at least 30 minutes at a time at least three times a day.
7. The most common cause of small bowel obstruction in patients with previous surgeries is adhesions.
8. Intussusception in adults usually occurs due to a solid lesion in the small intestine, not from a functional cause.
9. Fluoroquinolone and metronidazole combination therapy is the first-line treatment regimen for diverticulitis.
10. Patients with adult polycystic kidney disease have a high incidence of diverticular disease and hepatic cysts.

17.49 Year 3—Week 16—Day 3

1. Nasal corticosteroids are first-line agent for patients with moderate to severe allergic rhinitis.
2. Cetirizine is an antihistamine agent which is associated with psychomotor impairment at doses at or above 10 mg daily.
3. Any patient presenting with hemolytic anemia that has history of liver disease and neuropsychiatric disorders must be worked up for Wilson's disease. The first lab test to get is the serum ceruloplasmin level.
4. The acute treatment of Wilson's disease is D-penicillamine which binds copper stores. The long-term copper binding treatment is zinc therapy.

5. Patients with hypoparathyroidism are noted to have increased bone density as PTH acts to increase bone turnover.
6. Alcohol use disorder patients will sometimes be noted to be with features of hypoparathyroidism due to magnesium deficiency due to wasting magnesium in urine (from alcohol effect on the kidneys). Magnesium is an essential cofactor for intact parathyroid function.
7. The most common anatomical abnormality found in patients with primary hyperparathyroidism is one single adenoma. Generalized hyperplasia of all glands is the second most common finding.
8. Most patients with MEN syndromes 1 and 2 have hyperparathyroidism, not parathyroid cancer. The most common pancreatic tumor with MEN 1 syndrome is the gastrinoma.
9. Patients with previous history of diabetes mellitus can develop insulinomas later in life.
10. Patients receiving oral itraconazole suspension for the treatment of histoplasmosis cannot take proton pump inhibitors or H2 receptor antagonists as these drugs interfere with the absorption of itraconazole, which requires an acidic environment in the stomach.

17.50 Year 3—Week 17—Day 1

1. Carcinoid syndrome can be associated with ectopic ACTH if lesions are located in the bronchial area.
2. Filariasis (*Wuchereria* or *Brugia* organisms) can cause chylous peritoneal effusions.
3. Chylous ascites can also be seen with lymphangioleiomyomatosis which is classically associated with chylous pleural effusions.
4. Patients with chylous ascites with a high lymphocyte component should have flow cytometry performed to rule out lymphoma as the cause.

5. T-cell lymphoma is associated with hypercalcemia more than the B-cell lymphomas.
6. Patients with recurrent chylous ascites or pleural effusions need a diet that is free of long chain triglycerides (use medium chain triglycerides as this bypasses the lymphatic system much more).
7. Gastric carcinoid is a lesion highly associated with pernicious anemia.
8. *Enterobius vermicularis* is the most common worm to cause acute appendicitis in the USA while *Strongyloides stercoralis* is the one most associated with recurrent gram negative bacteremia states.
9. Hepatic artery embolization is part of the treatment regimen for patients with carcinoid lesions in the liver.
10. The portal vein needs to be patent to perform hepatic artery embolization.

17.51   Year 3—Week 17—Day 2

1. Tigecycline has action against both gram-positive and gram-negative organisms but with no significant activity against Pseudomonas or Proteus organisms.
2. Polymyalgia rheumatica patients can present with a symmetrical arthritis. Although these patients state they are "weak," they have preserved strength on individual muscle testing and suffer more from pain and stiffness particularly at the shoulders and the hips.
3. There is a high association between hepatitis B and polyarteritis nodosum. Cryoglobulins can be seen in both hepatitis B and hepatitis C (usually with positive rheumatoid factor). Porphyria cutanea tarda is highly associated with hepatitis C with findings of milia and hypertrichosis in patients.
4. Consider alveolar hemorrhage in a patient with known history of SLE who is presenting with hemoptysis and shortness of breath and has diffuse infiltrates present on CXR. Treatment is usually with Cytoxan.
5. Patients with recurrent lobar pneumonias should be excluded for obstruction with bronchoscopy.

6. If bronchoscopy yields no answers in a patient with recurrent pneumonias, one should consider immunoglobulins testing.
7. The first step in management of a patient suspected of having multiple myeloma is to perform a SPEP and UPEP. 20% of myelomas are SPEP negative and UPEP positive. The second step in management is then to perform immune fixation (quantitative immunoglobulins) to further classify the M-protein spike.
8. Risks of cyclophosphamide include hemorrhagic cystitis, bladder cancer, and an increased risk of lymphoma.
9. Transplant medications such as sirolimus can lead to secondary lymphomas that can be quite aggressive. Interestingly, the management of some of these patients is to stop the medication and not give chemotherapy. Most patients with bulky disease will get chemotherapy and the patients who need to still be on transplant medications will at least have the daily dose of the transplant medication lowered from usual value.
10. Rheumatoid arthritis can cause secondary lymphomas regardless of whether a patient is on disease modifying anti-rheumatic drugs.

17.52   Year 3—Week 17—Day 3

1. When one sees a glucose value in pleural fluid under 40 mg/dL, one should consider either infection, rheumatoid arthritis, or aggressive malignant involvement of the pleural space.
2. Among one of the more missed causes of pancreatitis is hypercalcemia, because when drawn in acute setting, the calcium level will drop to the normal value. This is due to the saponification of fat due to pancreatic necrosis and this sequesters calcium. The time to check the calcium level again is 3–4 weeks after discharge.
3. One of the common causes of hypercalcemia is hyperparathyroidism. The most common cause of primary hyperparathyroidism is a single adenoma.

4. Pancreas divisum is seen in about 7% of the general population but does not cause significant disease in but about 10% of patients with the finding. One episode of pancreatitis in these patients is not enough to warrant intervention.

5. Ovarian cancer is staged as a stage III if only ascites is seen and the prognosis is usually better than other adenocarcinomas with malignant ascites.

6. HTLV- 1 virus causes tropical spastic paraparesis and can cause lymphoma.

7. The organ system most at compromise in a patient with erythroderma is the cardiovascular system.

8. The organ system that best responds to phlebotomy in patients with hemochromatosis is the heart.

9. The treatment of acute Wilson's disease is D-penicillamine. Chronic treatment is with zinc usually.

10. Smoking will markedly worsen the lung disease of a COPD patient with alpha-1 antitrypsin disease.

17.53 Year 3—Week 18—Day 1

1. A widened mediastinum on CXR should raise concern for aortic dissection and anticoagulation should be withheld until this entity is ruled out.

2. Treat initially for aortic dissection with esmolol (beta-blocker) and then use nitroprusside for additional blood pressure control once beta-blockade is in place.

3. U1-RNP values are elevated in patients with mixed connective tissue disease.

4. Ovarian cancer is linked to paraneoplastic presentations of scleroderma, dermatomyositis, and polymyositis.

5. Methotrexate has been linked with oral ulcers, alopecia, hair loss, and nausea. Folic acid may help ameliorate those symptoms.

6. Fludrocortisone is not needed to be given to primary adrenal insufficiency patients who are receiving hydrocortisone in doses above 100 mg daily.

7. Recurrent episodes of optic neuritis and trigeminal neuralgia should raise concern for multiple sclerosis.

8. Isoproterenol is an anti-arrhythmic agent that can be used in the treatment of refractory torsades des pointes (polymorphic ventricular tachycardia).

9. T-wave inversions that involve lead AVL and lead I can be seen in association with acute anterior myocardial infarctions.

10. Patients with recent gastrointestinal bleeding and clean based ulcers noted on endoscopy can be discharged home from the hospital safely.

17.54 Year 3—Week 18—Day 2

1. If a pregnant patient develops scabies, the treatment is permethrin not Lindane. Lindane can cause fetal neurotoxicity.

2. If a pregnant patient develops hyperthyroidism, one treats with propylthiouracil (PTU) not methimazole. Methimazole can cause facial aplasia in the fetus.

3. Ace-inhibitors can cause fetal renal agenesis and thus are contraindicated during pregnancy. Fluoroquinolones are also contraindicated during pregnancy due to potential cartilage problems in the fetus.

4. Absolute contraindications to pregnancy include the Eisenmenger complex/syndrome and primary pulmonary hypertension.

5. The requirements for insulin and thyroid hormone in a patient with diabetes and hypothyroidism will continue to increase from trimester to trimester.

6. Among the causes of extrinsic restrictive lung disease are the following: obesity, kyphoscoliosis, ALS, myasthenia gravis, and Guillain-Barre syndrome.

7. Among the causes of intrinsic restrictive lung disease are the following: rheumatoid lung, idiopathic pulmonary fibrosis, sarcoidosis, and silicosis.

8. Beta-blockers are contraindicated in asthma but not in patients with COPD.
9. Uremic patients might bleed due to platelet dysfunction. DDAVP, infusion of platelets, and hemodialysis are options in treatment.
10. Differential diagnosis for gynecomastia includes the following: use of cimetidine (is anything good ever mentioned about this drug), use of spironolactone, Klinefelter's syndrome, and large cell lung carcinoma.

17.55 Year 3—Week 18—Day 3

1. Pregnancy is a relative contraindication to the use of thrombolytic agents.
2. The most common cause of secondary amenorrhea is pregnancy.
3. Lithium use during pregnancy is associated with Ebstein's anomaly, which is a displacement of the tricuspid valve into the right ventricle causing an "atrialized" hypoplastic right ventricle.
4. Ace-inhibitors are to be avoided in pregnancy as they can cause fetal renal agenesis.
5. Tetracycline is to be avoided in pregnancy as it can cause hypoplasia of tooth enamel in the fetus and permanent yellow-brown discoloration of future deciduous teeth of the fetus.
6. Coumadin use during pregnancy is contraindicated in most instances as it can lead to nasal hypoplasia and stippled bone epiphysis in the fetus but it is still used in pregnant patients with history ofcatastrophic anticardiolipid/antiphospholipid syndrome and mechanical heart valves.
7. Fluoroquinolones are contraindicated during pregnancy due to possible cartilage developmental problems of the fetus.
8. Valproic acid is the least preferred of the anticonvulsants during pregnancy as it has a high association with open neural tube defects in the fetus.
9. Heparin use during pregnancy can lead to osteoporosis in the treatment of DVT. Calcium and vitamin D replacement should be given.

10. A woman who develops hypertension after the 20th week of pregnancy is said to have pregnancy-induced hypertension.

17.56 Year 3—Week 19—Day 1

1. Metformin is initiated at small doses to prevent as best possible the side effect of diarrhea that can occur with the medication.
2. Percutaneous liver biopsy is the gold standard for the diagnosis of autoimmune hepatitis and primary biliary cirrhosis.
3. Small hyperechogenic kidneys are a common finding in patients with history of chronic renal failure.
4. Cogwheel rigidity, micrographia, hypokinesia, and difficulty in making turns are hallmark features of Parkinson's disease.
5. Embolic phenomenon to the brain can occur in patients with left atrial myxoma disease.
6. Patients with adrenal insufficiency can exhibit eosinophilia, normocytic normochromic anemia, hyperkalemia, hyponatremia, and hypercalcemia in their laboratory findings.
7. High-dose IV acyclovir can lead to acute renal insufficiency.
8. Frequent turns of the patient while recumbent during hospitalization help decrease the incidence of ileus.
9. A spinal cord tumor can lead to the finding of hyperreflexia or even clonus on physical examination.
10. Widening of the QRS complex occurs most often in tricyclic antidepressant poisoning and portends a poor prognosis if aggressive systemic alkalinization is not begun in patients.

17.57 Year 3—Week 19—Day 2

1. Patients with IgA deficiency are at higher risk for obliterative bronchiolitis and bronchiectasis complications involving

the lung along with Giardia infections of the GI tract.

2. Glutamic acid decarboxylase antibodies are found in patients with Stiff Person's syndrome and with type 1 diabetes mellitus.

3. Patients with constipation should have calcium and TSH levels checked to rule out hypercalcemia and hypothyroidism.

4. Niacin is the drug of choice to lower elevated levels of lipoprotein(a) and can lead to a drug induced gout state.

5. Ace-inhibitors can lead to abdominal pain not only by pancreatitis but also by inducing angioedema of the small bowel with a usual duration of episodes lasting about 1–3 days.

6. The ackee fruit of Jamaica is known to cause vomiting and can lead to hypoglycemia.

7. Patients with Gilbert's syndrome will have elevated levels of indirect bilirubin at times of stress, such as viral syndrome or interactions with medicine.

8. Hutchinson's sign is a term that has been used in the following two clinical scenarios: (a) describing the finding in melanoma where there is pigmentation past the nailbed into the skin and (b) describing an vesicle at the tip of the nose in the setting of a patient with herpes zoster (as they would have involvement of the nasociliary ganglion).

9. Patients with diabetes mellitus are at higher risk of emphysematous cholecystitis. The most common offending organism is *Escherichia coli.*

10. Patients with endocarditis can have both splenic and renal infarctions.

17.58 Year 3—Week 19—Day 3

1. Patients on danazol for hereditary angioedema need to discontinue this medicine when they become pregnant.

2. Thalidomide use during pregnancy is associated with bilateral limb anomalies of the fetus.

3. The drugs of choice in hypertension of pregnancy are still alpha-methyldopa and hydralazine.

4. Asymptomatic bacteriuria in pregnancy (seen in 2 urine samples hours apart) requires treatment due to increased risk of development of pyelonephritis.

5. A premenopausal patient with intermenstrual bleeding or a postmenopausal patient who continues to bleed after 6 weeks of initiation of hormone replacement therapy will need an endometrial biopsy.

6. The risk of unopposed estrogen hormone replacement therapy in postmenopausal women without hysterectomies is endometrial hyperplasia which can lead to endometrial cancer.

7. The lab abnormality most closely associated with menopause is an elevated FSH.

8. Nitrofurantoin use during pregnancy has been associated with a pneumonitis. Also, tocolytic-induced pulmonary edema should be recognized in the appropriate clinical scenario.

9. The vaginitis associated with the highest pH (6–7) is trichomoniasis. It is also associated with the strawberry cervix finding. The term "frothy" is used with this type of vaginitis.

10. The infectious vaginitis associated with the lowest pH is candidiasis (4–5). The character of the secretions is thick and curdy. It is seen often in patients with diabetes mellitus.

17.59 Year 3—Week 20—Day 1

1. There is a strong association between hepatitis B and polyarteritis nodosum (PAN) such that antiviral medications such as entecavir should be started before immunosuppressive therapy for PAN is begun.

2. Patients with granulomatosis with polyangiitis can present with hearing loss and with foot drop as these are signs of mononeuritis multiplex.

3. Patients with diabetes mellitus can have microinfarctions of nerve fibers leading to such findings as cranial nerve palsy (with intact pupillary reflexes) and foot drop (common peroneal nerve involvement).

4. Patients with leptospirosis are at risk of clinical hepatitis as part of their disease presenta-

tion unlike systemic brucellosis where clinical hepatitis is rarely part of that disease process.

5. Dapsone can be used only as single agent drug for *Pneumocystis* prophylaxis (unlike toxoplasmosis prophylaxis where it must be combined with at least twice weekly pyrimethamine) in patients who cannot tolerate sulfa based medication.

6. Still's disease is a common cause of fever of unknown origin and is marked by a transient evanescent rash and a very elevated serum ferritin level with sore throat and cervical lymphadenopathy being common early symptoms in the disease process.

7. The most common type of arthritis found in hemochromatosis patients is osteoarthritis.

8. There is an increased incidence of pseudogout in patients with primary hyperparathyroidism and hemochromatosis.

9. Calcification of the triangular ligament can be seen in patients with pseudogout.

10. Suspect tenosynovitis in patients with pain upon wrist extension, and this finding can be seen in gonorrhea infections.

17.60 Year 3—Week 20—Day 2

1. Dysphagia to solids only and not to liquids over a period of months to years is very worrisome for a slow growing tumor in the esophagus.

2. Achalasia present with dysphagia to both solids and liquids. Patients sometimes report improvement in swallowing when performing a Valsalva maneuver.

3. Aortic stenosis and hypertrophic cardiomyopathy are the two conditions during which an extra-systolic beat will increase a systolic murmur.

4. Tricuspid regurgitation murmur best increases with inspiration (usually a holosystolic murmur).

5. Isometric handgrip most reliably increases the murmur of mitral regurgitation.

6. Purtscher's retinopathy is an acute visual loss that occurs in patients with acute pancre-

atitis due to aggregated granulocytes affecting the posterior retinal artery.

7. The serum trypsinogen level is a useful test in making the diagnosis of chronic pancreatitis as the cause of steatorrhea.

8. Cefotaxime is the first-line drug in treatment of spontaneous bacterial peritonitis.

9. There is an increased incidence of emphysematous cholecystitis in elderly men and in patients with diabetes mellitus.

10. *Escherichia coli* is the most common pathogen causing both emphysematous cholecystitis and emphysematous pyelonephritis.

17.61 Year 3—Week 20—Day 3

1. Isolated gastric varices can result from splenic vein thrombosis.

2. A patient with portal hypertension due to splenomegaly from splenic vein thrombosis should have splenectomy.

3. Cladribine (2-chlorodeoxyadenosine) is the treatment of hairy cell leukemia.

4. Always rule out platelet clumping as the cause of a low platelet value in an otherwise asymptomatic person.

5. Von Willebrand's disease may cause prolongation of the PTT in coagulation testing in about 2/3 of cases.

6. A platelet function assay has taken the place of "bleeding time" in the workup of patients with von Willebrand's disease as it is much less labor intensive than the bleeding time laboratory testing.

7. Patients with von Willebrand's disease type 2b will present with thrombocytopenia and will not usually respond to DDAVP but rather to aminocaproic acid or tranexamic acid (antifibrinolytic agents).

8. DDAVP can be used as a temporizing measure while awaiting dialysis in patients with uremic bleeding.

9. Patients with vocal cord dysfunction will have a flattening out of their inspiratory portion of their flow-volume loops.

10. Heliox (combination of helium and oxygen) has been used in the treatment of patients with vocal cord dysfunction.

17.62   Year 3—Week 21—Day 1

1. Acute cluster headaches can present with Horner's syndrome. Treatment is 100% oxygen.
2. Horner's syndrome is also seen in patients with lateral medullary infarction (Wallenberg's syndrome) and with Pancoast tumor (bronchogenic cancer at apex destroying sympathetic plexus).
3. Post-herpetic neuralgia will not respond to acyclovir. Use agents such as gabapentin for treatment.
4. There is an association between aortic stenosis and angiodysplasia.
5. Patients with hamartomatous polyps in the colon do not need to have their surveillance for colon cancer changed compared to an individual with no polyps.
6. Patients with multiple gastric polyps noted on EGD should be screened for vitamin B12 deficiency if the histology proves to be gastric carcinoid.
7. Patients with vitamin B12 deficiency can present with pancytopenia.
8. When looking for folate deficiency, order the red cell folate lab value as it is most reflective of long-term folate stores.
9. Patients with hemolytic anemia diseases will develop folic acid deficiency (such as sickle cell anemia, hereditary spherocytosis, or autoimmune hemolytic anemia).
10. Patients placed on methotrexate for rheumatological conditions can develop folic acid deficiency and oral ulcerations may be found on physical exam along with diffuse abdominal pain complaints.

17.63   Year 3—Week 21—Day 2

11. Clue cells (bacteria adherent to epithelial cells) are seen with bacterial vaginosis. Mixing of gray-white secretions with 10% KOH will free amines that may be detected by their "fishy" smell.
12. Hormonal contraceptives prevent pregnancy by blocking the pulsatile secretion of FSH and LH from the pituitary gland.
13. Oral contraceptive users have a decreased incidence of endometrial and ovarian cancer, benign breast and ovarian disease, and pelvic infections. They are at small risk for formation of benign liver adenomas.
14. Hepatitis E carries the highest mortality rate for acute viral hepatitides during pregnancy.
15. Progestin-only oral contraceptive pills (OCP) have a higher failure rate than combination OCP and have a higher incidence of acne.
16. The lower dose of estrogen (ethinyl estradiol and mestranol to be specific) in OCP has led to a reduction in thromboembolic disease but is associated with higher rate of intermenstrual bleeding.
17. The most common cause of dysmenorrhea in young adolescents is excessive prostaglandin production.
18. Smoking and use of OCP above age 35 is associated with a higher rate of thromboembolic disease.
19. The most common cause of infertility in the USA is now felt to be asymptomatic Chlamydia infections.
20. There is felt to be an increased incidence of cervical cancer in patients who are sexually active beginning before age 16 due to the human papilloma virus (specifically types 16, 18, 31, 33, 35).

17.64   Year 3—Week 21—Day 3

1. Patients taking dilantin (phenytoin) or phenobarbital for prolonged periods of time are at risk of osteoporosis. This is also seen in patients taking heparin or low molecular weight heparin for an extended period of

time. Steroids are not the only drugs as you can see that can lead to osteoporosis problems.

2. Patients with hypogonadism are at risk for osteoporosis.

3. Pott's disease refers to the involvement of bone by tuberculosis.

4. Think of Pneumocystis carinii pneumonia in patients who present with an infiltrate and pneumothorax.

5. The top 3 diagnoses to consider in patients with periorbital edema are the following: trichinosis, hypothyroidism, and nephrotic syndrome.

6. Patients who undergo biliary manometry for sphincter of Oddi dysfunction have a 30% chance of having post-procedure pancreatitis (much higher than ERCP).

7. Valproic acid is associated with pancreatitis, LFT abnormalities, weight gain, thrombocytopenia, and alopecia.

8. Dapsone should be given within 48 h of a brown recluse spider bite to limit necrosis of the skin. The medication limits the action of sphingomyelinase.

9. Struvite stones can become so large that they are called staghorn calculi. Patients have had nephrectomies for these calculi.

10. Distal RTA (type 1) is seen commonly in patients with Sjogren's syndrome and has a high association with kidney stones.

17.65 Year 3—Week 22—Day 1

1. Human papilloma virus types 6 and 11 are associated with genital warts (condyloma acuminatum).

2. Menstruation is triggered by an involution of the corpus luteum with concomitant decline in plasma levels of progesterone.

3. Hirsutism and virilization are classified as androgen excess disorders.

4. Women with polycystic ovarian disease (Stein-Leventhal syndrome) have an increased LH to FSH ratio.

5. Diethylstilbestrol administration to a pregnant mother is associated with risk in fetus of development of clear cell adenocarcinoma of the vagina.

6. Over 90% of vulvar carcinomas are squamous cell cancers.

7. Cigarette smoking is felt to be a risk factor for development of cervical cancer (strongest association of all the OB/GYN cancers).

8. A patient who is found to have atypical squamous cells of undetermined significance (ASCUS) should have repeat Pap smears every 4–6 months until 3 smears in a row are normal. In postmenopausal patients, a short course of vaginal estrogen can be administered with repeat Pap smear after course. In either situation, if a repeat smear again shows ASCUS, then the next step in management is colposcopy.

9. Most cases of mild dysplasia on Pap smear (CIN 1–3, and low-grade squamous intraepithelial neoplasia) can be managed with repeat Pap smear if 4–6 months with colposcopy if repeat Pap is abnormal. High grade squamous intraepithelial neoplasia on a Pap smear is next managed with a colposcopy with endocervical curettage and directed biopsies (don't send these patients for repeat Pap smears unlike ASCUS and CIN 1–3/LGSIL). A colposcopy (which uses acetic acid to "whiten" lesions with increased nuclear/cytoplasmic ratio due to dysplasia) is adequate only if the entire squamocolumnar transformation junction is visualized as 95% of cervical cancers form there. If adequate visualization is unsatisfactory, the next step in management is cervical conization. Cervical conization is also necessary if there is a "two-step" discrepancy (such as CIN 1 on colposcopy versus HGSIL on Pap smear).

10. Atypical glandular cells of undetermined significance on Pap smear should be followed up with repeat Pap within a month with endocervical brush and most authorities would also do an endometrial biopsy. If this is negative, a cone biopsy may need to be pursued.

17.66 Year 3—Week 22—Day 2

1. Manifestations of acute pancreatitis include lobular panniculitis, Grey-Turner's sign, and Cullen's sign (periumbilical hemorrhage).
2. Essential thrombocytosis is associated with erythromelalgia (redness and burning of the extremities that is relieved with aspirin).
3. Syphilis is associated with generalized LAD and oral mucous patches when it is secondary. Treatment is benzathine penicillin G for three treatments (separated by 1 week).
4. Lemierre's syndrome is associated with Fusobacterium infections marked by septic pulmonary emboli and internal jugular vein thrombophlebitis.
5. Discoid lupus is associated with alopecia and follicular plugging of ears.
6. Multiple sclerosis can cause blurry vision with hot showers due to decreased nerve conduction with heat.
7. Lichen planus is associated with a pruritic rash usually at the wrists but patients can have oral lesions and lower extremity lesions with this condition.
8. Parvovirus infections can be seen with livedo reticularis similar to patients with antiphospholipid antibody syndrome.
9. Parvovirus infections are associated with aplastic anemia and giant pronormoblasts can be seen in the bone marrow aspirate/biopsy.
10. Myasthenia gravis has an association with thymoma and thymic hyperplasia. CT of thorax should be done in these patients.

17.67 Year 3—Week 22—Day 3

1. Patients with AML-M4 can present with gingival hyperplasia and CNS involvement.
2. The three most common drugs to cause gingival hyperplasia are dihydropyridine calcium channel blockers, cyclosporine, and dilantin (phenytoin).
3. Patients with AML-M4 with inversion of chromosome 16 and bone marrow eosinophilia can have a good prognosis. Another

one to remember with even better prognosis is AML-M2 with translocation of 8,21 (t 8,21).
4. Patients receiving all-trans retinoic acid can develop a pulmonary infiltrate syndrome (retinoic acid syndrome) that responds to steroids and temporary cessation of medication.
5. L-Asparaginase is a chemotherapeutic drug used in many treatments for ALL that is classically linked to drug-induced pancreatitis.
6. Every patient with ALL should be considered for lumbar puncture and chemotherapy (intrathecal) CNS prophylaxis if LP shows no malignancy.
7. Patients with multiple myeloma are more susceptible to contrast induced renal failure compared to the rest of the population.
8. Patients with Waldenstrom's macroglobulinemia do not get bone fractures/pain typically but are susceptible to hyperviscosity states.
9. Smudge cells are seen with CLL. One would see a cell that seems to be being squeezed out by surrounding red cells. There would be numerous small mature lymphocytes in the same slide as well.
10. Patients with hairy cell leukemia and myelofibrosis not uncommonly have a "dry" bone marrow tap.

17.68 Year 3—Week 23—Day 1

1. *Yersinia pestis* (plague) infections first-line treatment consists of aminoglycoside (streptomycin on standardized testing but gentamicin is most commonly used), doxycycline, and fluoroquinolone therapy. Beware of physical examination findings ranging from ulcerations to buboes to rales from pneumonia on exam.
2. Tuberculosis medications most commonly causing a thrombocytopenia are rifampin and ethambutol. Ethambutol and pyrazinamide will cause drug-induced gout. Rifampin will increase ("rev up") the cytochrome P4503a4 system and thus consume drugs like dilantin heavily.

3. Histoplasmosis is known to cause posterior mediastinitis, skin lesions that can resemble molluscum contagiosum, meningitis and splenic lesions. Treatment of mild to moderate disease usually involves itraconazole.
4. Methotrexate can cause small joint nodulosis, interstitial lung disease, and oral ulcerations (the latter one if folic acid not being taken daily).
5. Dermatomyositis lesions tend to fall directly over the joints of the hand and are known as Gottron's sign if flat and Gottron's papules if elevated lesions.
6. Painless oral ulcerations are common with systemic lupus erythematosus. Painful oral lesions are seen with Behcet's disease especially involving the tongue.
7. EBV and HIV are the two viruses that have synergy in the disease state known as oral hairy leukoplakia.
8. Patients with SLE (lupus) are noted to have interphalangeal erythema with sparing of the skin directly over the joint surface of the hands.
9. HIV and hepatitis C are the two most common infections causing nephrotic syndrome with focal segmental glomerulosclerosis pathology.
10. Odynophagia is an uncommon symptom of patients with dermatomyositis and polymyositis. IVIG has a role in the treatment of dermatomyositis disease.

17.69 Year 3—Week 23—Day 2

1. The first-line treatment of choice for patients with trigeminal neuralgia is carbamazepine.
2. Optic neuritis and trigeminal neuralgia are often herald signs of underlying multiple sclerosis especially when occurring in recurrent fashion.
3. Carbamazepine can be associated with a Steven–Johnson/toxic epidermal necrolysis syndrome which often occurs within the first 7–14 days of initiation of the medication.
4. The most common drug eruption is a morbilliform exanthematous drug eruption (measles-like appearance) which can be delayed up to 2 weeks after the last dose of

the medication and can be seen with multiple medications to include short course oral antibiotics (macrolides, fluoroquinolones).
5. Patients with rheumatological disease should be discontinued from their biological treatment agent (such as TNF-alpha receptor inhibitor) at least one cycle before the planned operation in order to promote best wound healing possible.
6. Serotonin selective uptake inhibitors (SSRI) can be tapered after one single major depressive disorder if side effects after the patient has noted improvement in major depression symptoms for at least 4–9 months on average. Such tapering may be needed for erectile dysfunction or hyponatremia as complications of therapy.
7. Multiple sclerosis is most common between the ages of 15 and 45 and is nearly unheard of after the age of 70. Vasculitis diseases such as temporal arteritis and CNS angiitis are misdiagnosed often as multiple sclerosis in patients above age 70 years old.
8. Treatment options in seborrheic dermatitis include low-dose topical steroids (5% or less hydrocortisone), 2% ketoconazole topical preparations and topical zinc.
9. Seborrheic dermatitis can present at a young age in patients with HIV disease and Hodgkin's disease.
10. Topical steroids will markedly worsen the rash of acne rosacea.

17.70 Year 3—Week 23—Day 3

1. Patients with lupus may present with hair loss from both a mechanism of alopecia areata and of telogen effluvium.
2. Patients with lupus will have lymphadenopathy on physical exam at times and may have lymphopenia on complete blood count.
3. Hydroxychloroquine is the first-line agent treatment of patients with subacute cutaneous lupus erythematosus.
4. Patients with hypothyroidism might present with periorbital edema. This finding can be

seen with patients with Trichinella spiralis infections and nephrotic syndrome as well.

5. Patients with disseminated gonorrhea can present with wrist pain due to tenosynovitis.

6. First carpometacarpal arthritis can be seen in patients with osteoarthritis disease. This is often found in patients who play many hours of video games daily.

7. Open lung biopsy is the next step in management when evaluating a patient with lung infiltrates to exclude bronchiolitis obliterans with organizing pneumonia.

8. High-dose steroid treatment is the first step in management of bronchiolitis obliterans with organizing pneumonia.

9. Patients with high-dose steroids being given for greater than 2 weeks course should be considered for prophylaxis against *Pneumocystis jirovecii* opportunistic infections.

10. *Nocardia asteroids* is an organism that often strikes in patients who have high-dose steroid treatments for prolonged periods. The disease can present with brain abscess, diffuse infiltrates, and disseminated subcutaneous nodules in the skin.

17.71   Year 3—Week 24—Day 1

1. Merkel cell cancer is a skin neuroendocrine cancer which requires wide margins on excision.

2. Thyroglobulin is a tumor marker for papillary and follicular thyroid cancer.

3. CEA level may be slightly elevated in smokers.

4. Calcitonin levels are useful when working up patients for medullary cancer of the thyroid. Always exclude pheochromocytoma before proceeding to surgery.

5. IGF-2 (insulin growth factor 2) levels will be markedly elevated in patients with paraneoplastic processes due to tumors especially the sarcomas.

6. A patient with recurrent episodes of optic neuritis should be worked up for underlying multiple sclerosis.

7. Hemicranium continuum is more common in females and attacks tend to linger for days (uncommon in cluster headaches).

8. Screen for acromegaly with somatomedin C level (IGF-1). Surgery is the treatment for acromegaly. Octreotide and radiation therapy are only used for surgery refractory disease.

9. Prolactinomas are always treated with medical therapy not surgical therapy first. Treat with cabergoline or bromocriptine (dopamine receptor agonist therapy).

10. Prolactin levels can be elevated between 40 and 200 mg/dL in situations such as pregnancy, phenothiazine use, severe hypothyroidism, and non-functioning adenomas that cause stalk effect.

17.72   Year 3—Week 24—Day 2

1. Superinfections with cytomegalovirus can occur in patients with recurrent exacerbation of ulcerative colitis.

2. Ulcerative colitis may involve the first couple of centimeters of the terminal ileum (backwash ileitis) but if there is widespread involvement of the terminal ileum, one should consider Crohn's disease as the diagnosis.

3. NSAID use is associated with lithium toxicity by promoting reabsorption of lithium at the level of the kidney.

4. D5W is the intravenous solution of choice for replacing free water in patients with hypernatremia due to lack of free water, as long as free water replacement by NG tube is refused by the patient (as that is the best route of replacement in compliant patients). One cannot use D5 W in diabetic patients with glycosuria noted (as D5 W would promote continued osmotic diuresis if glycosuria is present).

5. Doxycycline and ciprofloxacin are among the treatment options in dealing with anthrax. There is a cutaneous anthrax that can be seen in hunters.

6. Anthrax should not cause pneumonia but rather hemorrhagic mediastinitis (which can present with hemoptysis).

7. The first-line agent of treatment of Yersinia pestis is streptomycin.

8. Aeromonas hydrophilia is a freshwater borne bacteria that can cause an aggressive cellulitis and even colitis in patients with end-stage liver disease (can occur in immunocompetent patients as well).

9. Penicillin is associated with a self-limited hemorrhagic colitis that usually occurs 3 days after PCN use.

10. Activated charcoal is to be used within the first 4 h of a toxic ingestion of acetaminophen. It can be given around the time that N-acetylcysteine administration has begun.

17.73   Year 3—Week 24—Day 3

1. Photonegative chest X ray finding opposite of what would be seen in CHF (congestive heart failure), eosinophilia, and diffuse peripheral wandering infiltrates are findings that raise the suspicion of chronic eosinophilic pneumonia as the underlying diagnosis.

2. Bronchiectasis is a cause of hemoptysis and can ensue from repeated pulmonary infections and if found in patients with recurrent COPD exacerbations, acute treatment of those COPD exacerbations would require fluoroquinolone therapy due to higher risk of *Pseudomonas* infections.

3. Lung abscesses are a cause of foul-smelling sputum in patients.

4. Nocardia, tuberculosis, and necrotizing streptococcus/staphylococcus infections are three bacterial causes of cavitary lung abscess.

5. Lambert-Eaton syndrome, ectopic ACTH syndrome, subacute cerebellar degeneration are three paraneoplastic processes of small cell lung CA.

6. Previous TB infection, cause of massive hemoptysis, may need angioembolization of bronchial artery are three things associated with aspergilloma.

7. Direct extension is the way it spreads, risk is not increased with smoking, and risk factor

is asbestos exposure are three things to know about mesothelioma.

8. Sand-blasting professional work is a risk factor for silicosis lung disease.

9. *Stenotrophomonas* infections are usually resistant to carbapenem therapy, especially imipenem.

10. Malignancy, empyema, and rheumatoid arthritis are three causes of a pleural effusion with a low glucose level.

17.74   Year 3—Week 25—Day 1

1. Numerous seborrheic keratoses forming in less than 6 months constitute the sign of Leser-Trelat which is associated with carcinomas, especially gastric cancer.

2. Risk for pancreatic cancer, small bowel hamartoma is most common finding, risk factor for colon cancer are three facts associated with Peutz-Jeghers syndrome.

3. Risk factor for colon cancer, autosomal recessive in inheritance in some literature models, associated with brain tumors are three facts associated with Turcot syndrome.

4. Jaw osteomas, skull osteomas, risk for colon cancer are three facts associated with Gardner's syndrome.

5. Cancer of the ampulla of Vater can cause silvery colored stools due to mix of bile and blood. These cancers are highly seen in Gardner's syndrome.

6. Calcium channel blockers are first-line therapy of diffuse esophageal spasm.

7. Medical therapy with calcium channel blockers or nitrates, surgical myotomy, and botulinum toxin injections are three treatment options for achalasia.

8. Primary sclerosing cholangitis is associated with an increased risk for cholangiocarcinoma.

9. Early treatment with ursodeoxycholic acid is effective in patients with primary biliary cirrhosis.

10. Antigen test for soluble liver specific antigen, anti-liver-kidney-microsomal antibodies, and smooth muscle antibodies are all lab

findings one sees with autoimmune hepatitis.

17.75 Year 3—Week 25—Day 2

1. Endocarditis, pneumonia, and acute liver failure are all manifestations of *Coxiella burnetii* or Q-fever.
2. Red blood cell inclusions are characteristic of *Babesia microti* infection.
3. White blood cell inclusions can be seen with Ehrlichiosis and Histoplasmosis infections.
4. Q-fever, Ehrlichiosis, Vibrio vulnificus, or parahemolyticus infections are three infections treated by doxycycline effectively.
5. *Sporothrix schenckii, Nocardia brasiliensis,* and *Mycobacterium marinum* are three infections associated with the pattern of nodular lymphangitis also known as sporotrichoid pattern.
6. HACEK endocarditis infections, advanced Lyme disease with advanced carditis and neurological signs, and disseminated gonorrhea are three conditions treated with IV ceftriaxone.
7. *Mycoplasma hominis, Ureaplasma urealyticum,* and *Chlamydia trachomatis* are three causes of nongonococcal urethritis.
8. *Campylobacter jejuni* and Mycoplasma infections are associated with Guillain-Barre syndrome.
9. Cold agglutinin disease, transverse myelitis, and bullous myringitis are three clinical manifestations of *Mycoplasma pneumoniae* infections.
10. Streptococcus, tuberculosis, and leprosy are three infections associated with erythema nodosum.

17.76 Year 3—Week 25—Day 3

1. Pancreatitis, normal D-dimer level, elevated fibrin split product can be seen with systemic fibrinolysis.
2. AML M3 leukemia can be associated with disseminated intravascular coagulation findings (DIC).

3. Splenomegaly, leukopenia, good result if treated with 2-CDA are three things associated with hairy cell leukemia.
4. Schistocytes, normal PT and PTT levels, and fever and confusion along with low platelets can be seen in TTP.
5. Hypoglycemia is a common finding in acute fatty liver of pregnancy along with a microangiopathic hemolytic anemia.
6. CLL, Wilson's disease, and inflammatory bowel disease are three states associated with autoimmune hemolytic anemia.
7. Giant platelets, defect in glycoprotein 1b-9, and thrombocytopenia are associated with Bernard-Soulier syndrome.
8. Treatment with cyclosporine and antithymocyte globulin (ATGAM) is used to treat aplastic anemia.
9. Treatment with IVIG is commonly used in patients with Parvovirus B 19 infections who have sickle cell disease with a crisis with decreased reticulocyte count.
10. Patients with Sweet's syndrome have an increased risk for AML over the next 5 years from onset of diagnosis.

17.77 Year 3—Week 26—Day 1

1. Titubation of the head is seen in essential tremor.
2. Horner's syndrome may be seen, treat with 100% oxygen acutely, lithium can be used for prophylaxis in cluster headaches.
3. Clonus, high fever, confusion are features of serotonin syndrome.
4. Horner's syndrome, ataxia, dysarthria can be seen with lateral medullary infarct syndrome or Wallenberg's syndrome.
5. Positive Romberg test, neutropenia, peripheral neuropathy can be seen with vitamin B12 deficiency.
6. Ataxia, confusion with confabulations, ophthalmoplegia can be seen with Wernicke's disease.
7. Lichenoid skin eruption, hypersensitivity syndrome, nystagmus are three things associated with dilantin (phenytoin) therapy.

8. Hepatotoxicity, weight gain, pancreatitis are possible side effects of valproic acid.
9. Metoclopramide can cause a drug-induced Parkinsonism state.
10. Carbidopa-Levodopa, ropinirole or pramipexole (dopamine receptor agonists), and entacapone or tolcapone (catechol-0-methyltransferase or COMT inhibitors) are three treatment regimens for Parkinson's disease.

17.78 Year 3—Week 26—Day 2

1. Patients with polycystic kidney disease will have hepatic cysts and diverticular disease onset at early age.
2. Two medications that will falsely elevate serum creatinine are trimethoprim-sulfamethoxazole and cimetidine.
3. Staghorn or magnesium ammonium phosphate stones are also struvite stones caused usually by Proteus urinary tract infections. Remember urine pH is usually above 8.0 value.
4. Kidney stones at young age, abnormality noted by IVP, and rare incidence of early onset renal failure are statements that should make one think of medullary sponge kidney disease.
5. Hearing loss along with early onset renal failure with family history of similar findings should make one think of Alport's disease.
6. Hematuria can be seen with the following states: stones, bladder cancer in smokers, and squamous cell cancer in patients with *Schistosoma haematobium* from swimming in the Nile River.
7. Focal segmental glomerulosclerosis can be seen in chronic heroin use, morbid obesity, and Fabry's disease.
8. Hodgkin's disease and HIV disease are associated with adult-onset minimal change disease.
9. The following diseases are associated with membranoproliferative glomerulonephritis: hepatitis B, hepatitis C, and Lupus.

10. Diffuse arthralgias and hemorrhagic necrotic rash with new onset renal insufficiency along with abnormal AST and ALT should make one think of acute Hepatitis B infection with features of serum sickness.

17.79 Year 3—Week 26—Day 3

1. The most common cause of retinal detachment in the general population is myopia.
2. Flashing lights, decreased vision, and increased floaters in visual field are all signs that a diabetic may be headed for acute retinal detachment.
3. Tinnitus, hearing loss, vertigo are all signs of Meniere's disease.
4. Low salt diet, thiazide diuretic therapy, radiofrequency ablation, and gentamicin ablation are all treatment options for Meniere's disease.
5. The most common cause of hearing loss in the elderly population is presbycusis.
6. The most common reason for acute visual loss in a patient taking methanol is optic neuritis.
7. The most common cause for acute loss of vision in patients with acute pancreatitis is posterior retinal small vasculature occlusion known as Purtscher's retinopathy.
8. The most common cause for acute vision loss in a patient with a cherry red spot in the macula is acute retinal artery occlusion.
9. The most common cause for acute vision loss in a patient with fundoscopic exam revealing widespread hemorrhage and edema (blood and thunder appearance) is acute retinal vein occlusion.
10. The most common causes of subconjunctival hemorrhage are protracted vomiting, coughing, or Valsalva maneuvers.

17.80 Year 3—Week 27—Day 1

1. Patients with refractory to treatment dermatomyositis may respond to IVIG therapy. Patients with polymyositis usually do not respond to IVIG.

2. Patients with inclusion body myositis will generally have minimal elevations of CPK and will not respond to steroids or other immunosuppressive agents.
3. Morphea is a term that has been used to describe very limited scleroderma.
4. Minocycline is still the preferred antibiotic to use in cases of acne that do not respond to topical therapy.
5. Secondary syphilis, SLE, and valproic acid are all associated with a nonscarring alopecia.
6. Hypertension is the most common systemic disease associated with epistaxis in the elderly.
7. Control of heart rate and blood pressure is as important as serial CT scanning in patients with aneurysms of the aorta that do not meet criteria for surgical treatment at time of first detection.
8. Patients with mixed connective tissue disease who present with high U1-RNP levels generally have favorable outcomes.
9. Consider reflex sympathetic dystrophy in the differential diagnosis of a patient who develops swelling of an extremity shortly after trauma in the face of lack of infection.
10. Contraction of the palmar fascial bands is the mechanism for Dupuytren's contracture.

17.81   Year 3—Week 27—Day 2

11. Asymptomatic bacteriuria in pregnancy (seen in 2 urine samples hours apart) requires treatment due to increased risk of development of pyelonephritis.
12. A premenopausal patient with intermenstrual bleeding or a postmenopausal patient who continues to bleed after 6 weeks of initiation of hormone replacement therapy will need an endometrial biopsy.
13. The risk of unopposed estrogen hormone replacement therapy in postmenopausal women without hysterectomies is endometrial hyperplasia which can lead to endometrial cancer.

14. The lab abnormality most closely associated with menopause is an elevated FSH.
15. Nitrofurantoin use during pregnancy has been associated with a pneumonitis. Also, tocolytic-induced pulmonary edema should be recognized in the appropriate clinical scenario.
16. Clue cells (bacteria adherent to epithelial cells) are seen with bacterial vaginosis. Mixing of gray-white secretions with 10% KOH will free amines that may be detected by their "fishy" smell.
17. Hormonal contraceptives prevent pregnancy by blocking the pulsatile secretion of FSH and LH from the pituitary gland.
18. Oral contraceptive users have a decreased incidence of endometrial and ovarian cancer, benign breast and ovarian disease, and pelvic infections. They are at small risk for formation of benign liver adenomas.

17.82   Year 3—Week 27—Day 3

1. Inpatient video EEG monitoring should be done as next step in all patients with history of questionable seizures, particularly if "pelvic thrusts" are part of the movements described in the seizure.
2. A serum ceruloplasmin measurement is the first step in management when suspecting a patient with Wilson's disease who has had seizures, liver disease, hemolytic anemia, and psychic overtones.
3. D-Penicillamine is the treatment of acute Wilson's disease. Zinc is the most common drug used to bind copper as chronic treatment.
4. Patients with progressive supranuclear palsy will present with a "Parkinson's plus" type picture with bradykinesia, cogwheel rigidity, difficulty making turns, and tremor.
5. A patient having a hemorrhagic cerebellar stroke should have urgent neurosurgical evaluation for a decompression surgery.
6. Look for "startle myoclonus" in patients with rapidly progressive dementia when suspecting Creutzfeldt-Jacob disease.

7. Look for progressive multifocal leukoencephalopathy (PML) in patients with HIV disease who have low CD 4 counts and present with mental status changes and visual field deficits with ataxia.
8. Metoclopramide can cause a myriad of neurological issues to include tardive dystonia, akathisia, and drug-induced Parkinsonism. Late onset Chediak-Higashi syndrome is also a cause of Parkinsonism type symptoms.
9. Dopamine agonist receptor drugs such as ropinirole or pramipexole can cause increased gambling behavior and mania-type symptoms (such as starting numerous jobs but never finishing any of them).
10. Patients who describe a TIA episode occurring on same day of presentation to ED (with resolution) should still be admitted for expedited workup (echocardiogram of heart, MRI/MRA brain, and carotid studies).

17.83   Year 3—Week 28—Day 1

1. Patients with primary adrenal insufficiency will often crave salt (due to mineralocorticoid deficiency).
2. Olanzapine is associated with hyperglycemia.
3. Ziprasidone can cause QT interval prolongation leading to torsades des pointes.
4. Mirtazapine has anticholinergic properties and can lead to weight gain.
5. Serum fructosamine levels are the test to check for long-term glycemic control in patients with hemoglobinopathies as the hemoglobin A1C will not be able to be interpreted correctly in these patients.
6. Trifascicular block involves left anterior fascicular block (LAFB), first-degree AV block, and right bundle branch block.
7. Lamotrigine can cause exfoliative dermatitis.
8. Herpes simplex virus type 1 is the most common cause for erythema multiforme.

9. Somatostatinoma can cause diabetes mellitus, diarrhea, gallstones, and even glossitis.
10. Most morbilliform exanthems due to medications usually occur about 1–3 weeks after starting therapy (thus, they may develop once the patient is off the medication).

17.84   Year 3—Week 28—Day 2

1. Patients with invasive head and neck carcinoma usually receive neoadjuvant chemotherapy with cisplatin and radiotherapy before being considered for surgical resection.
2. Adrenal cancer is a very rare phenomenon, most common cause of a malignancy involving the adrenal gland is metastatic lung cancer.
3. 10% of pheochromocytomas are bilateral, and 10% are malignant.
4. Risk factors for squamous cell cancer of the esophagus include lye ingestion, Plummer-Vinson syndrome (iron deficiency anemia and esophageal webs/cysts), tylosis, and alcohol/smoking abuse.
5. Squamous cell cancer of skin usually arises from an actinic keratosis.
6. The metastatic potential of squamous cell cancer of the skin is greatest when it is from the lower lip or from the ears.
7. Two skin conditions associated with HIV disease are eosinophilic folliculitis and seborrheic dermatitis.
8. Besides HIV disease, think of Parkinson's disease in patients with seborrheic dermatitis affecting them at a very young age (as in the 20's–40's).
9. Embryonal cell carcinoma of the testes is treated after orchiectomy with chemotherapy involving bleomycin, etoposide, and cisplatin.
10. Bleomycin can cause pulmonary fibrosis, Raynaud's phenomenon, and sclerodactyly.

17.85 Year 3—Week 28—Day 3

1. Dupuytren's contracture is associated with chronic liver disease, carpal tunnel syndrome, RA, diabetes mellitus, and epilepsy.
2. There is a syndrome usually seen in elderly gentlemen known as remitting severe symmetric synovitis with pitting edema, usually affecting the hands, wrists, ankles, and feet. Treatment is with NSAIDs, diuretics, or low-dose prednisone. Cause is unknown.
3. Angioid streaks is a disruption of Bruch's membrane of the eye that can be associated with choroidal neovascularization and macular degeneration and can be seen with systemic disorders such as pseudoxanthoma elasticum, Paget's disease, and hemoglobinopathies.
4. Women are two to three more times likely to develop an arthritis syndrome from gonorrhea than are men.
5. Atypical mycobacteria can cause periarticular bone lesions at the same time as causing a "septic arthritis" picture.
6. Synovial biopsy is needed frequently in patients with unexplained recurrent arthritis flares with negative joint fluid examinations.
7. If full flexion (and extension for that matter) can be retained at an elbow that is swollen and erythematous, then the likely diagnosis is bursitis rather than arthritis.
8. Normal synovial fluid generally contains less than 180 cells per MM3, most of which are mononuclear cells.
9. At a WBC count at or above 3000 cells/mm^3, the diagnosis of osteoarthritis is rather unlikely.
10. The first-line treatment of osteoarthritis is still acetaminophen therapy maximized to 3–4 grams daily in patients with normal liver function testing.

17.86 Year 3—Week 29—Day 1

1. Neurosarcoidosis usually does not present in isolation but rather with other findings of sarcoidosis, such as hilar lymphadenopathy, pulmonary symptoms, uveitis, and cardiac conduction block abnormalities.
2. Pituitary adenomas should not cause posterior pituitary problems such as central diabetes insipidus.
3. Lymphocytic hypophysitis is a state that usually affects young females, sometimes after pregnancy and can be associated with posterior pituitary problems.
4. Propranolol has been noted to cause loss of mental sharpness or intellect among many patients (it crosses into the CSF barrier). In patients with essential tremor and this complaint, use primidone instead.
5. Beta-blockers as a class may be associated with nightmares.
6. Tricyclic antidepressants may be associated with decreased effective action of central acting hypertensive agents such as reserpine and clonidine.
7. The classic side effect of reserpine is depression. This medication is rarely used nowadays for hypertension.
8. The worst prognostic factor in a tricyclic antidepressant overdose is QRS width prolongation.
9. Patients with TCA poisoning should be managed with alkalinization with the pH of the arterial blood gas followed to titrate effect.
10. Dextromethorphan can interact with SSRI agents and lead to increased risk of serotonin syndrome.

17.87 Year 3—Week 29—Day 2

1. Patients with fear of exposure to influenza type B will not get any protective effects from amantadine.
2. Amantadine is associated with mental status changes and hallucinations, and the drug can cause hyponatremia.
3. Imipenem and high-dose penicillin intravenously are associated with a risk for seizures.
4. Patients with episcleritis can be observed for resolution of symptoms for 2 weeks or so.

Patients with scleritis should be seen by an eye doctor as soon as possible.

5. Patients with immunosuppression who have marked cranial nerve palsies unilaterally should be worked up for cavernous sinus thrombosis.

6. Acute angle closure glaucoma can present with abdominal symptoms first before the patient develops a red eye.

7. Severe myopia remains as the most common cause of retinal detachment.

8. A diabetic patient with new eye "floaters" requires an urgent to emergent referral to an eye doctor to rule out retinal detachment.

9. Anterior communicating artery aneurysms can cause third cranial nerve palsies.

10. Diabetes mellitus is a frequent cause of painless third cranial nerve palsies with the finding of the affected eye in a "down and out" position.

17.88 Year 3—Week 29—Day 3

1. Consider tuberculosis, sarcoidosis, and cryptococcus in cases of basilar meningitis.

2. Add disopyramide to beta-blockade therapy in patients with recalcitrant hypertrophic cardiomyopathy.

3. Use itraconazole as first-line treatment of sporotrichosis and histoplasmosis.

4. Use primidone as the second-line agent for essential tremor if beta-blockade fails.

5. Use alpha blockers as second-line agent for Raynaud's phenomenon if calcium channel blockers fail.

6. The three cardinal signs of Behcet's syndrome are oral ulcers, genital ulcers, and uveitis.

7. Patients with Marfan's syndrome need to be followed regularly by eye doctors due to risk of lens dislocation, usually posterior in nature.

8. Patients with homocystinuria are also at risk of lens dislocation usually anterior in nature.

9. Severe myopia remains the most common cause of retinal detachment.

10. New onset floaters in a diabetic's visual field require urgent eye clinic referral.

17.89 Year 3—Week 30—Day 1

1. Patients receiving recurrent over the counter pharmacological enemas for constipation may be at risk of hyperphosphatemia.

2. Hypophosphatemia is one of the causes of rhabdomyolysis.

3. Hypothyroidism, when severe, can cause elevations of both the AST and ALT as these are released as well with myopathies.

4. Proximal myopathy differential should include hypothyroidism, steroid use (not the anabolic ones), and inclusion body myositis.

5. Inclusion body myositis responds very poorly to immunosuppressive therapy.

6. Hypophosphatemia may arise as one is treating the acidosis in a patient with diabetic ketoacidosis. The risk factor of severe hypophosphatemia involves rhabdomyolysis (as noted above) and diaphragmatic dysfunction that could lead to respiratory failure.

7. Patients with liver disease and diabetes mellitus are at risk of Dupuytren's contracture.

8. Keep in mind both acromegaly and amyloidosis in the differential diagnosis of a patient presenting with carpal tunnel syndrome.

9. One of the more unusual symptoms in temporal arteritis involves tongue infarction where a patient can present with a loss of taste. One also usually sees jaw claudication in this setting.

10. Indomethacin is the drug of choice for treatment of chronic paroxysmal hemicranium headaches.

17.90 Year 3—Week 30—Day 2

1. Patients with acute glaucoma can present with a wide range of symptoms including an acute abdomen presentation (yes, usually they have the red eye at the same time).

2. Timolol can actually cause significant bradycardia and even congestive heart failure has

been reported once the medication was started.

3. Latanoprost has been associated with significant myalgias as a side effect. Consider switching to another class of agents for treatment of glaucoma if the symptoms are intractable.

4. The pupil may be constricted in patients presenting with acute anterior uveitis and there may also be a whitish layer of cells present known as hypopyon iritis.

5. Roth's spots occur mostly in association with endocarditis but similar lesions have been noted to occur in patients with fungemia and with acute leukemia.

6. Central retinal artery occlusion is manifested by a cherry red spot in the macula and can be seen with hypercoagulable states or infectious states.

7. Central retinal vein occlusion is noted by a fundoscopic exam noting "blood and thunder" throughout the retina.

8. Rheumatoid arthritis patients can get a variety of eye disorders including corneal melt, corneal ulcers, and scleromalacia perforans, as well as scleritis and episcleritis.

9. Angioid streaks are disruptions of Bruch's membrane that can be visualized on fundoscopic exam and can be seen in diseases such as acromegaly, Paget's disease, pseudoxanthoma elasticum, sickle cell disease, and Ehlers-Danlos syndrome.

10. Sunflower cataracts and Kayser-Fleischer rings (involving Descemet's membrane) are among the ocular manifestations of Wilson's disease.

17.91   Year 3—Week 30—Day 3

1. A common mistake in missing celiac sprue is failing to order the IGG isotypes of the antibodies (such as tissue transglutaminase) as this condition may be accompanied by IGA deficiency.

2. Washed RBCs can be used in transfusion of patients with IGA deficiency to decrease chance of reaction.

3. Consider IGA deficiency testing in patients who have an anaphylactic reaction to fresh frozen plasma.

4. The best blood product to give to a patient who has a very low VWF level and needs surgery is cryoprecipitate, not fresh frozen plasma.

5. Celiac disease should be considered in patients with unexplained iron deficiency anemia and unexplained sensory polyneuropathy.

6. Among the diseases/states associated with celiac sprue are Addison's disease, alopecia areata, migraine disease, cerebellar ataxia, idiopathic dilated cardiomyopathy, Sjogren's disease, iron deficiency anemia, and osteoporosis.

7. Behavioral therapy (such as bladder training techniques) is preferred over oxybutynin or tolterodine as initial treatment of urge incontinence.

8. Oxybutynin is an anticholinergic agent, so be wary of mental status changes in the elderly.

9. West-Nile virus encephalitis can present with poliomyelitis type symptoms due to disease affecting the anterior horn cells of the spinal cord.

10. Small bowel T-cell lymphoma is associated with celiac disease.

17.92   Year 3—Week 31—Day 1

1. Osteomalacia should be considered in patients with complaints of bone pain with an increased alkaline phosphatase and negative workups for multiple myeloma and metastatic disease to bone.

2. The five most common tumors to metastasize to bone are prostate, breast, kidney, lung, and thyroid.

3. AL amyloid is seen with multiple myeloma and with primary amyloidosis.

4. Sputum cytology can be helpful in the diagnosis of lung cancer in a patient with newly discovered lung mass.

5. There is an increased incidence of *Staphylococcus aureus* lung infections in

patients post-influenza. The most common bacterial organism post-influenzae is still *Streptococcus pneumoniae*.

6. The best fluoroquinolone for treatment of *Streptococcus pneumoniae* (pneumonia or meningitis) is levofloxacin.
7. Active alveolitis may appear as a ground glass infiltration on a high resolution CT scan. Steroids are usually indicated with this finding.
8. The only agent indicated in mild persistent asthma is inhaled corticosteroids.
9. A subtle sign of asthma is the scalloping of the descending phase of the expiratory side of the flow volume loop.
10. Most patients with mild asthma have normal spirometry and would be found only with methacholine challenge test.

17.93 Year 3—Week 31—Day 2

1. Pancreatitis can lead to splenic vein thrombosis. The treatment is splenectomy.
2. Azathioprine and 6-mercaptopurine are used as steroid-sparing agents in Crohn's disease. Both agents can lead to drug-induced pancreatitis.
3. Gynecological cancers are associated with Lynch syndrome (hereditary non-polyposis coli) and with Peutz-Jeghers syndrome.
4. Patients with IgA deficiency are at increased risk of *Giardia lamblia* infections with recommended treatment of metronidazole or nitazoxanide.
5. *Isospora belli* is an opportunistic agent that can lead to diarrhea in HIV positive patients, but unlike other similar parasites, it can be treated with an oral antibiotic (usually sulfa-based antibiotic).
6. Check for iron deficiency anemia in patients with restless leg syndrome.
7. Patients with vocal cord dysfunction will be misdiagnosed as having asthma. Check a flow volume loop which will reveal a spastic, chaotic inspiratory flow limb in vocal cord dysfunction.

8. Acute hepatitis B usually occurs within the first six months that a patient is exposed to the virus with most patients only have a mild form of the disease at the time.
9. Acute retroviral syndrome might resemble infectious mononucleosis and should be sought after especially in patients with a morbilliform exanthem that spares the palms and soles.
10. CMV is the most common viral pathogen in adults presenting as a mononucleosis after EBV has been ruled out.

17.94 Year 3—Week 31—Day 3

1. Carbamazepine is used for treatment of complex partial seizures. The frontal lobe variety of this seizure can lead to "freezing" episodes.
2. Nimodipine is used to treat vasospasm post-subarachnoid hemorrhage in setting of cerebral aneurismal bleed. This medication should be given for 21 days in all patients in this situation.
3. Iron deficiency anemia can be found in patients with restless leg syndrome and oral iron helps with symptoms.
4. Amantadine and benztropine can be used in Parkinson's disease patients whose main feature of disease is isolated tremor. Watch out for hyponatremia and mental status changes with amantadine (even hallucinations can occur).
5. Propranolol is the preferred beta-blocker agent to use in patients with essential tremor.
6. Lamotrigine is a medication that can be used as an adjunct with carbamazepine in treatment of complex partial seizures.
7. The features of internuclear ophthalmoplegia as can be seen in multiple sclerosis include weakness of the adducting eye and nystagmus of the abducting eye on lateral gaze.
8. Other common phrases that can be seen in questions or cases involving multiple sclerosis are optic atrophy, afferent papillary defect (Marcus-Gunn pupil), central scotoma, transient paresthesia in arms and legs with neck flexion (Lhermitte's sign), and worsening of

neurological function with heat or fever (Uhthoff's phenomenon).

9. The Jarisch-Herxheimer reaction describes fevers, arthralgias, rash after getting penicillin due to death of spirochetes.

10. The prozone phenomenon describes a state of having too much spirochete antigen such that the RPR can come back falsely negative.

17.95 Year 3—Week 32—Day 1

1. The paraneoplastic process of hypercalcemia is usually due to PTH-related peptide in solid tumors such as squamous cell lung cancer. About one-third of non-Hodgkin's lymphomas can have hypercalcemia mediated by calcitriol.

2. The anti-Yo antibody is helpful in detecting subacute cerebellar degeneration in patients with breast and ovarian cancer, and less useful for detecting this entity in patients with small cell lung cancer.

3. The anti-Hu (anti-neuronal antibody 2) is used to detect limbic encephalomyelitis which may afflict patients with Hodgkin's disease, small cell lung cancer, and testicular cancer.

4. Calcitonin may be used in the first 24 h to treat extreme elevations of serum calcium but its effect is nowhere near as potent as IV hydration with normal saline and concomitant Lasix.

5. Patients with normal pressure hydrocephalus may present with lower extremity Parkinsonism.

6. Polymyalgia rheumatica can present initially as a seronegative symmetrical polyarthritis before its more usual presentation of hip and shoulder stiffness.

7. Enthesopathy is inflammation at insertion point of tendon or ligament into bone, and it can be seen in such diseases as ankylosing spondylitis, reactive arthritis, psoriasis, and arthritis associated with inflammatory bowel disease.

8. There has been epidemiological evidence linking hidradenitis suppurativa and spondyloarthropathies.

9. Samter's syndrome is the triad of bronchial asthma, nasal polyposis, and intolerance to aspirin.

10. Patients with silicosis are at high risk of developing tuberculosis.

17.96 Year 3—Week 32—Day 2

1. Acrodermatitis enteropathica is the acral rash associated with zinc deficiency. Consider this in patients with poor nutrition or chronic alcoholism.

2. Non-small cell lung cancer is the neoplasm associated with hypertrophic pulmonary osteoarthropathy.

3. Ectopic ACTH syndrome, subacute cerebellar degeneration, limbic encephalitis, and Lambert-Eaton syndrome are among the paraneoplastic processes associated with small cell lung carcinoma.

4. Tuberculosis and histoplasmosis are amongst the diseases that have an affinity for infection of the adrenal glands.

5. Consider adrenal hemorrhage as a possible cause of hypotension in patients with Capnocytophaga canimorsus infections developing hypotension.

6. Hypertriglyceridemia is the most common lipid abnormality in patients with chronic renal failure.

7. Arsenic has been used in refractory cases of AML and its main side effect is QT interval prolongation.

8. Normal septal depolarization is noted on an EKG by a small Q-wave in lead V6. Loss of this Q-wave in lead V6 might imply an old septal infarct.

9. Folinic acid needs to be given to patients in treating methanol toxicity.

10. The urine chloride level is the most reliable test to get in patients with metabolic alkalosis to see if there will be a response to normal saline.

17.97 Year 3—Week 32—Day 3

1. Theophylline is notorious for causing drug-induced multifocal atrial tachycardia, even at therapeutic levels.
2. Trapped lung syndrome leads to transudative pleural effusions. Malignant involvement of pleural lining leads to exudative pleural effusions.
3. Aneurysms from syphilis most commonly occur in the ascending aorta.
4. Anatomical areas where chondrocalcinosis can occur include the symphysis pubis and triangular ligament of the wrist. Chondrocalcinosis can be an asymptomatic finding or be seen in association with pseudogout.
5. Generally, doses of prednisone start at 1 mg/kg daily when treating a patient with severe bullous pemphigoid.
6. Vancomycin is the most notorious antibiotic to cause exacerbation of linear bullous IGA disease.
7. Patients with lupus panniculitis or lupus profundus will respond to hydroxychloroquine.
8. Hypertension is common in patients with adult polycystic kidney disease. Only about 10% of patients will develop berry aneurysms.
9. Homocystinuria leads to dilation of the aorta and pulmonary arteries and is also associated with lens subluxation and osteoporosis.
10. Osteomalacia is adult vitamin D deficiency and can present with significant bone pain and pseudofractures on X-rays.

17.98 Year 3—Week 33—Day 1

1. AZT-associated myopathy in HIV disease is lower than previously seen in the past due to lower dosing of the medication in current regimens.
2. Nucleoside reverse transcriptase inhibitors are associated with acute ascending neuropathy and possible lactic acidosis. In this setting, the patient must be taken off the medication immediately.
3. Efavirenz is associated with CNS side effects such as insomnia and delirium.
4. Abacavir can lead to an acute hypersensitivity reaction marked by fevers, lymphadenopathy, morbilliform rash, hepatitis, abdominal pain, and shortness of breath.
5. Paroxysmal nocturnal hemoglobinuria (PNH) is associated with defects in the RBC membrane at CD-55 and CD-59 and can lead to thrombosis of major vessels and of hemolytic anemia.
6. TTP is now felt caused by antibodies to the metalloproteases of the von Willebrand factor (which do not allow the large multimers of VWF to be broken down).
7. HIV-associated myelopathy (vacuolar) may mimic B-12 deficiency.
8. Distal symmetrical polyneuropathy is probably the most common neurological manifestation of HIV disease and is highly associated as well with HIV antiretroviral drugs, such as DDI, DDC, and D4T.
9. Foscarnet can be used to treat CMV disease. It is associated with renal insufficiency and hypophosphatemia.
10. Cranial nerve palsy may be the presenting sign of tuberculosis. Treatment of CNS manifestations of tuberculosis includes corticosteroids in addition to antibiotics against tuberculosis.

17.99 Year 3—Week 33—Day 2

1. Systemic mastocytosis can progress to mast cell leukemia. Prognosis is poor at this stage.
2. Patients on beta-blockers still receive epinephrine first in cases of anaphylaxis (do not go to glucagon as first-line agent, but rather use it if no response to appropriate epinephrine dosing).
3. Nasal ipratropium is the drug of choice for gustatory rhinitis.
4. Serum sickness of mild to moderate intensity can be treated with NSAID and/or antihistamine therapy rather than corticosteroid therapy.
5. Differential for low complement levels and active worsening renal disease includes Cholesterol emboli syndrome, active lupus with renal disease, cryoglobulinemia, and other causes of rapidly progressive glomerulonephritis such as vasculitis syndromes.
6. The acute treatment of Goodpasture's disease is plasmapheresis as it is an antibody driven process namely the anti-glomerular basement membrane antibody.
7. *Neisseria meningitidis* recurrent infections should lead to testing for late complement deficiency (C5b-C9).
8. Avoid mango in patients with excessive reactions to poison ivy.
9. Avoid banana, kiwi, avocado, and chestnut in patients with excessive latex allergies.
10. Desensitization cannot be done in patients who have history of hypersensitivity reactions to medications, such as abacavir or dilantin.

17.100 Year 3—Week 33—Day 3

1. Skin patch testing cannot be done in patients with history of dermatographism or active erythroderma or those who have had a severe allergic reaction to an exposure.
2. Erythroderma can be seen with psoriasis and T-cell lymphoma.

3. The organ system most vulnerable to damage in patients with erythroderma is the cardiovascular system.
4. In patients with hemochromatosis, phlebotomy helps cardiovascular symptoms the most.
5. Churg-Strauss vasculitis presents with adult-onset asthma, allergic rhinitis symptoms, eosinophilia, and mononeuritis multiplex.
6. Ipratropium is only used in asthma treatments for severe acute exacerbations not responding to normal treatment.
7. It is safe to use beta-blockers on most patients with COPD.
8. Patients with recurrent pneumonias and sinusitis with normal immunoglobulin levels should be tested for IGG subclass deficiencies.
9. Patients with common variable immunodeficiency have an increased risk of non-Hodgkin's lymphomas.
10. The most common cause of syncope in a young patient is vasovagal syncope. Lifting legs above level of heart to improve venous return is first step of action.

17.101 Year 3—Week 34—Day 1

1. Wedge-shaped appearing "infiltrates" on chest X-rays might actually represent lung infarction in the setting of pulmonary emboli.
2. Posterior myocardial infarctions demonstrate with various findings such as tall R-wave in lead V1 or significant ST-segment depression along leads V1–V2.
3. Afterload reduction is crucial in the treatment of aortic insufficiency and mitral regurgitation.
4. Heart rate control is crucial in treating patients with mitral stenosis and when these patients go into tachycardia, they are at risk of pulmonary edema.
5. When patients with aortic stenosis become symptomatic, then they should have surgical valve replacement.

6. Lactic acid levels and LDH levels may be normal in patients with ischemic and necrotic bowel.
7. Suspect mesenteric ischemia when there is focal small bowel dilation on plain X-rays with little or no abnormalities of the large intestine.
8. Patients with new onset left bundle branch block and chest pain should be treated as are those patients with ST-segment elevation.
9. Patients on steroids and morphine for pain control may not manifest abdominal pain in the setting of visceral perforation.
10. Patients with rapid atrial fibrillation due to Wolff–Parkinson–White syndrome will generally not demonstrate any delta waves in the QRS complex (slurring of upstroke of QRS complex).

17.102 Year 3—Week 34—Day 2

1. Patients with Parkinson's disease will generally exhibit the classic triad of tremor, rigidity, and bradykinesia. They will also have subtle changes before these three conditions manifest such as trouble rising from a chair, trouble turning in bed, personality changes, non-specific pain complaints, autonomic dysfunction, and postural instability.
2. Levodopa will induce dyskinesias within 5–7 years of treatment. Dopamine receptor agonists are associated with less incidence of dyskinesias.
3. Levodopa does not treat dementia, autonomic dysfunction, postural instability, or the freezing episodes associated with Parkinson's disease.
4. Levodopa should be administered at least 1 h apart from meals as dietary protein will compete with the uptake of levodopa from the gut.
5. If the dose of levodopa exceeds 1000 mg per day and there is still no clinical effect, then the patient likely has Parkinsonism rather than true Parkinson's disease.

6. Causes of Parkinsonism include trauma, cerebrovascular accident, hydrocephalus, and drug-induced causes. Metoclopramide (Reglan) and phenothiazines are the most common causes of drug-induced Parkinsonism.
7. Ergot-derived dopamine receptor agonists (bromocriptine) are rarely used anymore in treating Parkinson's disease as they have side effects that include erythromelalgia (redness and burning of digits), retroperitoneal fibrosis, Raynaud's phenomenon, and coronary vasospasm.
8. Non-ergot derived dopamine receptor agonists used in the treatment of Parkinson's disease include ropinirole and pramipexole. Side effects include nausea, vomiting, hypotension, hallucinations, confusion, and peripheral edema.
9. Supraventricular arrythmias are a much more common cause of syncope than ventricular arrythmias.
10. Seizure drop attacks may be a cause of syncope. These may respond well to lamotrigine therapy.

17.103 Year 3—Week 34—Day 3

1. Osteoporosis circumscripta is a finding in patients with Paget's disease on bone and is clearly seen on skull X-rays.
2. The two most common lab findings in patients with Paget's disease are an elevated alkaline phosphatase level and an elevated urinary hydroxyproline level.
3. Bisphosphonate therapy is considered in treating patients with Paget's disease who have pain unresponsive to NSAIDS.
4. Hypercalcemia occurs in Paget's disease only when a patient is immobilized for a long period of time.
5. Primary hyperparathyroidism may be associated with a slight elevation in alkaline phosphatase level but will be clearly recognized by accompanying low phosphorus and high calcium levels.

6. Vitamin D deficiency can cause a slight elevation in the alkaline phosphatase level.

7. The alkaline phosphatase level needs to be monitored every 6 months in patients with Paget's disease to make sure that an occult osteosarcoma does not arise.

8. Erythroderma and Paget's disease are associated with high output heart failure.

9. Paget's disease may lead to hearing loss due to compression of cranial nerve eight.

10. Patients with Paget's disease may get angioid streaks of the eye (disruption in Bruch's membrane).

17.104   Year 3—Week 35—Day 1

1. The most common cause of kidney stones in the general population is idiopathic hyperoxaluria.

2. Excessive vitamin C intake could lead to calcium oxalate stone formation.

3. Use folic acid in the long-term treatment of patients with chronic hemolysis.

4. Patients with common variable immunodeficiency are at increased risk of Giardia infections.

5. Patients with common variable immunodeficiency may be at increased risk of lymphoma of small bowel as well as non-Hodgkin's lymphomas in other anatomical locations.

6. Patients with celiac sprue may present with arthritis and with a rash known as dermatitis herpetiformis.

7. Patients with pernicious anemia are at increased risk of gastric carcinoid polyps.

8. Patients with recurrent broncho-pneumonias are at increased risk of bronchiectasis, which may lead to hemoptysis.

9. The most common organism infecting patients with COPD and pneumonia is *Streptococcus pneumoniae*.

10. The second most common pathogen infecting patients with COPD and pneumonia is *Haemophilus influenzae*.

17.105   Year 3—Week 35—Day 2

1. Fabry disease is a lysosomal storage disorder marked by deficiency of alpha-galactosidase A.

2. Burning acroparesthesias, particularly made worse in febrile episodes, is the usual first sign of Fabry's disease.

3. Enzyme replacement biweekly with alginase is the treatment of Fabry disease.

4. 70% of females that carry the disease of Fabry disease will develop clinical symptoms. Acroparesthesias do not tend to be as severe in females as they do in males.

5. The usual heart complication in patients with Fabry disease is hypertrophic cardiomyopathy with diastolic dysfunction.

6. Fabry disease can cause corneal involvement, renal involvement, abdominal pain, and cryptogenic stroke.

7. Angiokeratomas can develop in patients with Fabry disease and can involve the penis and scrotum in male patients.

8. Relief of gastrointestinal symptoms is usually the first effect of enzyme replacement in patients with Fabry disease.

9. Long term, the greatest benefit of enzyme replacement in Fabry disease will be the chronic neuropathic pain and the peripheral neuropathy symptoms.

10. Paget-Schrotter's disease or effort-induced DVT occurs in patients with repetitive activity that involves bringing the arm above the head, such as baseball pitchers.

17.106   Year 3—Week 35—Day 3

1. False cervical ribs are a common cause of thoracic outlet syndrome. Surgery is the treatment of choice (removal of false first ribs).

2. Catheter-directed thrombolysis provides the greatest initial relief of symptoms in patients with Paget-Schrotter's disease. Anticoagulation for 3 months usually follows and then followed by surgical resection

of any correctible anatomical malformations.

3. Beta-blockers should not be used pre-operatively in patients with low risk for cardiac events.

4. Propranolol is the preferred beta-blocker historically in patients with liver disease to prevent variceal bleeding.

5. Adrenal insufficiency might cause isolated oral hyperpigmentation without skin hyperpigmentation.

6. Lab abnormalities in primary adrenal insufficiency include eosinophilia, hypercalcemia, metabolic acidosis, and hyperkalemia.

7. Babesiosis causes red blood cell inclusions and hemolytic anemia in clinical presentation.

8. Ehrlichiosis causes WBC inclusions along with thrombocytopenia, AST and ALT elevation, and splenomegaly.

9. Doxycycline is the first-line therapy for *Ehrlichiosis.*

10. Histoplasmosis *is* the other classic infection that can lead to WBC inclusions.

17.107 Year 3—Week 36—Day 1

1. The most common location for a carcinoid tumor is the small bowel and appendix.

2. Carcinoid tumors can metastasize aggressively to the liver and can cause iron deficiency anemia.

3. There is targeted chemoembolization of carcinoid tumors that have metastasized to the liver. Liver involvement with carcinoid will lead to facial flushing, similar to carcinoid bronchial involvement.

4. A complication of embolization chemotherapy or surgical resection of carcinoid is carcinoid crisis, which involves hypotension, profound flushing, confusion, and hyperthermia.

5. Severe right-sided heart failure can arise in patients with carcinoid syndrome.

6. Anticoagulation for DVT prophylaxis in patients with spinal cord injury is usually only needed for about 4–6 months after the acute injury.

7. Among the reasons for decreased DVT risk in SCI patients after 6 months. (a) The arterial atrophy in the paralyzed limbs that then leads to venous atrophy and paradoxical improvement in stagnation of blood and (b) the development of high muscle tone that is accompanied by spasms which improves the "calf muscle pump."

8. Seborrheic keratosis do not generally form at the palms and soles.

9. Basal cell carcinomas are nearly unheard of being found in the upper eyelid of patients.

10. Asteatotic eczema with "tapioca-seated" vesicles can occur in patients washing hands on numerous occasions.

17.108 Year 3—Week 36—Day 2

1. Development of new onset diabetes mellitus in elderly patients should concern providers about a possible development of pancreatic cancer.

2. Obstructive jaundice remains the most common initial presentation of pancreatic cancer.

3. Criteria for surgical resection of pancreatic cancer include besides no evidence of metastasis the following: (a) patency of the portal vein and superior mesenteric vein confluence and (b) absence of celiac axis or superior mesenteric artery involvement.

4. Tumor involvement of the portal vein or of the superior mesenteric vein is not considered a contraindication for resection of pancreatic cancer.

5. Gemcitabine monotherapy is an accepted chemotherapy of choice for metastatic pancreatic cancer.

6. Vasculitic neuropathy is estimated to affect about 10% of patients with rheumatoid arthritis.

7. Sjogren's disease can present first with an asymmetric chronic peripheral neuropathy years before the classic dry eyes/dry mouth (sicca syndrome) symptoms present.

8. There is no data concerning the use of GM-CSF or G-CSF for non-chemotherapy induced agranulocytosis states.

9. Methimazole, captopril, propylthiouracil, sulfasalazine, and carbamazepine are among the most common medications to induce agranulocytosis.

10. It generally takes about 10 days after discontinuation of a culprit drug to see the resolution of agranulocytosis.

17.109 Year 3—Week 36—Day 3

1. Sphingomyelinase toxin of the brown recluse spider bite (causing necrosis) can be attenuated by use of dapsone within 48 h.

2. Community-acquired MRSA infections can mimic the appearance of a brown recluse spider bite.

3. Infliximab is used in the treatment of pyoderma gangrenosum.

4. Patients with Ehlers-Danlos syndrome are prone to recurrent hernias and GI bleeds.

5. Kayser-Fleisher rings are the classic finding in Wilson's disease on eye exam and involve copper deposition in Descemet's membrane.

6. Erythrasma is caused by *Corynebacterium minutissimum* and is treated with erythromycin.

7. Avoid dapsone and trimethoprim-sulfamethoxazole in patients with G6PD deficiency.

8. Gilbert's syndrome is the most common cause of an elevated bilirubin in the general population.

9. Patients with first episode of pancreatitis should not undergo any endoscopic or surgical therapy in general if pancreas divisum is found (wait for second episode before launching corrective action).

10. Adenosine is the drug of choice for initial drug therapy of supraventricular tachycardia.

17.110 Year 3—Week 37—Day 1

1. All patients using methotrexate must be on folic acid to prevent megaloblastic anemia changes.

2. Leflunomide can cause hepatotoxicity similar to methotrexate.

3. Methotrexate is the first-line drug of choice for erosive rheumatoid arthritis.

4. Methotrexate is also the first-line drug of choice for patients with erosive psoriatic arthritis.

5. Among the anterior mediastinal masses, do not forget substernal thyroid goiter as one of the causes.

6. Myasthenia gravis is associated with a thymoma in about 15% of cases.

7. Avoid aminoglycoside therapy in all patients being admitted with a myasthenia gravis exacerbation.

8. Metronidazole can cause delirium, especially in patients with renal dysfunction.

9. Differential diagnosis for patients with Horner's syndrome should include Pancoast tumor, cluster headaches, and Wallenberg syndrome (lateral medullary infarction).

10. Patients with ectopic endometrial tissue in the lung can suffer bleeding as well as pneumothorax.

17.111 Year 3—Week 37—Day 2

1. The antibody of choice in a patient with primary biliary cirrhosis is the antimitochondrial antibody.

2. The antibody of choice in a patient with autoimmune hepatitis is the anti-smooth muscle antibody. The second most common is the anti-liver-kidney-microsomal antibody.

3. Li-Fraumeni syndrome involves a deletion in the p53 tumor suppressor gene and can cause tumors in the adrenal gland, brain, and breast along with increased propensity for leukemias.

4. Hereditary non-polyposis coli does involve transformation of a polyp into a carcinoma.
5. Inflammatory bowel disease is the only mechanism to get colon cancer without a polyp, and namely this occurs through dysplasia.
6. Pyoderma gangrenosum is most highly associated with ulcerative colitis as the underlying disease.
7. The best treatment of pyoderma gangrenosum is to treat the underlying disease.
8. The treatment of a patient with ulcerative colitis who has even mild dysplasia noted on screening colonoscopy is to have a total proctocolectomy.
9. 5-ASA medications remain the standard initial drug of choice for ulcerative colitis.
10. Beware of the drug-induced pancreatitis that might occur when using azathioprine to treat inflammatory bowel disease.

17.112 Year 3—Week 37—Day 3

1. Patients with type 2 diabetes mellitus may have anemia due to erythropoietin deficiency even with normal renal function.
2. Consider obtaining a celiac sprue panel in patients with iron deficiency anemia and no occult blood loss to explain the state.
3. Ceftriaxone needs to be used in treating Lyme disease when there is severe carditis and when there are severe neurological symptoms (otherwise use doxycycline or amoxicillin if allergic to doxycycline).
4. West-Nile virus needs to be considered in patients with flu-like illness with weakness pattern resembling poliomyelitis. A high protein value will be obtained in CSF analysis.
5. Recombinant factor VIIa or purified porcine factor 8 can be used in treating patients with factor 8 inhibitor.
6. Patients with diabetes mellitus can have increased incidences of rashes such as granu-

loma annulare and necrobiosis lipoidica diabeticorum.
7. Caution needs to be used with thyroid replacement in the elderly as over-correction may lead to atrial fibrillation and osteoporosis.
8. It is vital to recognize signs of hypothyroidism such as worsening hypertension, lipid panels (particularly LDL), early onset alopecia, constipation and weight gain.
9. Among the causes of sudden death due to the circulatory systems are anomalous coronary artery, atherosclerotic CAD, coronary artery hypoplasia, coronary aneurysm, intramyocardial coronary bridge, and coronary dissection.
10. Other causes of cardiac sudden death in young adults include bicuspid aortic stenosis, embolic myocardial infarction, and various cardiomyopathy states.

17.113 Year 3—Week 38—Day 1

1. Patients with chronic renal disease who become pregnant have a greater risk of pre-eclampsia than those with no history of renal insufficiency that become pregnant.
2. Among the clues for renal artery stenosis are (1) the presence of a systolic-diastolic abdominal bruit, (2) difficult to treat hypertension (more than 2 agents), and (3) onset of significant hypertension over a relatively short period of time (1–2 years) in a patient above age 50.
3. The sulfosalicylic acid test will be positive in patients with multiple myeloma, while the urine dipstick for albumin will be negative.
4. The most common histology seen in patients with HIV disease who have nephrotic syndrome is focal and segmental glomerulonephritis.
5. HAART therapy can have an impact in the kidney function of patients with HIV chronic kidney disease.

6. An alkaline phosphatase level over 1000 mg/ dL with an elevated GGT level and minimal transaminitis and total bilirubin elevation should raise suspicion of a space-occupying lesion in the liver (infiltrative process, malignancy, etc.).

7. *Plasmodium malariae* can cause nephrotic syndrome.

8. Patients with sickle cell disease are LESS prone to get malarial infections compared to the general population.

9. The biggest risk factor for dengue hemorrhagic fever is previous infection to any dengue virus.

10. Patients with *Strongyloides stercoralis* can have super-infection with gram-negative organisms (think of this in unusual clinical situations such as a patient with *E. coli* meningitis for instance).

17.114   Year 3—Week 38—Day 2

1. Recall that there is no demonstratable weakness in patients with polymyalgia rheumatica.

2. One can have polymyalgia rheumatica and even temporal arteritis with a normal sedimentation rate.

3. Cyclophosphamide has potential risks of urinary bladder squamous cell cancer and well as systemic lymphoproliferative disorders that can arise with use of the medication remains the first-line therapy of patients with Wegener's granulomatosis.

4. Oral contraceptive therapy may lead to the skin finding of erythema nodosum.

5. When sarcoidosis initially presents with erythema nodosum, this is a good prognostic sign.

6. Uveitis might be seen in patients with ankylosing spondylitis and sarcoidosis.

7. Anterior ischemic optic neuropathy is the usual ophthalmologic finding in patients with temporal arteritis.

8. Myopia is the most common cause of retinal detachment in the general population.

17.115   Year 3—Week 38—Day 3

1. Erythromelalgia refers to redness and burning of a patient's digits in underling myeloproliferative disease and relief is acquired in about 30 minutes after a dose of aspirin.

2. Chronic myelogenous leukemia (CML) is treated with imatinib mesylate as first-line therapy.

3. Bone marrow transplantation is the treatment of choice in young patients with myelodysplastic disease.

4. Aminocaproic acid is the drug of choice in treating primary fibrinolysis.

5. Ceftriaxone is the treatment of Kingella species endocarditis infections.

6. Consider Behcet's disease as the underlying diagnosis in a patient with bilateral pulmonary emboli and history of pulmonary artery aneurysms.

7. Chlorambucil is the drug of choice to treat the vascular complications of Behcet's disease.

8. Plasmapheresis is the treatment of choice in a patient with acute Goodpasture's syndrome.

9. The anti-glomerular basement membrane antibody is the one most commonly seen with Goodpasture's syndrome.

10. Nitrofurantoin can be used in the third trimester of pregnancy to treat a urinary tract infection.

17.116   Year 3—Week 39—Day 1

1. There is a hemorrhagic variant of dengue fever which can be quite severe.

2. Carbamazepine is the drug of choice for controlling partial complex seizures.

3. Carbamazepine is associated with leukocytosis, leukopenia, and hyponatremia.

4. Lamotrigine is the anti-epileptic drug most linked to the side effect of exfoliative dermatitis.

5. Valproic acid is the anti-epileptic drug most effective for generalized seizure disorders and is most linked to side effects of weight gain, pancreatitis, and hair loss.

6. A patient having a seizure from alcohol withdrawal does not need anti-epileptic therapy.
7. Vasovagal syncope can have tonic-clonic activity associated with it that resembles seizure. No need for anti-epileptic therapy in those cases.
8. Vasovagal syncope is the most common cause of syncope.
9. Squatting increases preload to the heart and thus will increase the murmurs of aortic insufficiency, mitral insufficiency (regurgitation), mitral stenosis, and aortic stenosis.
10. The murmur of hypertrophic cardiomyopathy gets louder with a Valsalva maneuver and with standing from a squatted position (standing in such fashion also increases murmur of mitral valve prolapse).

17.117 Year 3—Week 39—Day 2

1. Left bundle branch block is the EKG finding most linked to paradoxical splitting of the second heart sound.
2. Right bundle branch block is the EKG finding most linked to persistent splitting of the second heart sound.
3. A second heart sound that is wide with a fixed split should raise suspicion of an atrial septal defect.
4. Most mechanical complications of myocardial infarction occur in patients who are having their first heart attack (no collateral circulation present). It should be noted that all of these complications are rare.
5. Free wall rupture is the post-MI mechanical complication most likely to result in death.
6. An emergent echocardiogram needs to be done in all patients suspected of having papillary muscle rupture or VSD formation post-MI.
7. A patient with chest pain and a new onset left bundle branch block should be treated as if the patient has ST-segment elevation.
8. Hydralazine can cause a reflex tachycardia. It is used with nitrate therapy in treating congestive heart failure.

9. Patients with right ventricular infarcts need normal saline to be able to keep up with their preload.
10. The treatment of acute aortic insufficiency is afterload reduction with ace-inhibitor and possibly nitroprusside therapy.

17.118 Year 3—Week 39—Day 3

1. Seminomas are radiosensitive similar to CNS dysgerminomas.
2. Seminomas should always be alpha fetal protein (AFP) stain negative.
3. All poorly differentiated midline carcinomas that have no characteristics of any tumor that can be identified should be treated as if they are germ cell tumors with bleomycin, etoposide, and cisplatinum as this is the most chance for cure for the patient.
4. Klinefelter's syndrome is associated with an increased risk of both male breast cancer and testicular cancer.
5. Diagnosis of Klinefelter's syndrome is made by karyotyping using material from a buccal smear.
6. Low ceruloplasmin levels along with neuropsychiatric history should raise concern for Wilson's disease.
7. Wilson's disease patients are treated with D-penicillamine for acute period and then switched over to zinc for chronic copper chelation therapy.
8. Lead poisoning can be treated with several agents, including succimer and EDTA.
9. ATN is marked by isosthenuria (inability to concentrate or dilute urine with specific gravity usually 1.010 value) and muddy brown casts in the urinalysis.
10. Urinary eosinophils are seen usually only in about 20% of cases of allergic interstitial nephritis, but you may notice a busy urinary sediment with leukocytes with lack of infection.

17.119 Year 3—Week 40—Day 1

1. Hypothyroidism can elevate CPK levels and LDH levels and present with proximal weakness and myalgias.
2. Hypothyroidism can also lead to an increased LDL level.
3. Brown's syndrome is the inability to gaze downward and in, which affects patients with rheumatoid arthritis due to tenosynovitis of the superior oblique muscle.
4. Patients with diabetes mellitus can also have problems accommodating their pupils leading to night vision problems.
5. Lofgren's syndrome involves sarcoidosis with features of ankle arthritis, bilateral hilar lymphadenopathy, and erythema nodosum.
6. Patients with psoriasis can have onycholysis in addition to nail pitting.
7. Patients with reactive arthritis can develop the manifestations of circinate balanitis, keratoderma blennorrhagica, and conjunctivitis.
8. Patients with ankylosing spondylitis get anterior uveitis which may lead to a layer of white cells in the anterior chamber of the eye (hypopyon iritis).

17.120 Year 3—Week 40—Day 2

1. Trimethoprim-sulfamethoxazole is the second-line agent to be used in patients with Listeria infection who cannot take ampicillin due to PCN allergy.
2. Trisomy 8 and Monosomy 7 are poor cytogenetic prognostic factors in dealing with patients with myelodysplasia.
3. Ertapenem does not cover *Pseudomonas* or *Acinetobacter* reliably. Use imipenem instead.
4. Adrenal insufficiency may present with subtle signs of pigmentation, such as pigmentation of the oral cavity with no other obvious pigmentation sites.
5. There must be greater than 90% bilateral adrenal destruction by tumor before adrenal insufficiency is likely to arise in a patient.

6. Besides CML, imatinib mesylate can be used in treatment of eosinophilic leukemias.
7. Thalidomide can be used in the treatment of multiple myeloma, severe lupus disease, and myelodysplastic syndromes.
8. Morning headaches can occur in patients with COPD who suffer from overnight hypoxemia while they sleep. These patients do not necessarily have obstructive sleep apnea.
9. Pemberton's sign involves the turning of a patient's facial skin into a reddish hue as he holds his arms above his head due to compression of a substernal goiter on central vasculature.
10. Propranolol, PTU, and dexamethasone are three drugs which block the peripheral conversion of T4 to T3.

17.121 Year 3—Week 40—Day 3

1. Plicatic acid is the material in Western Cedar wood that activates complement and leads to allergy formation.
2. Aspirin allergic patients can safely be given choline, magnesium, or sodium salicylates, as well as tartrazine.
3. Epinephrine lowers overall placental blood flow and can have teratogenic effects; thus, it should be avoided in pregnant patients with asthma.
4. Farmer's lung is usually due to thermophilic actinomycetes.
5. The usual component in cement causing allergic conditions is chromium.
6. T-helper cells subset 1 (TH1) produce gamma interferon and IL-2. In contrast, T-helper cells subset 2 produce IL 4 and IL 5 which are involved in eosinophil production. HIV patients have increased TH2 to TH1 ratios, which may explain why they commonly have blood eosinophilia and eosinophilic folliculitis.
7. Thymomas are seen in pure red cell aplasia and in myasthenia gravis. About 15% of patients will have thymomas in myasthenia

gravis but the rest will have thymic hyperplasia in which thymectomy is also indicated.

8. The diagnostic test of choice for sinusitis is a limited coronal CT scan of the sinuses. This test gives a good view of the ethmoid sinuses which were notoriously missed on Waters view (plain X-ray) of the sinuses.

17.122 Year 3—Week 41—Day 1

1. The most reliable end point in assessing the screening efficacy in a randomized trial involving oncology is the cause-specific cancer mortality.
2. Generalizability is a confounding effect that is not addressed by randomization in a definitive cancer-screening trial of volunteer study subjects with cancer mortality end points.
3. When a spectrum of a disease is not considered in the randomization of patients, then the study is susceptible to the confounding effect of length bias.
4. Overdiagnosis is an extreme form of length bias.
5. Randomized, controlled trials with cancer mortality end points are the best way to avoid lead-time bias, because they measure mortality in both screened and non-screened patients from the same point of time, namely when they enter the study rather than when they were diagnosed with the cancer.
6. Trials performed using volunteers are called efficacy studies.
7. Trials performed on POPULATION-BASED subjects are called effectiveness studies.
8. A cohort would have study subjects categorized based on the exposure or lack of exposure of a risk factor, and then followed to determine if a particular outcome results.
9. A clinical trial is a prospective study in which an intervention is applied.
10. Oral contraceptive therapy with estrogen is contraindicated in patients with migraine with aura.

17.123 Year 3—Week 41—Day 2

1. Aminoglycosides can cause hearing loss by causing cochlear cell dysfunction and loss.
2. Thyroid hormone requirements are expected to increase as a pregnancy advances.
3. All patients with chronic liver disease who have negative hepatitis A and hepatitis B serologies need to be vaccinated for these two viruses.
4. If a patient has received the hepatitis A vaccine more than 1 month before exposure to hepatitis A, there is no need to give passive hepatitis A immunoglobulin.
5. The treatment of granulomatosis with polyangiitis involves cyclophosphamide and steroids but failure of those agents should prompt a trial of rituximab therapy in these refractory cases.
6. The initial treatment of polymyositis and dermatomyositis is IV steroids. These patients then are weaned off steroids after addition of azathioprine.
7. The first-line treatment of osteoarthritis is acetaminophen.
8. The treatment of temporal arteritis is 1 mg/kg of oral steroids initially, with gradual weaning occurring. A late complication of temporal arteritis is aortic dissection.
9. Azathioprine should not be initiated in patients until checking thiopurine methyltransferase (TPMT) activity.

17.124 Year 3—Week 41—Day 3

1. Allergic bronchopulmonary aspergillosis is associated with "brown hamburger meat" sputum and will have positive skin tests to mold spore extracts. This condition is associated with fleeting pulmonary infiltrates and will commonly require initiation of steroids or increase of current steroid dose when symptoms worsen (not unlike the situation of worsened warm hemolytic anemia in inflammatory bowel disease where steroids are increased).

2. Nasal ipratropium is the first line agent of treatment of gustatory rhinitis which presents within minutes of ingestion of offending agent but is not associated with pruritis or sneezing in usual cases.

3. Rhinitis medicamentosa refers to drug-induced rhinitis most commonly caused by nasal oxymetazoline, but also could be caused by alpha-blockers and estrogen-containing compounds.

4. The aspirin allergy triad is of asthma, nasal polyps, and aspirin/NSAID intolerance.

5. The definitive treatment of all allergic rhinitis conditions is the use of steroids. Steroids reduce mucus and nasal blood flow.

6. GERD should be in the differential of chronic cough and treatment-resistant asthma.

7. The first-line treatment of non-allergic perennial rhinitis is low-dose decongestants.

8. In the differential for unilateral sinusitis, tumor needs to be included. Tumors that can cause this condition include adenoid squamous cell cancer, lymphoma, angiofibromas (especially in adolescents that notice some bleeding as well), and inverted papillomas. Rhinoscopies and CT scans should be done quicker in patients with unilateral sinusitis.

9. The peak flow is a measurement derived from FEV1 and is to be followed in all patients with asthma symptoms. All patients with asthma should have a peak flow meter at home and educated about what to do when the peak flow numbers begin to drop from baseline.

17.125 Year 3—Week 42—Day 1

1. Hepatitis E carries the highest mortality rate for acute viral hepatitides during pregnancy.

2. Progestin-only OCP (oral contraceptives) have a higher failure rate than combination OCP and have a higher incidence of acne.

3. The most common cause of infertility in the USA is asymptomatic Chlamydia infections.

4. There is felt to be an increased incidence of cervical cancer in patients who are sexually active beginning before age 16 due to the human papilloma virus (types 16, 18, 31, 33, 35).

5. Human papilloma virus types 6 and 11 are associated with genital warts (condyloma acuminatum).

6. Menstruation is triggered by an involution of the corpus luteum with concomitant decline in plasma levels of progesterone.

7. Hirsutism and virilization are classified as androgen excess disorders.

8. Women with polycystic ovarian disease (Stein-Leventhal syndrome) have an increased LH to FSH ratio.

9. Diethylstilbestrol administration to a pregnant mother is associated with risk in fetus of development of clear cell adenocarcinoma of the vagina.

10. Cigarette smoking is felt to be a risk factor for development of cervical cancer.

17.126 Year 3—Week 42—Day 2

1. The Churg-Strauss syndrome is a vasculitis with presenting signs of eosinophilia and asthma. Obviously, the vasculitis affects the lung. Mononeuritis multiplex may occur in these patients to include hearing loss, cranial nerve palsy, or foot drop.

2. Cromolyn sodium is an effective therapy in the treatment of exercise-induced asthma.

3. Among the hypersensitivity reactions that are anaphylactoid (non-IGE mediated) are radiocontrast dye reaction, hypersensitivity pneumonitis, sulfite reaction, and reaction to yellow dye No. 5.

4. Urticaria pigmentosa is marked by mast cell infiltration of the skin and presents with Darier's sign (stroking of a macule causes formation of a wheal over the macule). Systemic involvement is termed systemic mastocytosis. This spectrum includes mast cell leukemia.

5. Type 1 reactions are immediate hypersensitivity and are mediated by IGE. Type 4 reac-

tions are delayed hypersensitivity (as in PPD test) and are mediated by helper T-cells.

6. Patients with sarcoidosis tend to be anergic in skin testing due to lack of CD4 cells in circulation. Paradoxically, in patients with lung disease, there will be increased CD4 to CD8 ratio in lymphocytes on bronchoalveolar lavage with noncaseating granulomas seen if biopsy of bronchial tissue is performed.

7. Hereditary angioedema has autosomal dominant inheritance and is usually caused by low levels of C1 inhibitor or defective C1 inhibitor.

8. Serum sickness can occur in patients being treated with anti-thymocyte globulin for aplastic anemia. That medication is commonly used with cyclosporine in aplastic anemia patients.

17.127 Year 3—Week 42—Day 3

1. Sickle cell disease patients are at risk of retinal hemorrhage which appears "sea-fan" or "shell" shaped on fundoscopic exam. Treatment is emergent photocoagulation.

2. Patients with Waldenstrom's macroglobulinemia have hyperviscosity and thus will have "sausage-linked" or "box-car" appearance to their vessels on fundoscopic exam.

3. The most common tumor in the retina is melanoma. The most common eyelid tumor is basal cell cancer.

4. Hyphema reflects blood in the anterior chamber of the eye.

5. Episcleritis refers to a limited inflammation of the superficial conjunctiva and runs a self-limited course with no referral needed to ophthalmology. Scleritis has the potential to erode through the sclera and needs to be urgently referred to ophthalmology.

6. Patients with Wilson's disease not only have Kayser-Fleisher rings due to copper deposition in Descemet's membrane but also are notorious for developing "sunflower" cataracts.

7. Patients with neurofibromatosis can develop Lisch nodules (hamartomas of the iris) if

they have NF-1 disease, whereas patients with NF-2 disease are at risk of a peculiar cataract known as juvenile posterior subcapsular lenticular opacity. NF-1 and NF-2 are carried on different chromosomes. Optic gliomas can be seen in both conditions but remember that the bilateral acoustic neuromas are seen in NF-2.

8. In Graves' disease, there is thickening of the extraocular muscles with sparing of the tendons. This differs from pseudotumor cerebri where the tendon is also thickened.

9. Hypopyon iritis refers to the pooling of white cells in the anterior chamber of the eye and can be seen in patients with Behcet's disease. Patients with this disease can have both posterior and anterior uveitis, and the disease is also marked by pulmonary artery aneurysms, skin pathergy, and thrombophlebitis. The eye disease and the arterial disease respond best to chlorambucil.

10. A slit lamp examination by an ophthalmologist is usually required in making the diagnosis of uveitis.

17.128 Year 3—Week 43—Day 1

1. *Trichinella spiralis* causes eosinophilia, myalgias, and periorbital edema. The diagnostic test is muscle biopsy. Treatment is mebendazole and steroids.

2. Treatment of tropical sprue is with high-dose doxycycline for 3–6 months until malabsorption picture has resolved. Folinic acid supplementation is needed in this situation.

3. *Ancylostoma braziliense* is the likely cause of cutaneous larval migrans in the Caribbean. Treat with thiabendazole orally or could even use topical form at leading edge of skin migration.

4. *Wuchereria bancrofti* (filariasis) can cause chyluria (milk-colored urine). This disease can only be acquired by repeated infection over a one-year time period at least (thus not a concern to tourists of area).

5. Praziquantel and niclosamide can be used to treat *Diphyllobothrium latum* infections,

which can cause megaloblastic anemia (by B12 and folate deficiency).

6. Mebendazole or albendazole and steroids are the treatment of choice for neurocysticercosis.

7. *Schistosoma haematobium* infection of the bladder leads to squamous cell carcinoma of the bladder. Treatment is with praziquantel.

8. Protozoans do not give eosinophilia, except rarely *Isospora belli* (which causes a diarrheal illness in patients with HIV; treat with Septra similar to Cyclospora). Thus, there is no eosinophilia noted in patients with malaria and Giardia.

9. Entamoeba histolytica infections should be treated with metronidazole and a luminal agent to eliminate cysts, such as paromomycin or iodoquinol.

10. Microsporidia infections can only be diagnosed by small bowel biopsy (ova and parasite will not reveal organism).

17.129 Year 3—Week 43—Day 2

1. Rheumatoid arthritis can cause scleritis, episcleritis, scleromalacia perforans, and corneal ulcers. Rheumatoid eye disease responds well to cyclosporine-A.

2. Glaucoma is marked by an increase in the optic cup to disc ratio, generally above 0.4 value.

3. A pale, swollen, almost "ghost-like" optic disc is seen in patients with temporal arteritis. Treatment is immediate high-dose steroids with bilateral temporal artery biopsy to be scheduled within a week. Biopsy should show giant cells with disruption of the internal elastic lamina but frequently the pathology is not seen as the disease tends to have skip areas.

4. Sjogren's disease patients have dry eyes and dry mouth with positive anti-RO (ss-a) and anti-LA (ss-b) antibodies. The diagnosis of Sjogren's can also be made from a minor salivary gland biopsy showing reticular lymphocytosis.

5. Macular degeneration is the most common cause of visual loss in this country and can have drusen seen in the macula on fundoscopic exam.

6. The treatment of proliferative diabetic retinopathy (neovascularization) is laser photocoagulation.

7. A Hollenhorst plaque seen on fundoscopic evaluation should trigger an atherosclerosis workup of the carotid arteries and the heart.

8. Diabetes mellitus can present with cranial nerve palsies (most commonly CN 3) that are usually painless and resolve with better control of underlying disease. Suspect if given clinical scenario with Hispanics or Pima Indians as both have increased incidence of diabetes.

9. Wernicke's disease in alcoholics can present with cranial nerve palsies along with ataxia. CN6 is the most common involved in this scenario.

10. An oculomotor palsy will leave the eye appearing "down and out." The lateral rectus is served by CN6 while the superior oblique is served by CN 4. A common scenario for patients with CN4 difficulties is a patient who gives a history of difficulty walking down the stairs due to vision.

17.130 Year 3—Week 43—Day 3

1. HSV (Herpes simplex virus) encephalitis causes changes in MRI usually at the temporal lobes or inferior frontal lobes.

2. The test of choice to diagnose HSV encephalitis is PCR for DNA of HSV. The first test may be initially negative so a second test may need to be ordered.

3. Treatment of HSV encephalitis will involve IV acyclovir every 8 hours with treatment regimen often lasting 10-14 days in severe cases.

4. WPW (Wolff Parkinson White) is associated with Ebstein's anomaly, where the right ventricle appears nearly as small as the right atrium due to abnormal displacement of the tricuspid valve.

5. Definitive treatment of WPW is radiofrequency ablation especially in patients with numerous episodes of rapid atrial fibrillation.

6. The first step in complete heart block management is to stop all AV-nodal blocking agents, such as beta-blockers or digoxin.

7. The best treatment for progressive multifocal leukoencephalopathy is to treat the underlying HIV disease with antiretrovirals.

8. Atovaquone can be used for *Pneumocystis jirovecii* and toxoplasmosis prophylaxis in patients with sulfa allergy.

9. If a patient with a sulfa allergy develops acute toxoplasmosis, then one could use pyrimethamine and clindamycin for treatment.

10. Intracerebral metastasis is much more common than leptomeningeal carcinomatosis in patients with solid tumors.

17.131 Year 3—Week 44—Day 1

1. Patients with multiple sclerosis commonly have an afferent pupillary defect termed a Marcus-Gunn Pupil.

2. Anisocoria that is long standing and present with less than 2 mm difference in the size of the pupils is usually a normal variant. A driver's license photo is a helpful tool in the ER when trying to distinguish whether the anisocoria is old or new if the patient is unaware.

3. Gonorrhea conjunctivitis is associated with extreme pain and very copious purulent discharge.

4. CMV retinitis can be treated with either daily IV foscarnet or ganciclovir or intraocular ganciclovir. Another way of treatment if the patient refuses all above choices is IV cidofovir once a week, which should be avoided in patients with marked chronic renal insufficiency. Fundoscopic exam of these patients will show marked hemorrhages reflecting a large exudative component to the disease.

5. Among the risk factors for open-angle glaucoma are HTN, diabetes mellitus, myopia, and increasing age. Smoking is not a risk factor for open-angle glaucoma.

6. Complications from cataract surgery include glaucoma, infection, vitreous loss, and retinal detachment.

7. The most common cause of uveal tract inflammation in the USA is idiopathic.

8. Supratemporal bilateral subluxation of the lens occurs in Marfan's syndrome. Homocystinuria is also associated with subluxation of the lenses but in a pattern different from Marfan's. The subluxation of the lens when unilateral will present as a monocular diplopia.

9. A chalazion is a firm nontender nodule in the upper eyelid due to chronic retention of meibomian gland secretions forming a lipogranuloma. Hordeolum is a term used to describe an acute inflammation of the eyelid that may be seen as an external swelling (usually involving a hair follicle) or an internal swelling on the conjunctival surface of the lid. Topical antibiotic therapy may have some role for hordeolum treatment but not for the treatment of chalazion. Hot compresses are used for the treatment of both conditions.

10. Bitemporal hemianopsia is a visual field deficit commonly seen in lesions of the pituitary that also affect the optic chiasm. When a homonymous hemianopsia is found, workup should be done by MRI to look for a posterior circulation stroke.

17.132 Year 3—Week 44—Day 2

1. Patients with involvement of the superior cervical ganglion will show the following: (a) miosis, (b) anhidrosis, and (c) ptosis.

2. Down's syndrome or Trisomy 21 has atrial septal defects as its main cardiac feature (notice difference from Edwards syndrome) and carries a high incidence of atlantoaxial subluxation. There is an increased incidence of amyloidosis in the brain over time and it is not uncommon to find lymphopenia which leads to increased infections. Most adults

that reach age 40–50 have the average IQ of no greater than a 10-year-old.

3. Klinefelter's syndrome, or XXY syndrome, has a high incidence of both breast and testicular carcinoma from the mechanisms of gynecomastia (for breast CA) and cryptorchidism (for testicular CA). Diagnosis can be made by buccal smear to test for karyotype.

4. Turner's syndrome, or XO syndrome, is marked by cardiac features of aortic stenosis, coarctation of the aorta, and bicuspid aortic valve (this one is the most common). Patients can also have horseshoe kidney, webbed neck features, short stature, primary ovarian failure, and lymphedema.

5. Osteogenesis imperfecta is marked by blue sclerae on physical examination and involves antibodies to type I collagen. These patients have brittle bones and pathological fractures.

6. Chediak-Higashi syndrome is marked by large lysosome vesicles in neutrophils on light microscopy and involves a defect in lysosomal emptying. There is a marked increase in Streptococcus and Staphylococcus infections.

7. In patients with diabetic ketoacidosis, insulin stimulates potassium to move from the extracellular space to the intracellular space and another way to remember this is as there is a rise in pH, Hydrogen ion moves out and potassium ion moves into the cell.

8. A patient with chronic granulomatous disease will have defective neutrophil phagocytosis which is reflected by a negative nitroblue tetrazolium dye test. Normal individuals thus will always have a positive nitroblue tetrazolium dye reduction test.

9. Patients with tuberous sclerosis (autosomal dominant inheritance) will show facial angiofibromas (known as adenoma sebaceous) and tumors in the heart known as cardiac rhabdomyomas. They will have mental retardation with tubers (atypical astrocytes) found in the cerebral cortex and the periventricular areas.

10. Secondary hyperparathyroidism leads to the following processes: (a) impaired calcium reabsorption, (b) impaired phosphate excretion, (c) impaired activation of vitamin D, and (d) hypocalcemia which stimulates parathyroid hormone release and leads to more bone turnover (seen with increased elevated alkaline phosphatase).

17.133   Year 3—Week 44—Day 3

1. Burkitt's lymphoma is marked by involvement of the c-myc chromosome 8 gene as well as the immune long chain of chromosome 14 and leads to nasopharyngeal carcinoma.

2. The most common non-ocular carcinoma to occur in a survivor of hereditary retinoblastoma is femoral osteosarcoma.

3. Bilateral renal cell carcinoma should raise suspicion of von Hippel–Lindau disease involving chromosome 3. Other tumors can be found in the adrenal medulla and the retina. Inheritance is autosomal dominant.

4. Ehlers-Danlos disease leads to early onset osteoarthritis and is caused by antibodies to type III collagen.

5. Goodpasture's disease which leads to kidney and lung disease is caused by antibodies to type IV collagen.

6. Adenovirus is the most likely virus to cause sore throat, conjunctivitis, rhinitis, and cough in young adolescents.

7. Wiskott-Aldrich syndrome is marked by eczema, thrombocytopenia, and recurrent pyogenic infections.

8. Neurofibromatosis 1 involves a chromosome 17 defect and is marked by lesions in the iris (Lisch nodules) and gliomas in the brain.

9. Neurofibromatosis 2 is marked by a defect in chromosome 22 and is found to have bilateral acoustic neuromas without any lesions in the iris.

10. The most common lesion found in patients with Sturge-Weber syndrome is a leptomeningeal angioma.

17.134 Year 3—Week 45—Day 1

1. MEN 1 and MEN 2 syndromes are inherited in autosomal dominant fashion.
2. Lead poisoning can cause gout to occur in children (saturnine gout) with the classic stippling of the red blood cell on a peripheral smear.
3. Arsenic poisoning is notorious for causing a keratosis skin eruption in patients.
4. Copper poisoning can lead to recurrent headaches and Parkinsonism manifestations (also seen in manganese poisoning).
5. There are two essential fatty acids that the body cannot perform synthesis and they are linolenic acid and linoleic acid.
6. There are eight essential amino acids that your body cannot perform synthesis and they are the following: leucine, lysine, isoleucine, phenylalanine, tryptophan, methionine, threonine, and valine.
7. Patients have inferior quadrilateral optic defects if they have a lesion affecting the superior optic radiations that come through the parietal lobe.
8. Patients have superior quadrilateral optic defects if they have a lesion affecting the contralateral Meyer's loop or the inferior optic radiations that go through the temporal lobe.
9. Patients infected with a "dimorphic fungus" have an entity that can demonstrate the ability to take form of septated hyphae and conidia at 25 degrees Celsius while being a cigar shaped yeast at 37°C.
10. The rate limiting step in bile synthesis is 7-alpha hydroxylase. A deficiency in apolipoprotein CII (cofactor for lipoprotein lipase) will lead to a marked increase in chylomicrons. Meanwhile, a deficiency in apolipoprotein E will lead to increased chylomicrons and increased VLDL levels.

17.135 Year 3—Week 45—Day 2

1. Scurvy deficiency is marked by perifollicular hemorrhages and excessive gum bleeding. Levels of ascorbic acid can be checked for the diagnosis, but skin biopsy can reveal changes consistent with diagnosis in much quicker fashion.
2. Parathion poisoning will lead to confusion, wheezing, vomiting, and excessive salivation along with generalized weakness. Treatment is with 2-Pralidoximine (2-PAM).
3. A type 1 hypersensitivity reaction is driven by the action of IGE on mast cells and basophils. Vasodilation can occur in very quick fashion.
4. Tetralogy of Fallot involves the components of VSD, over-riding aorta, right ventricular hypertrophy, and pulmonary stenosis.
5. Patients with varicoceles have an abnormal dilation of the pampiniform venous plexus of the spermatic cord as can be seen in young patients with left-sided renal vein thrombosis from renal cell carcinoma.
6. The most common finding in acetaminophen poisoning is centrilobular necrosis on pathology. These patients can have a marked rise in lactate dehydrogenase levels.
7. Patients with hypertrophic cardiomyopathy will have accentuation of their systolic murmur after a premature ventricular complex due to increased gradient that occurs across obstruction from increased contractility.
8. Patients with acne rosacea can have flares of their disease if treated with topical steroid therapy over their affected areas.
9. Patients with molluscum contagiosum can be treated with cryotherapy. The disease is caused by poxvirus.
10. The next step in management of a patient with an inflamed seborrheic keratosis is cryotherapy.

17.136   Year 3—Week 45—Day 3

1. Manifestations of acute pancreatitis include lobular panniculitis, Grey-Turner's sign, and Cullen's sign (periumbilical hemorrhage).
2. Essential thrombocytosis is associated with erythromelalgia (redness and burning of the extremities that is relieved with aspirin).
3. Syphilis is associated with generalized lymphadenopathy and oral mucous patches when it is secondary. Treatment is generally benzathine penicillin G for three treatments (separated by 1 week).
4. Lemierre's syndrome is associated with Fusobacterium infections marked by septic pulmonary emboli and internal jugular vein thrombophlebitis.
5. Discoid lupus is associated with alopecia and follicular plugging of ears.
6. Multiple sclerosis can cause blurry vision with hot showers due to decreased nerve conduction with heat.
7. Parvovirus infections are associated with aplastic anemia and giant pronormoblasts can be seen in the bone marrow aspirate/biopsy.
8. Myasthenia gravis has an association with thymoma and thymic hyperplasia. CT of thorax should be done in these patients.

17.137   Year 3—Week 46—Day 1

1. Verner-Morrison syndrome is another name for VIPoma, one of the functional tumors that can cause diarrhea.
2. In a patient with beta-thalassemia trait who has a normal hemoglobin A2 fraction (after previously being elevated), suspect iron deficiency anemia has ensued.
3. It is expected that the MCV lab value will rise in patients being treated with hydroxyurea and lack of such rise will usually imply non-compliance with the medication.
4. Tularemia is transmitted by the Dermacentor ticks and also by Amblyomma americanum (the Lone star Tick).

5. Amantadine has uses in Parkinson's disease (for tremor) and in multiple sclerosis (for chronic fatigue syndrome).
6. MEN syndromes are inherited in autosomal dominant fashion. Hypoglandular autoimmune syndromes are inherited in autosomal recessive fashion.
7. Beta-blockers are the first-line therapy for patients with hypertrophic cardiomyopathy and for patients with prolonged QT syndrome.
8. Niacin is felt to cause flushing through a G protein receptor on Langerhans cells in the epidermis which leads to a release of prostaglandins.

17.138   Year 3—Week 46—Day 2

1. Yellow nail syndrome is marked by bronchiectasis, sinusitis, pleural effusions that can be chylous in nature, and, of course, yellow nails on physical exam.
2. *Serratia marcescens* is a gram-negative rod that can cause pneumonia and can produce a reddish pigment that appears as if it was bloody sputum.
3. Pheochromocytoma of the bladder should be considered in patients with palpitations and piercing headaches just before, during, and after micturition.
4. Acute vertigo occurring immediately after pressing on the tragus portion of the ear should raise suspicion for perilymphatic fistula.
5. Irritated/inflamed seborrheic keratosis are treated with cryotherapy ablation.
6. Disopyramide cannot be used in patients with history of acute angle closure glaucoma due to its anticholinergic properties.
7. Propafenone is the only anti-arrhythmic with the side effect of taste disturbance. This drug cannot be used in patients with structural heart disease.
8. The three types of atrial septal defects are ostium primum, ostium secundum, and sinus venosus.

17.139 Year 3—Week 46—Day 3

1. Episcleritis refers to a limited inflammation of the superficial conjunctiva and runs a self-limited course with no referral needed to ophthalmology. Scleritis has the potential to erode through the sclera and needs to be urgently referred to ophthalmology.
2. Patients with Wilson's disease not only have Kayser-Fleisher rings due to copper deposition in Descemet's membrane but also are notorious for developing "sunflower" cataracts.
3. Patients with neurofibromatosis can develop Lisch nodules (hamartomas of the iris) if they have NF-1 disease, whereas patients with NF-2 disease are at risk of a peculiar cataract known as juvenile posterior subcapsular lenticular opacity.
4. In Graves' disease, there is actually thickening of the extraocular muscles with sparing of the tendons. This differs from pseudotumor cerebri where the tendon is also thickened.
5. Hypopyon iritis refers to the pooling of white cells in the anterior chamber of the eye and can be seen in patients with Behcet's disease. Patients with this disease can have both posterior and anterior uveitis and the disease is also marked by pulmonary artery aneurysms, skin pathergy, and thrombophlebitis. The eye disease and the arterial disease respond best to chlorambucil.
6. Rheumatoid arthritis can cause scleritis, episcleritis, scleromalacia perforans, corneal melt, corneal ulcers, and perforation of the eye globe. Rheumatoid eye disease responds well to cyclosporine-A.
7. A pale, swollen, almost "ghost-like" optic disc is seen in patients with temporal arteritis. Treatment is immediate high-dose steroids with bilateral temporal artery biopsy to be scheduled within a week. Biopsy should show giant cells with disruption of the internal elastic lamina but frequently the pathology is not seen as the disease tends to have skip areas.
8. Sjogren's disease patients have dry eyes and dry mouth with positive anti-RO (SS-A) and anti-LA (SS-B) antibodies. The diagnosis of Sjogren's can also be made from a minor salivary gland biopsy showing reticular lymphocytosis.

17.140 Year 3—Week 47—Day 1

1. Patients with porphyria cutanea tarda can actually have Wood's lamp fluorescence of their gums due to deposition of the porphyrins in that location.
2. Consider acute intermittent porphyria in patients with histories of acute abdomen episodes with no organic cause found. One should order 24 h porphyrin studies in these patients.
3. Three disease states to remember as possibly causing transudative pleural effusions include pulmonary embolus, hepatic hydrothorax, and hypothyroidism.
4. Erythema ab igne is a rash that may appear in patients using chronic heating pads.
5. Cholesterol emboli syndrome patients with underlying cause of aortoiliac unstable plaque disease should be treated with HMG COA reductase inhibitors and antiplatelet agents.
6. Dexamethasone should be employed in the treatment regimen of patients with high-altitude cerebral edema.
7. Calcium channel blockers can be used in the treatment of high-altitude pulmonary edema as they help bring down pulmonary artery pressures.
8. High resting pulmonary artery pressures might be associated with tricuspid regurgitation on an echocardiogram and tall R-waves in Lead V1 on an EKG.
9. Urticaria pigmentosa is the skin-limited condition associated with underlying mastocytosis. Stroking such a lesion on the skin will lead to wheel and flare reaction of the lesion which is known as Darier's sign.

17.141 Year 3—Week 47—Day 2

1. The treatment of proliferative diabetic reti-nopathy (neovascularization) is laser photocoagulation.
2. Diabetes mellitus can present with cranial nerve palsies (most commonly CN 3) that are usually painless and resolve with better control of underlying disease. Suspect if given clinical scenario with Hispanics or Pima Indians as both have increased incidence of diabetes.
3. Wernicke's disease in alcoholics can present with cranial nerve palsies along with ataxia. CN6 is the most common involved in this scenario.
4. An oculomotor palsy will leave the eye appearing "down and out." The lateral rectus is served by CN6, while the superior oblique is served by CN 4. A common scenario for patients with CN4 difficulties is a patient who gives a history of difficulty walking down the stairs due to vision.
5. Patients with multiple sclerosis commonly have an afferent pupillary defect termed as Marcus-Gunn Pupil.
6. Anisocori has multiple causes from benign entities such as migraine headaches and medications such as scopolamine to more worrisome causes such as acute meningitis infection and brain aneurysm.
7. Gonorrhea conjunctivitis is associated with extreme pain and very copious purulent discharge.
8. Among the risk factors for open-angle glaucoma are HTN, diabetes mellitus, myopia, and increasing age. Smoking is not a risk factor for open-angle glaucoma.

17.142 Year 3—Week 47—Day 3

1. Patients with severe leptospirosis infections (with usual liver and kidney involvement) should be treated with IV penicillin.
2. Patients with actinomycosis infections can present with fistula formation and should be treated with penicillin.

3. Patients with Nocardia asteroids infections can present with brain abscess, disseminated skin nodules, and pulmonary infiltrates. Treatment is with Septra first line for up to 6 months to a year, with second-line therapy being minocycline.
4. Patients with Listeria infections should be treated with IV ampicillin. Trimethoprim-sulfamethoxazole could be used if a patient had severe PCN allergy. Cephalosporins will not work.
5. In patients with HACEK endocarditis infections, ceftriaxone is the drug of choice and the organism may not grow for up to 5-10 days in blood cultures.
6. Patients with permanent lines (ports) found to have Corynebacterium jeikeium infections should have those lines removed.
7. Patients with *Candida krusei* will not respond to fluconazole and should be treated with voriconazole or amphotericin B.
8. Patients with streaking cellulitis due to streptococcus could be treated with IV penicillin at high doses and IV clindamycin to bind the toxin.
9. Patients with septic pulmonary emboli on lung X-ray with internal jugular thrombophlebitis should be treated with penicillin and are most likely to have *Fusobacterium*.
10. Malassezia furfur causes a "spaghetti and meatballs" appearance on KOH and is treated with topical ketoconazole or systemic therapy if severe.

17.143 Year 3—Week 48—Day 1

1. Methotrexate is indicated as first-line treatment of rheumatoid arthritis (RA) in patients with erosive bone disease, which tend to have positive rheumatoid factor and active deformities.
2. Spinal stenosis patients have pain worse with hyper-extension, while patients with sciatica tend to have pain worse with hyper-flexion.
3. A very high rheumatoid factor may be a clue to rheumatoid lung disease or rheumatoid

vasculitis, and it tends to be also associated with rheumatoid nodule formation.

4. The most common vasculitis is a drug-induced vasculitis, and it tends to be at the level of the post-capillary venule.

5. Among the findings in Felty's syndrome (RA, neutropenia, and splenomegaly) are an association with large granular lymphocyte (LGL) syndrome, pretibial hyperpigmentation, and malleolar ulcers.

6. In over 90% of cases with *Staphylococcus aureus* septic joint (the most common cause of septic arthritis in RA and the general population), the organism will grow from synovial cultures.

7. Hemochromatosis is associated with an arthritis of the second and third MCP joints. The joint pain does not tend to improve even after phlebotomy.

8. Polyarteritis nodosa is a vasculitis associated with mononeuritis multiplex (commonly seen as foot drop), microaneurysms in a mesenteric angiogram in patients with abdominal pain, and with sparing of the lung. Testicular tenderness is unique to this vasculitis due to the microaneursymal aortic disease leading to testicular artery insufficiency.

9. Acute intermittent porphyria is associated with abdominal pain, hyponatremia, urine that turns dark on prolonged exposure with light.

10. The deficit in polymyalgia rheumatica is pain and stiffness but classically there is no weakness. Steroid use of no more than 15 mg daily should bring about relief. Higher dose of steroids (usually 1 mg/kg daily in early stages of disease) is used in temporal arteritis.

17.144 Year 3—Week 48—Day 2

1. Progesterone is associated with a vasculitis and angioedema syndrome.

2. Celiac sprue has a link between IGA deficiency and diabetes mellitus type 1 likely through HLA associated mechanisms.

3. Prednisone may be used in patients in short term fashion who are refractory to the gluten free diet in patients with celiac sprue.

4. Dapsone is used to ameliorate the pruritis of dermatitis herpetiformis which may be seen in patients with celiac sprue and location includes predominantly extensor surfaces of the knee and elbows, as well as the buttocks.

5. Early post-op prosthetic valve endocarditis should be treated with vancomycin, rifampin, and gentamicin.

6. Most pleural effusions associated with tuberculosis are non-bloody.

7. Pulmonary emboli can cause large pulmonary effusions, which can be either transudative or exudative in nature and they tend to resolve with anticoagulation therapy.

8. Hypothyroidism is associated with either exudative or transudative pleural effusions. The pleural effusion may have a moderately high triglyceride level as well usually at a level of 65-110 mg/dl but not usually entering levels seen with chylous states.

17.145 Year 3—Week 48—Day 3

1. Sudden death in patients with prolonged QT syndrome can be triggered by states of emotion or exercise. Fever is also associated with a higher risk of death in patients with underlying Brugada syndrome from lower threshold for arrhythmia. Brugada syndrome patients need aggressive treatment with acetaminophen to lower febrile states.

2. Patients with prolonged QT syndrome with symptoms refractory to beta-blockers could be considered for left-sided cardiac sympathetic denervation, AICD placement, or pacemakers depending on the clinical situation.

3. Patients with CLL have increased risk of infection with encapsulated organisms making pneumococcal vaccination a priority in these patients as an outpatient prevention strategy.

4. Recurrent pneumonias in patients with common variable immunodeficiency may lead to the development of bronchiectasis.

5. There may be benefit to IVIG infusion in patients with CLL who have low serum IGG levels (below 3 gm/dL) and who have history of recurrent significant infections of the lung and sinuses.

6. Besides Giardia infection, there is an increased risk for *Campylobacter jejuni* and Yersinia infections in patients with IGA deficiency.

7. Dilantin can lower IgA levels within 3–4 months of starting therapy and lead to complete deficiency in about 5 percent of patients (this is reversible by stopping the medication).

8. There is a marked risk of lymphoma in patients who have common variable immunodeficiency.

17.146 Year 3—Week 49—Day 1

1. Yellow deposits called drusen can be found in patients with dry macular degeneration.

2. The prevalence of macular degeneration increases with age and is the most common cause of visual loss with advancing age.

3. Macular degeneration patients typically normal peripheral vision while having trouble seeing at a distance, recognizing faces, and distinguishing between colors.

4. Wet macular degeneration is less common than the "dry" form and is marked by subretinal fluid accumulation with neovascularization, retinal pigment epithelial detachment, and subretinal hemorrhage possible. Symptom onset is typically rapid.

5. Among the possible side effects of systemic carbonic anhydrase inhibitors (such as dorzolamide), which are topically used for glaucoma, are bitter taste, headaches, nausea, and even the rare description of kidney stones.

6. Among the sympathomimetic topical agents for glaucoma, brimonidine works similar to clonidine and is contraindicated in patients taking MAO-inhibitors.

7. Loss of color vision is among the earliest signs of ethambutol toxicity when being used for treatment of tuberculosis.

8. Band keratopathy has been described in patients with chronic hypercalcemic states as well as patients with juvenile rheumatoid arthritis.

17.147 Year 3—Week 49—Day 2

1. Sulfasalazine, cyclosporine, and infliximab are treatment options for pyoderma gangrenosum which should never be debrided locally as it will worsen its current state.

2. Streptococcus is the most common infectious agent to cause erythema nodosum. Other infectious causes include Yersinia, coccidiomycosis, and tuberculosis while non-infectious causes are sarcoidosis, oral contraceptive use, and inflammatory bowel disease.

3. Aphthous ulcers can be seen in patients with inflammatory bowel disease although the most common reason for these ulcers is an idiopathic state in young adults which only requires local therapy care.

4. Acrodermatitis enteropathica is the rash that is seen with zinc deficiency while pellagra causes a photosensitive rash that is prominent around the neck given that the skin is exposed above the shirt (that finding has been named Casal's necklace).

5. Scurvy is seen with perifollicular plugging and corkscrew hair formation. Treatment is ascorbic acid and complications include severe bleeding episodes, infections and left ventricular dysfunction systolic heart failure.

6. Dermatitis herpetiformis and lichen planus lesions are pruritic. Dermatitis herpetiformis is usually found on extensor surfaces while lichen planus is found on flexor surfaces usually.

7. Tissue transglutaminase is felt to be the most sensitive and most specific antibody to detect celiac sprue but one must obtain both IGA and IGG levels as celiac sprue is highly asso-

ciated with IGA Deficiency and thus falsely negative results will return in patients with IGA deficiency.

8. Oral beta-carotene is the treatment of variegate porphyria, which demonstrates features of both porphyria cutanea tarda and acute intermittent porphyria, but excessive dosing of oral beta carotene will lead to a diffuse orange-yellow discoloration of the skin.

9. Cryoglobulinemia has also been noted in HIV disease, multiple myeloma, Sjogren's syndrome, and systemic lupus erythamatosis.

17.148 Year 3—Week 49—Day 3

1. Conditions such as atrial septal defect, aortic insufficiency, and left ventricular hypertrophy may make a patient with cardiac tamponade not demonstrate pulsus pardoxicus.

2. Hepatitis C is the least likely of the viral hepatitides to present with acute fulminant liver failure.

3. The treatment of *Vibrio vulnificus* and parahemolyticus infections is with doxycycline as first-line agent.

4. Patients with liver disease can get a fulminant cellulitis from freshwater exposure from both Aeromonas infections and Plesiomonas infections. Plesiomonas infections can be treated with penicillin therapy similar to Aeromonas.

5. Ciprofloxacin will not cover *Streptococcus pneumonia*. Moxifloxacin and levofloxacin are effective treatments for that organism in the fluoroquinolone drug class.

6. If a patient is found to have Listeria meningitis by lumbar puncture, treatment should be de-escalated to IV ampicillin with discontinuation of vancomycin and Ceftriaxone.

7. Consider West-Nile virus encephalitis in patients returning from hunting trips with mental status changes particularly if they have markedly elevated CSF protein levels.

8. Do not use colchicine to treat acute gout attacks in patients with advanced renal failure (use prednisone instead).

17.149 Year 3—Week 50—Day 1

1. Creutzfeldt-Jacob disease patients have rapid mental decline and have startle myoclonus.

2. If a transplant patient is allergic to sulfa antibiotics, those patients will be desensitized as this is a situation where it is crucial to be able to use sulfa-based antibiotic therapy for prophylaxis against *Pneumocystis jirovecii* infections.

3. All adrenal masses must be ruled out for pheochromocytoma before surgical removal ensues. Failure to do so may result in a hypertensive crisis during a surgical or interventional procedure that could be life threatening.

4. Adult polycystic kidney disease patients have a high incidence of hepatic cysts by age 50 (over half the patients will have this finding by that age).

5. Workers in the aerospace industry are at risk of berylliosis which presents with hilar lymphadenopathy and reticulonodular opacities and the diagnosis can be proven via a lymphocyte transformation test.

6. Breast cancer may present with persistent irritation of the nipple area (Paget's disease of the breast).

7. Patients with the aspirin triad cannot be given any NSAIDS ideally for pain treatment (salsalate is the safest of them all if one must be used).

8. Patients with Lewy body disease present with impressive visual hallucinations early on in their dementia course.

17.150 Year 3—Week 50—Day 2

1. *Erysipelothrix rhusiopathiae* is the organism that causes erysipeloid and this condition will not respond to vancomycin.

2. Splenomegaly can be detected at times on a plain film of the abdomen.

3. Loss of a psoas shadow on a plain abdominal film should raise the suspicion of psoas abscess.

4. Persistent unilateral serous otitis media in a patient with smoking history should raise suspicion of a squamous cell carcinoma in the nasopharynx.

5. Collapse of a vertebral disc with compromised disc space on plain films of the back should raise suspicion for vertebral body osteomyelitis.

6. Chronic drug users who are "skin poppers" are at risk for amyloidosis and central clearing of an area of skin popping with surrounding hemorrhage is suggestive of cocaine as the drug being used for skin popping.

7. Up to 10% of acute subarachnoid hemorrhage will be missed on a CT scan of the head.

8. Deep inverted T-waves can be seen in the setting of subarachnoid hemorrhage.

9. Cryptococcal infections can lead to chronic CSF pressure elevation as these organisms and their subsequent scarring/inflammation lead to blockage of CSF reabsorption in the arachnoid granulation area.

10. Cryptococcus can present as a primary infection of the lung with large lesions mimicking primary lung cancer or metastatic disease to lung.

17.151 Year 3—Week 50—Day 3

1. Acute aortic dissection can lead to a diastolic decrescendo murmur that is best heard over the right sternal border.

2. Aortic regurgitation, mitral valve prolapse, and acute aortic dissection are among the cardiac manifestations of Marfan's syndrome.

3. Disopyramide has strong anticholinergic properties and should be avoided in patients with urinary retention issues and in patients with acute delirium.

4. Atrial tachycardias can be associated with increased nocturia due to release of atrial natriuretic peptide.

5. Always suspect digoxin toxicity in patients with long-standing chronic atrial fibrillation who present acutely ill with regular rhythms

on auscultation and EKG's particularly if they are junctional rhythms in nature.

6. Brugada syndrome is demonstrated on EKG with a RBB pattern with chronic ST-segment elevation in leads V1, V2, and V3. This syndrome has been associated with risk of sudden death.

7. Sneddon syndrome is manifested by livedo reticularis with history of multiple cerebral ischemic insults.

8. Dapsone is the first-line agent for treating leprosy which is notorious for causing lesions that demonstrate anesthesia and which if left untreated in facial area can transform a patient to have "leonine facies".

9. Dapsone may also be used in hemolytic anemias as an adjunct to prednisone. It has also been used to reduce sphingomyelinase toxin in patients with brown recluse spider bites but the efficacy of this indication is within 48 h of the bite.

17.152 Year 3—Week 51—Day 1

1. Consider checking a CPK level if there is an isolated AST elevation without elevated GGT level in a patient's lab as the AST may be elevated from muscle damage.

2. Hyperthyroidism has been noted to increase the AST and ALT without specific liver injury. Also, with very elevated AST and ALT levels, and concomitant high LDH and alkaline phosphatase levels, consider ischemic hepatitis.

3. One condition to consider when the ALT to AST ratio is greater than 4:1 is Wilson's disease. The next test would be a ceruloplasmin level although consider that up to 20 percent of patients may have a low normal ceruloplasmin level and would need 24 hour copper assay for definitive diagnosis.

4. In central vertigo, there is no latency before the onset of vertigo when performing a Dix-Hall-Pike maneuver, whereas peripheral vertigo will have a latency anywhere from a few seconds out to about half a minute.

5. The duration of nystagmus during such a test as described in #4 is usually less than 1 minute in peripheral vertigo but may be longer than a minute in central vertigo.
6. Modified Epley maneuvers are employed to overcome the vertigo in benign positional vertigo.
7. Levodopa may give a false positive glucose test on a urinalysis in a patient with no hyperglycemia.
8. Phenazopyridine may give a false positive bilirubin test in the urine in patients with normal bilirubin levels.

17.153 Year 3—Week 51—Day 2

1. The most common deficiency noted in patients with warfarin induced skin necrosis is protein C deficiency.
2. The second most common deficiency noted in patients with warfarin induced skin necrosis is protein S deficiency.
3. Patients with methotrexate chronic use can develop a small nodulosis of the joints of the hands despite having concomitant improvement of joint pain and stiffness symptoms. Treatment should be continued as those lesions are not of concern clinically.
4. The most common side effect of leflunomide therapy has been noted to be an elevation of the AST and ALT levels of the liver.
5. Patients with polymyalgia rheumatica should have marked improvement in the pain and stiffness of their shoulders and hips after a few days of low-dose steroid therapy. Serological markers such as elevated C Reactive protein should drop acutely with therapy.
6. Ptosis and hoarseness associated with myasthenia gravis worsens as the day progresses as does general fatigue in these patients.
7. Beta-2 microglobulin levels are a predictive factor as far as the prognosis of patients with multiple myeloma.

8. Patients with multiple myeloma and other plasma cell dyscrasias can have high output heart failure states very similar to Paget's disease.
9. Dermatitis herpetiformis, linear bullous IGA dermatosis and bullous disease manifestations of systemic lupus erythematosus are all treated with dapsone therapy.
10. The formation of a rash (most commonly a morbilliform exanthem but Stevens Johnson has been reported as well), weight gain, insomnia, methemoglobinemia and a mononucleosis like syndrome that usually occurs in the first 2-6 weeks of therapy (known as the dapsone syndrome) are all side effects of dapsone therapy.

17.154 Year 3—Week 51—Day 3

1. Three important atypical bacteria that commonly cause acute bronchitis are *Bordetella pertussis*, *Chlamydia pneumoniae*, and *Mycoplasma pneumoniae*. For antimicrobial treatment of atypical bacterial infections, macrolides such as azithromycin are recommended.
2. Vocal cord dysfunction frequently mimics persistent asthma and is often treated with high-dose inhaled and/or systemic corticosteroids, bronchodilators, and multiple emergency department visits w/ extensive workups.
3. Vocal cord dysfunction is caused by abnormal adduction of the vocal cords during the respiratory cycle (especially during the inspiratory phase) which causes airflow obstruction at the level of the larynx.
4. Diagnosis of vocal cord dysfunction is made w/ laryngoscopy which shows paradoxical vocal cord motion. A "chink deformity" is noted or with flow-volume loops which show inspiratory loop flattening.
5. The antiphospholipid antibodies include: anticardiolipin, lupus anticoagulant, and anti-β-2 microglobulin.

6. The drug tPA increases the conversion of plasminogen to plasmin in the presence of fibrin, so it is a more specific lytic agent than urokinase or streptokinase which cause a systemic lytic state.

7. The thiazolidinediones (TZD) work as agonists of the PPAR-γ receptor (peroxisome proliferator activated receptor) and help preserve insulin sensitivity.

8. Side effects of TZDs include weight gain, fluid retention, and risk of congestive heart failure exacerbation.

9. Patients with pseudohyponatremia present with a low serum sodium but a normal plasma osmolality. This can be due to hyperlipidemia or hyperproteinemia.

10. Baclofen intrathecal therapy is the treatment of choice for spasticity due to traumatic brain injury or spinal cord trauma injury.

17.155 Year 3—Week 52—Day 1

1. Bernard-Soulier (giant platelet) syndrome is an autosomal recessive condition in which patients have decreased platelet adhesion because of an absence of glycoprotein Ib which normally binds to vWF. These patients tend to have a low platelet count.

2. Glanzmann thrombasthenia is due to a deficiency in glycoprotein IIb/IIIa, so fibrinogen cannot cross-connect. Platelet count is usually normal in patients with this abnormality.

3. An acquired factor X deficiency can develop in patients with amyloidosis.

4. DIC (disseminated intravascular coagulation) is the most common acquired coagulopathy.

5. If there is a dramatic drop in platelets from 1 day to the next day, suspect artifact as the EDTA anticoagulant in collection tubes can cause platelet clumping and give a falsely low platelet count.

6. Von Willebrand disease (VWD) is the most common inherited bleeding disorder (1% of the population).

7. VWD is usually inherited in an autosomal dominant pattern.

8. Treat mild to moderate cases of VWD with DDAVP which induces a release of von Willibrand factor and factor VIII from the endothelial cells. Active bleeding with a low VWF activity may require cryoprecipitate therapy.

17.156 Year 3—Week 52—Day 2

1. Two GI conditions associated with thyroid cancer are the following: (1) Cowden's disease and (2) Familial adenomatous polyposis (FAP).

2. Cowden's disease is an autosomal dominant condition in which patients are at increased risk of breast, thyroid, uterine, and brain tumors.

3. Specifically, the cribriform–morular variant of papillary thyroid carcinoma is the type of thyroid cancer most associated with familial adenomatous polyposis. (Present in approximately one-fourth to one-third of cases).

4. Familial adenomatous polyposis results from germline mutations in the *APC* tumor suppressor gene on chromosome 5.

5. Screening with flexible sigmoidoscopy for colonic polyps and cancer is recommended annually for all family members of patients with familial adenomatous polyposis (FAP) starting at the age of 12 years. If the results are consistently normal, the screening program can be stopped at the age of 40 years.

6. One hundred percent of MEN-2 variants are associated with the development of medullary thyroid cancer. MEN-2 syndrome results from germline mutations in the *RET* oncogene.

7. In patients w/ aortic dissection, it is important to achieve good BP control; however, direct vasodilators such as hydralazine should be avoided b/c they can increase shear stress and provide less accurate and less reversible BP control.

8. Lateral femoral cutaneous nerve syndrome should be considered in any patient with ascites presenting with anterolateral thigh pain, numbness, tingling or burning.

9. Calciphylaxis (calcific uremic arteriolopathy) is a condition typically seen in patient receiving renal replacement therapy. The disorder manifests as small vessel calcification with necrosis of subcutaneous fat secondary to under perfusion.

10. Gingival hypertrophy can be caused by many medications, most notably the following: phenytoin, calcium channel blockers, cyclosporine, and D-penicillamine.

17.157 Year 3—Week 52—Day 3

1. Alopecia can be an early presenting sign of hypothyroidism in young patients and usually follows a telogen effluvium pattern.

2. Mucha-Haberman syndrome is a dermatological syndrome that appears like pityriasis rosea but has vasculitic lesions present. It is also known as pityriasis lichenoides et varioliformis acuta.

3. Fluoroquinolones are associated with spontaneous tendon rupture usually described in elderly female patients in the medical literature.

4. Rifampin is associated with orange discoloration of sweat and urine and can acutely lower the levels of dilantin through its action on cytochrome P450 3A4 system.

5. Ortner's syndrome is the hoarseness associated with mitral stenosis and subsequent impinging of the recurrent laryngeal nerve by an enlarged left atrium. Hoarseness in patients with rheumatoid arthritis should cause concern for cricoarytenoid joint disease.

6. Wallenberg's syndrome is the lateral medullary infarct syndrome associated with dizziness, dysarthria, Horner's syndrome, loss of ipsilateral pain and temperature on the face, and contralateral loss of pain and temperature in the rest of the body.

7. Pellagra is notorious for a photosensitive rash that can often be seen around the neck of patients. This finding was termed Casal's necklace. There is also diarrhea and dementia-like syndrome which has been associated with pellagra (which has niacin or vitamin B-3 deficiency).

8. Amyloid causes a "starry sky" or "speckled" heart echocardiogram along with low voltage on an EKG. Amyloid also is associated with "pinch purpura" and thickening of body appendages such as the tongue. It is associated with the "shoulder pad" sign.

9. "Wolf-man" appearance can come from excess hair in the facial area in patients with porphyria cutanea tarda.

Further Reading

Bouchama A, Knochel JP. Heat stroke. N Engl J Med. 2002;346(25):1978–88. https://doi.org/10.1056/NEJMra011089.

Brent GA. Clinical practice. Graves' disease. N Engl J Med. 2008;358(24):2594–605. https://doi.org/10.1056/NEJMcp0801880.

Brisman JL, Song JK, Newell DW. Cerebral aneurysms. N Engl J Med. 2006;355(9):928.

Brunzell JD. Clinical practice. Hypertriglyceridemia. N Engl J Med. 2007;357(10):1009–17. https://doi.org/10.1056/NEJMcp070061.

Clarke-Pearson DL. Clinical practice. Screening for ovarian cancer. N Engl J Med. 2009;361(2):170–7. https://doi.org/10.1056/NEJMcp0901926.

Cooper LT Jr. Myocarditis. N Engl J Med. 2009;360(15):1526–38. https://doi.org/10.1056/NEJMra0800028.

Darnell RB, Posner JB. Paraneoplastic syndromes involving the nervous system. N Engl J Med. 2003;349(16):1543–54. https://doi.org/10.1056/NEJMra023009.

de Berker D. Clinical practice. Fungal nail disease. N Engl J Med. 2009;360(20):2108–16. https://doi.org/10.1056/NEJMcp0804878.

El-Serag HB. Hepatocellular carcinoma. N Engl J Med. 2011;365(12):1118–27. https://doi.org/10.1056/NEJMra1001683.

Fishman JA. Infection in solid-organ transplant recipients. N Engl J Med. 2007;357(25):2601–14. https://doi.org/10.1056/NEJMra064928.

Fleming RE, Ponka P. Iron overload in human disease. N Engl J Med. 2012;366(4):348–59. https://doi.org/10.1056/NEJMra1004967.

Gabrielli A, Avvedimento EV, Krieg T. Scleroderma. N Engl J Med. 2009;360(19):1989–2003. https://doi.org/10.1056/NEJMra0806188.

Gines P, Cardenas A, Arroyo V, Rodes J. Management of cirrhosis and ascites. N Engl J Med. 2004;350(16):1646–54. https://doi.org/10.1056/NEJMra035021.

Hendley JO. Clinical practice. Otitis media. N Engl J Med. 2002;347(15):1169–74. https://doi.org/10.1056/NEJMcp010944.

Hesketh PJ. Chemotherapy-induced nausea and vomiting. N Engl J Med. 2008;358(23):2482–94. https://doi.org/10.1056/NEJMra0706547.

Hidalgo M. Pancreatic cancer. N Engl J Med. 2010;362(17):1605–17. https://doi.org/10.1056/NEJMra0901557.

Koplan BA, Stevenson WG. Ventricular tachycardia and sudden cardiac death. Mayo Clin Proc. 2009;84(3):289–97. https://doi.org/10.1016/S0025-6196(11)61149-X.

Kumar A, Cannon CP. Acute coronary syndromes: diagnosis and management, part I. Mayo Clin Proc. 2009;84(10):917–38. https://doi.org/10.1016/S0025-6196(11)60509-0.

Ledford DK. Immunologic aspects of vasculitis and cardiovascular disease. JAMA. 1997;278(22):1962–71. https://www.ncbi.nlm.nih.gov/pubmed/9396659.

Lembo A, Camilleri M. Chronic constipation. N Engl J Med. 2003;349(14):1360–8. https://doi.org/10.1056/NEJMra020995.

Pappas G, Akritidis N, Bosilkovski M, Tsianos E. Brucellosis. N Engl J Med. 2005;352(22):2325–36. https://doi.org/10.1056/NEJMra050570.

Paulson WD. Case study: from acid-base disorders to clinical diagnosis. J Crit Illn. 2000;15(2):113.

Peleg AY, Hooper DC. Hospital-acquired infections due to gram-negative bacteria. N Engl J Med. 2010;362(19):1804–13. https://doi.org/10.1056/NEJMra0904124.

Pirzada NA, Ali II. Central pontine myelinolysis. Mayo Clin Proc. 2001;76(5):559–62. https://doi.org/10.4065/76.5.559.

Rosenfield K, Jaff MR. An 82-year-old woman with worsening hypertension: review of renal artery stenosis. JAMA. 2008;300(17):2036–44. https://doi.org/10.1001/jama.300.13.jrr80009.

Shoback D. Clinical practice. Hypoparathyroidism. N Engl J Med. 2008;359(4):391–403. https://doi.org/10.1056/NEJMcp0803050.

Strasberg SM. Clinical practice. Acute calculous cholecystitis. N Engl J Med. 2008;358(26):2804–11. https://doi.org/10.1056/NEJMcp0800929.

Swanson DL, Vetter RS. Bites of brown recluse spiders and suspected necrotic arachnidism. N Engl J Med. 2005;352(7):700–7. https://doi.org/10.1056/NEJMra041184.

Taieb A, Picardo M. Clinical practice. Vitiligo. N Engl J Med. 2009;360(2):160–9. https://doi.org/10.1056/NEJMcp0804388.

Tolwani A. Continuous renal-replacement therapy for acute kidney injury. N Engl J Med. 2012;367(26):2505–14. https://doi.org/10.1056/NEJMct1206045.

Trapnell BC, Whitsett JA, Nakata K. Pulmonary alveolar proteinosis. N Engl J Med. 2003;349(26):2527–39. https://doi.org/10.1056/NEJMra023226.

Van Hattem S, Bootsma AH, Thio HB. Skin manifestations of diabetes. Cleve Clin J Med. 2008;75(11):772. https://doi.org/10.3949/ccjm.75.11.772.

Vassallo R, Ryu JH, Colby TV, Hartman T, Limper AH. Pulmonary Langerhans'-cell histiocytosis. N Engl J Med. 2000;342(26):1969–78. https://doi.org/10.1056/NEJM200006293422607.

Wakim-Fleming J. Hepatic encephalopathy: suspect it early in patients with cirrhosis. Cleve Clin J Med. 2011;78(9):597–605. https://doi.org/10.3949/ccjm.78a10117.

Walport MJ. Complement. Second of two parts. N Engl J Med. 2001;344(15):1140–4. https://doi.org/10.1056/NEJM200104123441506.

Watkins H, Ashrafian H, Redwood C. Inherited cardiomyopathies. N Engl J Med. 2011;364(17):1643–56. https://doi.org/10.1056/NEJMra0902923.

Weaver LK. Clinical practice. Carbon monoxide poisoning. N Engl J Med. 2009;360(12):1217–25. https://doi.org/10.1056/NEJMcp0808891.

Weiler CR, Bankers-Fulbright JL. Common variable immunodeficiency: test indications and interpretations. Mayo Clin Proc. 2005;80(9):1187–200. https://doi.org/10.4065/80.9.1187.

Weiss G, Goodnough LT. Anemia of chronic disease. N Engl J Med. 2005;352(10):1011–23. https://doi.org/10.1056/NEJMra041809.

Yuki N, Hartung HP. Guillain-Barre syndrome. N Engl J Med. 2012;366(24):2294–304. https://doi.org/10.1056/NEJMra1114525.

Ziegler TR. Parenteral nutrition in the critically ill patient. N Engl J Med. 2009;361(11):1088–97. https://doi.org/10.1056/NEJMct0806956.

Zimmerli W. Clinical practice. Vertebral osteomyelitis. N Engl J Med. 2010;362(11):1022–9. https://doi.org/10.1056/NEJMcp0910753.

Index

© The Editor(s) (if applicable) and The Author(s), under exclusive license to Springer Nature
Switzerland AG 2024
J. Lezama, *Internal Medicine Learning A to Z and 1, 2, 3*,
https://doi.org/10.1007/978-3-031-57546-4